➤ PRAISE FOR *BIKE FOR LIFE* ➤

"I love riding my bike. But I *really* love riding my bike with Roy Wallack, a pleasure I've enjoyed a few times over the years. Sure, we fall into rhythms and enjoy the scenery. But riding with Roy is really about listening to stories, and he has a million of them. That's what sets *Bike for Life* apart from any other bicycle book. Roy Wallack is the most entertaining writer on two wheels you'll ever have the pleasure of reading. Enjoy the training tips and the sage advice and the inspiration. But also settle back and enjoy the ride. Read about Roy's honeymoon on a tandem, his ride with a kick-butt, one-armed mountain biker, his ride up the world's steepest sea-to-summit mountain, his encounters with legendary cyclists—and cyclists who deserve to be legends. Roy fits that latter category. He's a legend in my mind—the rare writer who can convey tons of practical information along with a deep appreciation for what makes cycling the ultimate pathway to fitness. It's the same thing that makes *Bike for Life* a great read: It's just plain fun."—ROBERT EARLE HOWELLS, former Editor-at-Large of *National Geographic Adventure* and 2009 Lowell Thomas Travel Journalist of the Year Silver Award

"True, the bike industry is made up of many strange creatures, but of us all, few are as strange as Roy Wallack. At the start of many a group ride, as the rest of us primp and use carpenter levels to ensure a solidly level saddle, Roy will be over in the corner stretching and breathing loudly through his nose. 'That dude is bizarre,' we reassure ourselves as we do our best to catch a reflection of our bikes in the mirror-like surfaces of our shaved legs.

But now here's a book with verifiable stories of old dudes riding their bikes well into their late 90s. It talks about how diet, stretching, and cross-training regimens will help. Apparently, our steady regimen of leg shaving brings nothing more valuable than group consciousness to our pedaling efforts. Imagine, riding into your 90s—ha, we should all be so lucky....

Maybe Roy is onto something with all that heavy breathing."—ZAPATA ESPINOZA, Editor, *Road Bike Action Magazine*, and Mountain Bike Hall of Famer

"Roy celebrated his 50th birthday on a team with me at the 2006 Primal Quest, a weeklong, round-the-clock 300-mile adventure race of mountain biking, white-water kayaking, backpacking, rappelling, rope climbing. He was 10 to 20 years older than the rest of us. We all broke down at one time or another—except him. Now, a decade later, still hammering hard, he lays out his plan here in *Bike for Life* to keep living life all-out for another 50 years. It involves a lot of hard work and enthusiasm but really comes down to what I call the 'Wallack Way': Don't slow down! Keep pedaling! Keep seeing the world! Keep pushing your limits! This engaging how-to book, suffused with inspirational adventures and profiles of older riders doing amazing things, can change your life, on the bike and off of it."—STEPHEN REGENOLD, Syndicated Columnist and Editor/Founder of GearJunkie.com

⋟ ABOUT THE AUTHOR ⋞

Roy M. Wallack says he owes it all to cycling. A 5,500-mile Seattle-to-Maine-to-Florida bike trip in 1982 led to his first published article and a career change to journalism. Dozens of bike trips around the world in the 1980s, including Alaska to Seattle, the length of the Mississippi River, and London to Moscow on the first-ever bike tour into the USSR (in 1988), led to his first book, *The Traveling Cyclist* (1991). His 1994 honeymoon tandem ride from Nice, France, to Rome led to the birth of his son—exactly nine months later. His career as a magazine editor (*California Bicyclist*, *Bicycle Guide*, and *Triathlete*), as a freelancer for national magazines (such as *Outside*, *Men's Journal*, and *Competitor*), and as a longtime fitness-gear columnist and feature writer for the *Los Angeles Times* has revolved around fitness and cycling.

A former collegiate wrestler, Roy began focusing his attention on athletic aging after he hit age 40, profiling successful older athletes and seeking out training strategies and studies that can impact healthy longevity. He broke the news on the dangerous link between cycling and osteoporosis; a deleterious training phenomenon called the "Black Hole"; the connection between human growth hormone (HGH) and strength/interval training; the injury-reduction potential of barefoot-style running, and the benefits of "butt-centric" riding form and strength training for cyclists. That research led to the first edition of *Bike for Life: How to Ride to 100*, published in 2005. A half-dozen books on fitness and running, all keying on fit aging, followed in the next decade.

As he pushed 50 and beyond, Roy pushed it harder than ever on the bike, racking up more epic bike trips—including New Zealand by tandem with his wife, circumnavigating Iceland's Ring Road, and (almost) tandeming from Portland to Yellowstone National Park with his teenage son. He also competed in some of the world's toughest endurance cycling, running, and adventure events: the 1,200-kilometer Paris-Brest-Paris randonnée, the 24 Hours of Adrenalin Solo World Championship, the weeklong Eco-Challenge and Primal Quest expedition races, the Badwater Ultramarathon and Himalayan 100 running races, and numerous mountain bike stage races, including the three-day La Ruta de los Conquistadores ride across Costa Rica (seven times) and the weeklong TransAlp Challenge, TransRockies Challenge, BC Bike Race, and Breck Epic races. In 2004, at the age of 48, he finished second in the obscure World Fitness Championship (only three people competed, and one guy couldn't swim). He was inducted into the 24 Hours of Adrenalin Hall of Fame in 2008.

Roy's goals, he says, are simple: Keep writing about how we can all stay fit and healthy, and keep seeing the world in the best way he knows how, by bike. He lives next to a bike path and a vast trail network in Irvine, California.

BIKE FOR LIFE

⚔ ALSO BY ROY M. WALLACK ⚔

The Traveling Cyclist: 20 Five-Star Cycling Vacations

Run for Life: The Injury-Free, Anti-Aging, Super-Fitness Plan to Keep You Running to 100

⚔ COAUTHORED BOOKS ⚔

Healthy Running Step by Step: Modern Methods for Injury-Free Running, Injury Prevention, and Rehab
with Robert Forster, PT

Fire Your Gym! Simplified High-Intensity Workouts You Can Do at Home
with Andy Petranek

Barefoot Running Step by Step: Barefoot Ken Bob, the Guru of Shoeless Running,
Shares His Personal Technique for Running with More Speed, Less Impact, Fewer Injuries and More Fun
with Ken Bob Saxton

Be a Better Runner: Real World, Scientifically Proven Training Techniques That Will
Dramatically Improve Your Speed, Endurance, and Injury Resistance
with Sally Edwards and Dr. Carl Foster

BIKE FOR LIFE

HOW TO RIDE TO 100—AND BEYOND

—REVISED EDITION—

ROY M. WALLACK

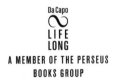

Da Capo
LIFE
LONG

A MEMBER OF THE PERSEUS
BOOKS GROUP

Designed by Jack Lenzo
Set in 11 point Whitman by the Perseus Books Group

Library of Congress Cataloging-in-Publication Data
Wallack, Roy.
  Bike for life : how to ride to 100 and beyond / Roy Wallack. -- Revised edition.
     pages cm
  Includes bibliographical references and index.
  ISBN 978-0-7382-1755-0 (paperback) -- ISBN 978-0-7382-1756-7 (e-book) 1. Cycling--Training. 2. Health. I. Katovsky, Bill.
II. Title.
  GV1048.W33 2015
  796.6--dc23

2014018589

First Da Capo Press edition 2014

Published by Da Capo Press
A Member of the Perseus Books Group
www.dacapopress.com

Note: The information in this book is true and complete to the best of our knowledge. This book is intended only as an informative guide for those wishing to know more about health issues. In no way is this book intended to replace, countermand, or conflict with the advice given to you by your own physician. The ultimate decision concerning care should be made between you and your doctor. We strongly recommend you follow his or her advice. Information in this book is general and is offered with no guarantees on the part of the authors or Da Capo Press. The authors and publisher disclaim all liability in connection with the use of this book.

Da Capo Press books are available at special discounts for bulk purchases in the US by corporations, institutions, and other organizations. For more information, please contact the Special Markets Department at the Perseus Books Group, 2300 Chestnut Street, Suite 200, Philadelphia, PA, 19103, or call (800) 810-4145, ext. 5000, or e-mail special.markets@perseus books.com.

10 9 8 7 6 5 4 3 2 1

To Marc, Martin, Bob, Larry, the Rev, Dad, Elsa,
Kennedy, Matta, Bell, Ed, and Joey—
Our epic bike adventures changed my life.

CONTENTS

INTERVIEWS

INTRODUCTION

"Russell—push it, man!" I yelled. "Come on, dude—you can do better than that! I can't do it alone! Give me some of that Olympic leg power!"

Suddenly, Russell Allen, the stoker on my tandem, kicked it into gear—and it was like a jet engine roared to life. Suddenly, he was that 19-year-old track rider on the 1932 US Olympic Team again. We stood up out of the saddle. I shifted into the big ring. We hit 25, 27, 30 mph. We passed hundreds of riders and hammered through the finish line of the 2006 LA Marathon bike ride, 22 miles long, in exactly one hour flat.

Russell was 93 years old.

"That was goddamn fast!" the last surviving member of the '32 team whispered to me when it was over, beaming like he'd won a gold medal. Halfway into his tenth decade of life, surrounded by photographers and gabbing away with three-time Olympic rider John Howard (1968, 1972, and 1976) in the VIP area afterward, he looked as happy as a 10-year-old kid.

Doing the tandem ride with Russell that day and seeing the childlike joy on his face was one of the greatest moments of my life. For me, it was also a testimony to the life-affirming and life-extending power of this magnificent machine, the

bicycle—and validated the promise of my 2005 book, *Bike for Life: How to Ride to 100*. It was another vivid example of how the bike literally can be a time machine—a fun, thrilling vehicle for anyone who wants to stay fit and functional at any age. Russell, an Olympic, professional, and lifelong cyclist, fitness buff, family man, car salesman, and

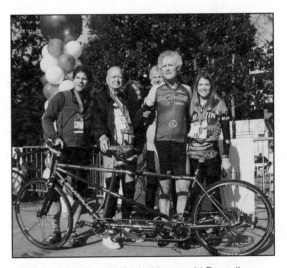

(l to r) Author Roy Wallack, 93-year-old Russell Allen, Jan and Bill McReady of Santana Tandems, John Howard, and Audrey Adler at the 2006 LA Marathon bike ride.

professional gambler—whom I actually met because of *Bike for Life* (as you'll read in a couple of minutes)—was proof of that.

Russell and other older riders have convinced me that the driving mission behind *Bike for Life* is completely realistic and doable. Yes, you can get fitter as you get older. At the very least, you can slow down and even stop the natural deterioration that hits everyone after about age 35.

And if everything goes as planned, you will indeed be able to, as *Bike for Life* promises, "Ride a century when you turn a century."

It'll just take lots of work—on and off the bike.

If you like riding bikes and love life, you are very lucky. Because cycling is simply one of the best—maybe *the* best—activities for functional, fit, and fun longevity.

Living to 100 used to be rare, but more and more, it will be common for those with good genes and healthy lifestyles. Tens of thousands of Americans will reach the century mark in the coming decades—advances in medical science will make sure of that. The question is: Do you want to be functional when you get there? Do you want to do the same stuff that you like doing now? If you're a cyclist, do you want to experience the triumph of conquering a steep hill, the thrill of the wind blasting your face on a winding descent—at age 80, 90, or 100? Wouldn't it be great to ride 100 miles at age 100?

Enter *Bike for Life*, a blueprint for longevity, health, and well-being. Cycling is a sport uniquely suited to long life, as it provides the potential for physical and mental challenge, superb cardiovascular fitness, adventure, relaxation, and social interaction—all at the same time. It works for all abilities, both sexes, and every age and demographic, so it's a great equalizer that can unify generations in fitness and fun.

Unfortunately, like all sports, cycling is not perfect. It does little for upper-body muscular strength, can wreck posture and bone density, and can unwittingly get you additcted to a destructive sugary/processed food habit that can leave you disease-prone and old before your time. Those issues are exacerbated in cyclists over the age of 35 or 40 as a result of the natural deterioration caused by aging. So cycling both giveth and taketh away—unless you train smart.

If you want to ride a century when you turn a century, you have to make two significant changes to your routine:

1. Add intensity to your rides: Shorter, more strenuous training sessions will help you maintain and build muscular power without wearing you out.

2. Get off the bike: Do some weight training, cross-training (run, swim, skate, play tennis, etc.), and flexibility/yoga exercises to protect your muscle mass, bone density, and posture.

This revised edition of *Bike for Life* is about 50 percent new content. It updates groundbreaking information about cycling-related osteoporosis, wrecked relationships, impotence, knee and back preventive care. It adds new, cutting-edge research about diet and training—both cardio and strength—that will have huge effects on achieving peak fitness, staying injury-free, and fighting the deterioration of aging. You'll get happy reading two colorful new chapters on cycling role models and ways to stay motivated. We don't skip the small stuff, either. In *Bike for Life*, you'll learn how to fight off a mountain lion, avoid and manage a car-bike accident, survive a bike-jacking, and deal with a dozen other "it-only-happens-to-someone-else" subjects that can throw your long-life plan off track.

Proudly, *Bike for Life* addresses some crucial topics largely ignored in the cycling press:

- **Bone loss:** Want to make sure you don't break a hip when you're 70? See Chapter 9: Cycling and Osteoporosis. *Bike for Life* broke the news on this crucial issue in 2005, and too many cyclists still are not paying attention to it. They should. If you only ride a bike for fitness, you are at risk—male or female. You'll learn why you need to hit the weight room, do some jogging and jumping jacks, and consume more calcium if you want to keep your skeleton as fit as your heart.

⅂ **Back pain:** Read Chapter 8: Prehab, long before you visit your chiropractor. Its unique Symmetry body-straightening, a leader in postural therapy, will save you time, money, and years of anguish.

⅂ **Power and endurance:** Want to be faster and go farther at age 40 than at 30, at 60 than 50? Check out the radical new "Maximum Overload" weight-training method in Chapter 2 and discover "butt-centric" riding in Chapter 8. These sections will help you hold power and form until the end of the longest rigdes and help you utilize the much-ignored—and highly powerful—gluteal muscles.

⅂ **Yoga for cyclists:** Cycling's unusual, not-found-in-nature position leads to imbalances that can cause on- and off-the-bike pain and poor performance. Renowned cycling and yoga coach Steve Ilg provides a 10-position yoga routine in Chapter 2 that will get your posture back in line.

⅂ **Reviving your reaction time:** Getting older, and afraid to ride because your reaction time has slowed so much that you can't avoid road hazards like you used to? Get back up to speed by reading Chapter 2, which describes explosive, rapid-contraction weight lifting, the only thing proven to re-suscitate your invaluable fast-twitch muscle fibers. A bonus: Doing so will also raise your flat-land speed, increase your fatigue-resistance on the hills, and restore youthful bulges to age-flattened muscles.

⅂ **The 5-to-1 relationship ratio:** Cycling is a demanding lover. Reconciling your significant other's and the sport's significant demands on your time will be a lot easier with the help of a mathematical plan from some of the world's foremost and fittest relationship psychologists. Find it in Chapter 12: Rolling Relationships.

⅂ **Staying motivated:** 90 percent of the challenge of staying fit is just getting up off the couch and doing it. The nine stories from the field in Chapter 11 will show you how to stay excited about cycling, including taking on crazy challenges, joining (or starting) a club, and turning a work trip into a memorable cycling vacation.

Cycling has a leg up on most other sports when it comes to long-term fitness and health. It's easier on joints and muscles than running. It's way more fun and far less monotonous than swimming. Unless your backyard backs up to a dock, it's a lot more convenient than paddling. With a $200 training stand, it's one of the rare workouts you can do while watching the evening news. And, best of all, cycling is one of the few sports you can do alone or in a group at any age. Some people start cycling in their 60s (see the first story in Chapter 10). Ever see a group of 60-year-old men play pickup football or basketball? Never. But on a century ride, a weekend charity ride, or a 24-hour mountain biking event, you'll see plenty of silver-haired men and women pursuing active retirement into their 70s. Riding is the best social security.

While pedaling into your seventh or eighth decade is commendable, why stop there? Why should age be a barrier to health? With a good strategy, age doesn't matter. Just take a look at hard-training cycling legends like John Howard and Ned Overend, who are deep into their 60s and 50s, respectively, as I write this. They have no intention of stopping—ever. Because the longer you do, the harder it is to get going again. If you are inactive now, don't wait another minute.

"It's not the older you get, the sicker you get, but the older you get the healthier you've been," said Dr. Thomas Perls, a geriatrician at Boston University, who was quoted in a *Time* magazine story entitled—get ready for this—"How to Live to Be 100."[1] The *Time* story confirmed my notions about longevity, but it also left me with one big question: Why stop there? A better tale, told in these pages, is "How to Ride to 100—and Beyond." I believe that the information compiled in *Bike for Life* can help you radically slow the deterioration that starts in your 30s and 40s and push the cycling odometer far into triple digits.

One of the best things about using cycling as your longevity tool is that it makes you part of a supremely positive culture that cuts across all racial, age, language, occupational, and socioeconomic groups. Being a cyclist makes you part of a team that celebrates adventure and goal achievement. If you've climbed the same hill as another cyclist, you're automatically bonded for life, even if you've barely met. I saw this

phenomenon firsthand when the first edition of *Bike for Life* helped reunite two cyclists who hadn't seen one another in 74 years: my LA Marathon tandem partner Russell Allen and his 1932 Olympic teammate, John Sinibaldi.

A year before that tandem ride, the original *Bike for Life* featured Sinibaldi, a member of the 1932 and 1936 US Olympic cycling teams, which competed in Los Angeles and Berlin, in a lengthy oral-history interview (which remains in this book). He was still riding, as was Allen. But they never met again after 1932, so each assumed he was the last survivor of the team.

Four months after the book came out in May 2005, a year before Allen and I rode the tandem together, I got a call out of the blue from Audrey Adler, a Los Angeles indoor-cycling instructor, who was also profiled in the book for her efforts to found a cycling-based charity.

"I just met Sinibaldi's teammate," she said. "His name is Russ Allen. He's handsome and fit, with sparkling blue eyes. We need to take him to Florida so he and Sinibaldi can meet."

Allen had walked into Adler's Los Angeles cycling class that day and asked if he could join. Noting his age, she mentioned that the class was very intense and that he might enjoy one of the club's senior classes instead.

"Oh, I can keep up," he said. "I ride on the beach bike path all the time. In fact, I even rode in the 1932 Olympic Games."

Adler was dumbstruck. "What? What's your name?" Upon hearing the name Russell Allen, she said, "Wait a minute. Do you remember John Sinibaldi?"

Allen got teary-eyed and sadly waved his hand in front of his face in a gesture of resignation. "Yeah, but he's gone," he said. "They're all gone. I'm the only one left."

"No you're not," said Adler, "I know for a fact that Sinibaldi is still alive. And I'm going to take you to see him."

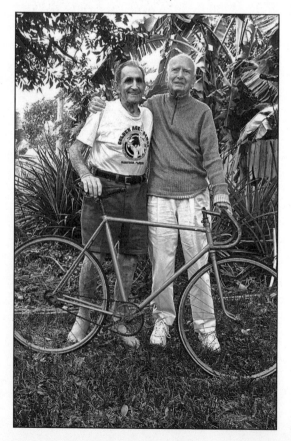

John Sinibaldi and Russell Allen with one of their 1932 Olympics–era bikes

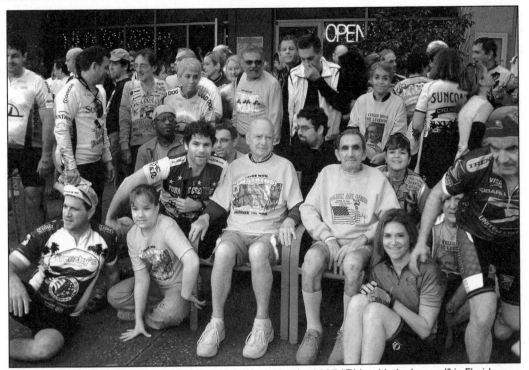

Allen and Sinibaldi, both in their 90s, take seats of honor at the 2005 "Ride with the Legend" in Florida.

Allen took her class (and had no trouble keeping up). A month later, Allen, Adler, and I flew to St. Petersburg, Florida, to meet his old teammate, Sinibaldi.

More than 500 other people from 15 states also showed up, joining us for a 25-mile ride officially dubbed "Ride with the Legend," which Sinibaldi's son and riding buddy, John Jr., had organized in his honor. Allen and Sinibaldi signed specially made "Legend" T-shirts for two hours. They signed books at my *Bike for Life* lecture. And the two Olympic teammates, who'd known each other—barely—for two weeks as 19-year-olds over seven decades earlier, were inseparable, posing for pictures, poring through photo albums, and talking non-stop. Joined at the hip for two straight days, both still sharp, they traded names and places like human Rolodexes.

It was amazing to see them go at it like two old pals, when in fact they had not seen each other since the Olympics. While Allen turned pro,

traveled the globe, and made big money doing six-day races until the start of World War II, Sinibaldi stayed amateur, went to the Berlin Olympics in 1936, and had then gone to work in a factory. After years off the bike, both continued cycling for decades. But they also credited their remarkable fitness and the spring in their steps to cross-training. Russell began lifting weights several times a week in the gym as a trainer during the war; Sinibaldi spent three hours a day digging and planting in his enormous garden.

Three weeks after Ride with the Legend, John Jr. called me. His dad had died. Sinibaldi Sr. had been diagnosed with terminal lung cancer right before I'd initially contacted him, a month before the party. "He was supposed to die in a week, the doctor told me," his son said. "What kept him alive was knowing that he was going to see Russell."

At the end of the phone call, John Jr. gave me instructions: "You must celebrate Russell, do for him what I did for my dad," he said.

So I did. I wrote a couple of big articles about Russell, did the LA Marathon tandem ride with him, and arranged to have him get a special "Legends" award at the Competitor Endurance Sports Awards gala. Adler and I would get together with Allen several times a year. His daughter started inviting us to all his birthday parties, and we became part of his large extended family.

At his 99th in March 2012, Russell looked frail but was excited to be flying to New Zealand the following week, where he was going to attempt to reclaim his record (originally set when he was 94) of being the oldest person to bungee jump off the famous bridge in Queenstown. He didn't make it. He died in his sleep the day before the flight.

Russell would be mad at himself for that. He was looking forward to being in my book as real proof that you actually could ride to 100. But 99's not so bad; it'll motivate the rest of us.

This edition of *Bike for Life* keeps the original book's interview with Sinibaldi and adds a large profile of Allen. You'll also find interviews and stories about venerable cycling champions and industry stalwarts, from three-time Olympian John Howard and mountain bike pioneer Gary Fisher to Specialized bike boss Mike Sinyard, all in their 60s, as well as reigning off-road endurance queen Rebecca Rusch and 1990s' mountain bike superstar Juli Furtado, both in their 40s. The book also profiles two notable age-80-plus riders: Don Wildman, fitness industry icon, 10-time Hawaii Ironman, and Malibu mountain bike legend; and UC–Berkeley professor emeritus Gerd Rosenblatt, who did 38 double-centuries after age 70 and was inducted into the California Triple Crown Hall of Fame.

Between the personality profiles and the technical chapters on training, diet, and technique, you will find a wealth of valuable lessons that you can apply to your own cycling longevity

plan. A reminder: Strength, flexibility, hard training, and recovery are the key threads. Going shorter is fine, as long as you go hard. The Golden Rule: Follow a hard day with a recovery day, as your body strengthens by adapting to the stress that you put on it. Any opportunity you get, challenge yourself, then rest. Most of all, just get on the bike and ride it.

A key: Goals. Weekly ones, yearly ones, and lifetime ones—they become self-fulfilling prophecies that force you to get on your bike when you don't feel like it, and remind you to do all the extra stuff that'll keep you riding. As a sport, nothing beats cycling for goal-setting, as it's replete with events that can keep you motivated year after year (see Chapter 14).

In my case, although I'm no mega-miler, it's endurance events. Since *Bike for Life* was first published in 2005, I've done six weeklong mountain bike stage races (TransRockies, BC Bike Race, Breck Epic, and three 3- and 4-day La Ruta de los Conquistadores races); half of the 1,200-kilometer Paris-Brest-Paris randonnée; hundreds of bike tours, century rides, one-day hill climbs; plus a mountain bike ride every Sunday with my buddies Kennedy and Matta. Although I was never a speed demon, I honestly can say I have not slowed at all from my 40s through my 50s, despite riding less. For that, I credit my ramped-up strength training, stretching, intervals, cross-training, a better diet—and the subtitle of my book. Because when you decide to tell the world "How to Ride to 100—and Beyond," it keeps you pretty motivated.

Do I really think you can ride to 100? Absolutely! In fact, I'm counting on it. See you in 2056 at the *Bike for Life* century ride.

Roy M. Wallack (age 58)
September 2014

THE CYCLING ANTI-AGING GAME PLAN

To stay young and injury-free at 40, 70, or 100, cycling's not enough.
You also have to strength-train, cross-train, and stretch.

September 2008,

Death Valley Inn, Death Valley, California

I'm lying face down on the massage table in an air-conditioned room after a 100-mile ride through the hottest place on Earth. This is Day 5 of the annual Specialized Bicycles ride to Interbike—a six-day bike trip from Specialized headquarters in Morgan Hill, California, 30 miles south of San Jose, to Las Vegas, Nevada, for the bike industry's giant yearly trade show. The 670-mile route traversed the Central Valley, Yosemite, the Sierra Nevada, and today Death Valley. The route, which I'd never done before in a lifetime of touring, is a beautiful, challenging tour of California. For me, however, it's more like a Tour de California—not a tour as I know it, but a race. Specialized executives, managers, and dealers, including some top age-group racers and company president Mike Sinyard, hunker down into pacelines the whole way, absolutely hammering.

It's their way, their culture; they ride every day at the Specialized lunchtime ride and after work. By contrast, I only ride on the weekends and do other stuff—running, swimming, yoga, CrossFit—during the week. Since I hate riding in pacelines and like to shoot pictures, I usually finish a good hour or two after the peloton. Other slowpokes were picked up by the van on this day, but I kept pedaling in the 120-degree heat. I do lots of crazy endurance events and have no hang-ups about finishing in the back of the

pack, as long as I finish. No surprise—I'm the last one into the massage room in Death Valley on this afternoon.

As I sprawl out on the table for my well-earned massage, the masseuse is astonished. "Wow, that's amazing," she says. "You can lay flat!"

"Huh?" I grunt. "What do you mean?"

"None of the other riders I've been working on this entire trip could do that," she replies. "They can't lay flat. Their backs and shoulders are sort of permanently hunched over—like crabs."

Crabs? Permanently hunched? That doesn't sound good.

January 1998,

Los Angeles, California, my bathroom mirror

Startled, I freeze at the sight of something so unexpected, so scary, that every thought is suddenly dominated by one haunting image: the desperate, dying Wicked Witch of the West in The Wizard of Oz, *shriveling into nothingness while screaming "I'm m-e-l-l-l-t-t-i-n-g!"*

It's my 41-year-old body. In the three months since I separated my shoulder at La Ruta de los Conquistadores—the crazy-hard, three-day, 200-mile Pacific-to-Atlantic mountain bike race across Costa Rica—it has morphed from "young" to "middle-aged." Former squared pecs have become shadow-casting man-breasts. A once-flat stomach now drips over my belt. With no upper-body exercise—the swimming, rowing, racquetball, and push-ups that have preserved my old college wrestler's physique—gravity has attacked. Daily Lifecycle-riding (all I can do) isn't enough; my torso is reverting to its true self, like a butterfly going back to a caterpillar. It's more than a blow to my vanity; it's a visual warning: For lifelong fitness, cycling isn't enough.

Fact: After age 35, flexibility naturally decreases, VO₂ max shrinks, and muscle mass shrivels—even in a cyclist's legs. Shoulders slump and posture corrodes. At any age, periods of inactivity cause a pronounced "detraining" effect. If you don't fight back with almost-daily aerobics and regular weight lifting and stretching, you might become one of those superfit 72-year-old cyclists who falls and breaks a hip because you lack the quick reaction time you need to avoid a car that has cut you off. Add the risk of osteoporosis (see Chapter 9), and your plan to roll into the sunset might be done in a wheelchair.

That image in the mirror was a wake-up call. Ever since, I've been cross-training, stretching, working on my posture, and lifting weights for 45 minutes in the gym at least twice a week. It's a hassle; you have to work harder to stay fit as you age. But it has paid off. Now pushing 60, I feel almost as fit as I was in my 20s. But I know I can't stop if I want to keep riding to 100.

By the way, the guys at Specialized got a wake-up call about flexibility. A few years ago, Mike Sinyard put in a gym with daily yoga classes at his company and attends religiously.

There's good news and bad news about riding your bike a lot, which the aforementioned stories are meant to illustrate. The good news is that you can stay really, really fit, developing a cardiovascular system that remains far "younger" than your chronological age. The bad news is

that the unusual, seated, non-weight-bearing position you take on a bike can exacerbate the normal deterioration of aging, leaving you with a bent-over posture, poor overall flexibility, no lateral agility, thinning bones, poor performance in bed, and shriveling muscle mass.

If you want to use your bike to stay young and ride to 100 and beyond, your strategy must maximize the good and minimize the bad. And that means you'll have to do a lot more than ride your bike.

Let's talk about the good news first: There are a lot of "old" people out there riding bikes, quite impressively.

On the aforementioned ride to Vegas in 2008, Specialized president Mike Sinyard was 62, easily hanging on in the middle of the pack, and he's still doing it as I write this six years later. In 2013, Tinker Juarez, two-time US Olympian and member of the Mountain Bike Hall of Fame, won his fifth 24-Hour Solo national championship; he was 52. Senior Games champion Don Wildman, 81, who kicked my butt mountain biking a couple of years ago (see Chapter 10), keeps up with serious athletes half his age; he's competed on two Race Across America teams in the past few years. John Howard, three-time Olympian and 1981 Ironman Triathlon winner, told me in late 2013 that he is as fast at 66 as he was a decade earlier, when I interviewed him for the first edition of this book.

"I have to work darn hard—and I might have lost a little snap, my explosive sprint," admits Howard. "But I am not slower. I can hang with hard-core unemployables in their 30s and 40s in a 70-mile race. It is fast. We're topping 30 mph on the flats."

You might be thinking that guys like Howard, Tinker, and Wild Man are freaks, but they aren't alone. Today, thousands of people over 40 are proving that high-level fitness is no longer merely the province of the young, and that longevity isn't simply based on lucky chromosomes. For the most part, the path to a long, fit life seems simple: You can stay amazingly fast at an "old" age—if you push it. Keep training—and training hard. This rule is not cycling-specific, but a baseline for anyone trying to stay young.

Researchers are finding that years of hard training in aerobic and strength activities can keep you young. They've discovered that the old rule of thumb—that we annually lose 1 percent per year in aerobic capacity (VO_2 max) and muscular strength after age 30 or 35—only applies to the sedentary; active people who maintain high training levels can cut the decline by half, or two-thirds, or more.

"What we thought was aging was really just inactivity," said athletics-and-aging researcher Joel M. Stager, PhD, professor of kinesiology and director of the Human Performance Laboratory at Indiana University, in a 2004 *New York Times* article.[1]

For average folk like me, who learn how to train better over the years, cycling is a true fountain of youth, as you can actually get faster. Today, at 58, I am actually faster on the bike than I was 20 years ago, a textbook example of the motivating effect of youthful mediocrity: We mediocre types can actually improve as we age, whereas the greats, with rare exceptions, such as Tinker Juarez and John Howard, can only get worse. That principle applies even more to non-athletes who get into cycling and other endurance sports later in life. Gerd Rosenblatt, University of California at Berkeley professor emeritus (see Chapter 10) and California Triple Crown Hall of Famer, never rode a bike seriously or did a century ride until age 67, or a double century until age 70. For the next seven years, until he crashed and broke a hip, he racked up 38 doubles and kept getting faster.

Does this mean that if you keep working out, you'll stay 25 forever? That if you just keep doing it—if you stay off the couch and keep riding, keep running, keep skating, doing Zumba, and whatever else makes you feel fit and healthy, and don't stop—blowing through 100 will be as easy as blowing out the candles on a birthday cake? That it all comes down to "use it or lose it"?

To a point. When you move, a host of good things happen that slow and delay the age-related deterioration of your body and brain, from enhanced circulation, hormone production, and calorie burn to all the basic cellular functions. And because cycling is far easier on your body than, say, running, a cyclist can tolerate year after year of hard training without injury far more easily than runners, who often end up with destroyed knee and hip joints. Cycling's so easy on the joints that it's often the preferred rehab for injuries from other sports. And it's so fun and exciting, unlike lap swimming, that it motivates you to get out there. Those facts alone are a big reason why it's such a great longevity sport—*if* you can minimize its bad aspects.

That's a big if. Every sport has gaps in its fitness benefits, due to the particular repetitive motion of the sport. Running's impact can wreck your knees; tennis's swing can wreck your elbows. The bad news is that cycling is not only deficient in many areas, but that those areas exacerbate the same deterioration that is linked to aging: *declining VO_2 max, postural integrity, bone density, sexual function, and muscle mass.*

Because of these issues, keeping "young" as a cyclist must involve more than time in the saddle. It involves a time-consuming, carefully balanced strategy that supports, protects, and replenishes those systems and structures of the body that deteriorate with age and neglect. "By your mid-30s, most people still look young, but are already experiencing the Big Three of aging: deteriorating lean muscle mass, worsening posture, and crumbling joints," physical therapist Robert Forster told me one day at his Santa Monica office, which is the unofficial meeting hall for West L.A.'s broken-down cyclists, triathletes, adventure racers, and gym rats. "Age-related decline hits sooner than you think."

Way sooner. Robert Wiswell, PhD, associate professor and expert on aging and exercise at the

University of Southern California's Department of Biokinesiology and Physical Therapy, told me that the typical man starts experiencing osteoarthritic changes (loss of smoothness) in his joints by his 20s, loses half a pound of muscle per year by the age of 35, and has been shrinking in height since he was 18 years old due to postural changes.

"The bad news is that you can't stop the decline," said Wiswell. "The good news is that you can slow it down and get injured less by thinking long-term."

A long-term anti-aging workout plan is part physical therapy and part cutting-edge exercise research. It is heavy on weights, hard aerobic workouts, stretching/flexibility drills, and recovery. Initially, it would baby your knees and shoulders with a lengthy, joint-lubricating warm-up. Next, it would keep your heart strong and your VO₂ max (ability to process oxygen) high, with hard efforts in your cycling and other aerobic activities at least a couple of times a week, and active recovery or cross-training in between. Finally, you hit the weight room twice a week, avoiding extreme range-of-motion exercises to protect connective tissue, building up vulnerable and neglected muscle groups, and then hammering your muscles with heavy weights and a blistering pace. The result: You revive flagging fast-twitch muscle fibers, snap a slumping spine to attention, expand your capillary and oxygen-processing network, and flood your bloodstream with youth-maintaining hormones. The workouts use jumping jacks, stretches, and the same weight machines and free weights you know and love, but require you to think—to protect your body with restraint and discipline before pushing it. No more winging it. All workouts fit into a logical, never-ending plan.

"Of course, it takes a lot more time to do all this stuff—time a lot of people with active social and work lives don't have," said Wiswell. "On the other hand, don't wait until you're 45 or 50 to integrate some of these elements. By then, you may have already done irreparable damage to your body and will be functionally much older than you ought to be."

In other words, if you want to ride a century when you turn a century, start now. Here's a guide on how to maintain and protect the five main problem areas of aging: VO₂ max (the body's maximum ability to take in and use oxygen), strength, joint integrity, flexibility, and posture.

PROBLEM 1: DECLINING VO₂ MAX/ AEROBIC FITNESS
Solution: Train frequently and rigorously, lift weights, cross-train, and integrate cycling into normal life activities.

Fitness guru Jack LaLanne, who died at age 96 in 2011, wasn't a cyclist. He was better known for chair push-ups and swimming handcuffed across San Francisco Bay on his birthday, not cycling. But the overriding message he promoted since the Depression remains the same and applies to anyone seeking longevity and fitness. "Don't stop working out," he told anyone who'd listen. "Inactivity kills your body."

It's a fact: The more you do nothing, the more you fall apart.

Past age 30 or 35, the heart and the other elements that contribute to VO₂ max start slipping about 1 percent a year in sedentary people. The muscles' oxygen-processing ability slips as muscle mass shrinks, the blood-carrying capillaries become less numerous, and mitochondria, the tiny intracellular engines that convert glycogen and fat into energy, become less numerous and powerful. The aging heart is socked two ways: declining maximum heart rate (its highest possible beats per minute, or bpm) and declining maximum stroke volume (the amount of blood in one pump of the heart). The result is a monstrous double whammy: A reduced volume of blood is pumped to shrinking muscles that are less capable of transporting oxygen, nutrients, and lymphatic waste products. The effect: You produce less energy than before, so you can't ride as fast or as long—or recover as quickly. If you want to slow or even reverse the VO_2 max decline, think of Jack. Jack up the intensity, lift weights, and don't stop, ever. Also, eat better. Natural foods and supplements (no sugar, refined grains, or processed food) mop up free radical and hormonal damage much better than processed ones, allowing better recovery and performance. Here are some details:

Solution 1a: Keep training—hard.

Message read on www.cyclingforums.com: *"I'm 40, started riding almost 3 years ago, and always finish in the top 5–10 percent of any event I ride in regardless of age. I attack every hill and pass a lot of younger riders regularly. On flats I can hold my own and can sprint up into the 32- to 39-mph range. Since I'm older and closer to death I take every ride seriously. I train like there's no tomorrow. How many 23-years-olds can say the same? —Rickw2, Arlington, Texas.*

Rickw2 is doing the right thing. Hard workouts can limit your deterioration to half the rate of the average person. Or more.

Numerous studies of runners and swimmers (there are few of cyclists) have found that older athletes who maintain vigorous endurance training experience a VO_2 max decrease of 0.05 percent per year—half that experienced by sedentary adults. That's an average; some see almost no ill effects of age at all. A landmark 1987 study by Dr. Michael Pollock, director of the Center for Exercise Science at the University of Florida, studied two dozen Masters champion athletes in several sports in 1971 and 1981. His findings: The VO_2 max levels of hard trainers barely declined at all in a decade (just 1.7 percent), but the results for those who slacked off in intensity declined an average of 12.5 percent. Low-intensity training did not increase capillary density.[2]

A study in *Swim* magazine that tracked Masters swimmers over a 15-year period reported similar results: The onset of VO_2 max decline was delayed from age 25 to the mid-30s, deterioration

was almost "imperceptible" into the swimmers' 40s, and it didn't reach 1 percent per year until they hit their early 70s. Non-athletes lost 25 percent of their physical capacity by age 50, and 50 percent by age 75, but competitive age-groupers who swam an hour a day declined only 3.5 percent by age 50, and 19.1 percent by age 75. "Another way to look at it," said study author Phil Whitten, PhD, "is that a 70-year-old competitive swimmer will have the strength and vitality of a 'normal' 45-year-old." The key, he said, is to never let yourself get out of condition.

Question: Why the decline at all? Why can't you maintain the same VO_2 max with hard training? Answer: Unfortunately, training apparently has no effect on one factor: the decrease in maximum heart rate. However, the other factors—declines in heart-stroke volume, density of capillaries and mitochondria, and even the production of creatine phosphate (an organic compound in muscle fibers that provides them with a quick source of energy when they need to move fast), can be reversed quickly with high-intensity exercise, with levels eventually potentially matching those of similarly trained younger athletes.

Bottom line: In theory, an older adult who trains at the same volume and intensity as a younger adult should be capable of very similar performances. Only the natural decrease in heart rate and consequential reduction in VO_2 max stands in the way of letting you stop time in its tracks.

Solution 1b: Lift weights.

Strength training boosts more than your strength, reflexes, and vanity. Bigger muscles expand your aerobic engine by processing more oxygen. Studies have proven that strength training builds up VO_2 max by increasing the density of capillaries and mitochondrial enzyme activity. See the next section ("Problem 2: Deteriorating Muscle Mass") for the strength benefits of weight lifting and the ideal lifting strategy.

Solution 1c: Cross-train like crazy.

Daily high-intensity riding is hard on any body—young or old, if you somehow have the time to do it. More likely, you don't—and fitness fades fast. If you skip several days in a row, a "de-training" effect starts to set in; skip three weeks, and your hard-won aerobic fitness is largely lost. By twelve weeks, you begin to lose musculoskeletal resiliency—the strength of your joints. By six months, so much joint strength, muscle tone and strength, and aerobic capacity is lost that you're back to being as unfit as someone who's been sedentary for years. The point: Avoid long periods of inactivity—whether caused by busy lives, bad weather, and injuries—at all costs.

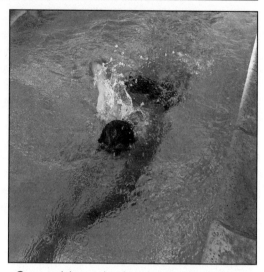

Cross-training: swimming

The easiest way to keep active is by broadening your athletic portfolio. Mix in running, swimming, rowing, the elliptical machine, jumping rope, salsa aerobics, VersaClimbing, or aerobic dance. Try the Trikke, the radical three-wheeled sensation that delivers a total full-body aerobic workout (I did the 2004 Long Beach Marathon on one in 2 hours, 13 minutes). Water-run in the pool with a flotation waist belt and resistance boots. Play your nephew one-on-one in basketball and win on pure hustle. If it gets your heart rate up and keeps it there for a while, it qualifies as cross-training.

You see, your VO_2 max isn't particular about which aerobic activities you do to develop it. Cross-training helps your body tolerate hard workouts, and it can't be beat for convenience. Two straight days of hard cycling is tough on your body, and one day of hard cycling followed by a hard swim session lets your legs recover while it works your upper body, but both blast your heart and lungs. Going on a business trip? Running shoes and swim goggles tuck into a suitcase. Tweak your knee on the bike? Kayak for a couple of days. Can't ride due to early nightfall or a January blizzard? Snowshoe or cross-country ski. Mixing up different activities—including road cycling *and* mountain biking—keeps you motivated, breaks up your routine, and helps

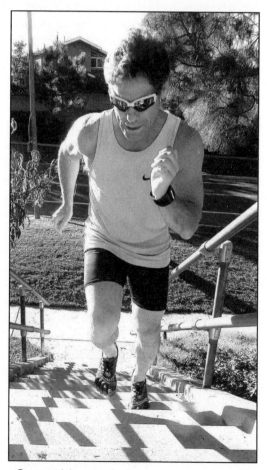

Cross-training: running

maintain wintertime fitness. As Ned Overend proved in his long, successful career (see interview on page 103), other sports not only don't hurt cycling, but provide variety that keeps you from getting bored with it.

Cross-training shouldn't be seen simply as a welcome off-season break from the saddle, to be set aside when springtime rolls around. Because it works all the muscles of the body rather than just a specific group, cross-training yields a smaller chance of chronic injury over the long term than any one single sport. And in the big picture, cross-training makes you fitter, enhancing VO_2 max by developing the oxygen-processing ability in all the muscles of your body, not just the ones in your legs.

"The definition of fitness is that it takes less effort for your body to do the same amount of work," said Dr. Herman Falsetti, an Irvine, California, cardiologist and consultant to the 1984 Olympic cycling team. "And if your body is fit all over—not just one part of it—your body's work goes that much easier."

Solution 1d: Integrate cycling into work and family time.

If playing with the kids, spending time with your spouse, and a thousand other things eat into your riding time, get creative. Do errands on your bike. Commute to work. Ride to family get-togethers. Buy a trailer, a Trail-a-Bike, or a kid-friendly tandem to combine babysitting and riding. With these items fairly cheap (I bought a Raleigh Companion tandem for $700—what some triathletes will pay for a wheel), you are shortchanging yourself without them.

PROBLEM 2:
DETERIORATING MUSCLE MASS
Solution: Pump weights fast and heavy. Then recover.

Weight lifting is underutilized by cyclists, and even scorned by some. "My legs get plenty of work already," some say. "Bulky arms and a big chest

will hurt me on the hills," say others. But from a pure health and longevity point of view, big, strong muscles are more functional and safer than smaller, weaker ones. They help aerobic performance by increasing your oxygen-processing capacity and provide the strength to push through headwinds and up hills. Which is why it is mildly upsetting to discover that muscle mass, like VO_2 max, also disappears at an average rate of 1 percent a year beginning in your 30s. And why it is downright scary to find, as researchers from Johns Hopkins and Boston universities did in 2002, that *power naturally falls off far faster than strength as you age.*[3]

The rapid drop-off in power is a big deal. It can cost you your life.

That's because power is defined as the ability to use your strength quickly—to respond to changing situations fast. Power gives you that instant reaction, the ability to make the microsecond adjustments that often mean the difference between success and failure—avoiding a fallen tree branch on a backcountry road; jumping a rock on a 30-mph downhill; swerving out of the way of cars that suddenly turn in front of you. Power is a key to survival.

Trainers have known for years that explosive weight training is necessary to keep pro athletes at the top of their game. Michael Jordan observed a rigorous explosive lifting program after age 30, as do many of this era's older pro athletes. What we didn't know until recently is that this power training is vital for average folks who want to *maintain* their speed and power—especially as they age. In other words, there is a very good argument for all of us to be weight training like professional athletes—especially after age 30 or 35.

A 40-year-old racquetball player, for example, might still be able to bench 250 pounds like he did a decade ago, but because his power is down 5 percent, he might lack the instant acceleration that allows him to retrieve that shot in the dead corner he used to get to. Further along the age

The Antioxidant "Cocktail" to the Rescue

Vitamins C and E can help reduce illnesses resulting from hard training

There is a downside to regular, hard exercise that you can easily minimize. In 2004, Dr. David Nieman and colleagues at California's Loma Linda University verified what marathon runners and endurance cyclists have long suspected: A long, arduous event or a day of sudden, hard training puts them at increased risk of illness and infection. Immune cells aren't weakened for a long period of time—21 hours in the case of Nieman's study—but that window is enough if you catch a chill or interact with someone who has a cold. An earlier study by Nieman of 2,000 Los Angeles Marathon runners found that those who trained 60 miles per week were twice as likely to get sick in the two months before the event than those who trained 20 miles per week. Conclusion: Your immune system, like your muscles, adapts to hard training, but also is initially weakened by it. So take care immediately following a hard workout.

Besides covering up and resting, taking antioxidant vitamins can help mitigate the short-term effects of hard workouts—and the longer-term damage some think may be caused by hard exercise. Dr. Kenneth Cooper of the Cooper Aerobics Center in Dallas, who invented the term "aerobics" in the 1970s and was the leading advocate of "the more, the better" school of thought, now believes that more than an hour per day of aerobic activity increases production of "free radicals," substances that can "oxidize" (damage) muscle tissue, particularly that of the heart. According to Cooper, the solution to this is regular doses of an "antioxidant cocktail" of vitamins C, E, and beta-carotene.

IT'S LIKE RUST-OLEUM FOR YOUR BODY

Free radicals are natural by-products of oxygen processing that, under normal circumstances, the body holds in check. Technically, they are unstable oxygen molecules (unstable because they lack some electrons in their outer core) that are constantly shooting about crazily in your body, crashing into, sticking to, and "oxidizing"—sort of rusting—other particles and tissues. This oxidation eventually can cause cancer, coronary artery disease, and other problems. Before excess free radicals get out of hand, however, the body dispatches built-in "antioxidant" enzymes to mop up the "oxidation" they cause. Unfortunately, your body can get out of whack; the antioxidants can be overwhelmed when free radicals multiply in response to pollution, cigarette smoke, food contaminants, depression, or excessive exercise. "They begin to run wild," said Cooper, "successfully attacking healthy as well as unhealthy parts of the body."

Since the publication of his 1994 book *The Antioxidant Revolution*, Dr. Cooper has advocated the use of a supplementary therapy based on consumption of vitamins C, E, and beta-carotene, antioxidants that bolster the body's natural free radical fighters. Vitamin C promotes cell growth, healing, and immunity; builds collagen (the main component of connective tissue such as tendons, ligaments, and skin, and abundant in cartilage, bones, blood vessels, the gut, and spinal discs); reduces the risk of some cancers and cataracts; and may lower cholesterol levels and increase immunity. Vitamin E is a blood-thinner that helps form red blood cells, reduces damage in muscle cells, protects against heart disease, and boosts immunity. Beta-carotene, the best known of the substances that make the yellow and orange color in apricots, sweet potatoes, and carrots, lowers the risk of cataracts, heart disease, and lung and other cancers. Taken together as a group, this "cocktail" protects muscles by keeping cell clumping, vessel clogging, and plaque formation in check; repairing cell membranes; and preserving them from rotting. Cooper claims the cocktail should be your main weapon in a war against a host of other age-old afflictions: cholesterol, heart attacks, strokes, cataracts, and some cancers. It even fights premature aging, he said.

(continues)

THE ANTIOXIDANT "COCKTAIL" TO THE RESCUE
(continued)

If you regularly work out hard for an hour or more a day, the latest research indicates that you need to take in far larger amounts of antioxidants than you can probably get from diet alone. Fifteen or 20 servings of fruit and vegetables per day may get you enough vitamin C and beta-carotene, but E is another story. It would take eight cups of almonds to get 400 IU (International Units) of E, the amount Cooper recommends for a moderate male exerciser in his 60s. It would take more than 15 oranges to get 1,000 milligrams (mg) of vitamin C and two or three carrots to get 25,000 IU of beta-carotene.

Dr. Cooper promotes a *four-step antioxidant plan* that includes supplements, moderate—not extreme—exercise, a low-fat diet, and limited environmental exposure:

1. Take a daily antioxidant "cocktail," which includes, for an active 50-year-old woman, 600 IU of vitamin E, 1,000 mg of vitamin C, and 50,000 IU of beta-carotene. If you are male or a more active woman, increase these amounts to 1,500 mg of vitamin C and 1,200 IU of E. A Tufts University study found that 800 IU of E reduced the amount of exercise-induced free-radical damage in muscle cells; there is evidence that higher doses fight cancer, Parkinson's, Alzheimer's, and heart disease. Nobel Prize winner Linus Pauling went to his grave at age 93 believing we should take 200 times the RDA (Recommended Dietary Allowance) of vitamin C (12,000 mg per day).

2. Limit consecutive days of hard-core, high-endurance training, which produces an abundance of *free radicals*. Cooper and other researchers have found a correlation between those with a history of marathon running and cancer and heart attacks.

3. Eat a natural-food diet, featuring whole (non-sliced) fruits and raw or steamed vegetables, lean meats, and limited processed grains and sugar. Sliced fruits lose vitamins when they are cut open and exposed to air; veggies lose vitamins when cooked or canned.

4. Limit exposure to radiation, electromagnetic fields, and pollution, all of which expose you to free radicals.

While not alll researchers agree on the efficasy of antioxidants, most are overwhelmingly positive. Some studies have even shown that making the antioxidant "cocktail" a daily habit may be a good idea whether you exercise hard, easy, or not at all. One study showed that antioxidants helped preserve mitochondrial density. Another indicated that they can have an immediate protective effect against a fatty meal, making your task literally this simple: Before you pig out on a Big Mac and fries or a couple of slices of double-cheese pizza, knock back a vitamin C and E cocktail—or at least a couple of oranges and a swig of wheat germ oil. That's advice derived from a study conducted by Dr. Gary D. Plotnick, a professor of cardiology at the University of Maryland School of Medicine, who subjected 20 test subjects to a combination of vitamin supplements, low-fat meals (Kellogg's Frosted Flakes, skim milk, and orange juice), and high-fat meals (McDonald's egg-and-sausage McMuffins and hash-brown patties). He found that pretreatment with vitamins C and E may indeed be akin to temporarily spraying Teflon on your tubes.

"Maybe McDonald's should serve McVitamins, too," he said.

While Plotnick warns that taking C and E is "no magic bullet"—a meal high in fat has other detrimental effects, such as increasing the risk for obesity and diabetes—his findings were clear: Protected by the vitamins, the inner lining of blood vessels stayed unchanged. By contrast, the vessels of test subjects who did not take the vitamins became "impaired" (and therefore open to a fatty buildup) for a full four hours, the length of time it takes a fatty meal to digest.

Incidentally, the finding that high-fat meals impaired vein-wall function for four hours raised Dr. Cooper's eyebrows when I told him about Plotnick's study. "That may explain why heart attacks and angina often occur just after a meal," he said.

he did 20 years earlier, but wipes out more on the descents, because his slower-reacting muscles can't avoid obstacles as quickly. A 75-year-old man might still give you an iron-grip handshake, since his strength still may be 80 percent of what it was decades earlier. But since his power is down by 50 percent, he might just lose his balance when he gets up from a table, falling and breaking his hip.

In a nutshell, lifting weights is good for everyone, and at every age. But for maximum benefits—to stay on top of your game—you've got to hit *heavy* weights *fast* and *frequently*. Here's how to stop muscle mass decline as you age.

Solution 2a: Hit fast-twitch fibers with fast contractions.

You may have heard of "superslow" weight lifting, whose proponents touted amazing health benefits from short sessions of agonizingly slow lifts; hundreds of copycat magazine articles promoted it in the early 2000s. Well, forget it. To restore size and power, do what every pro and college trainer tells his athletes: Go "superfast." The aforementioned 2002 Boston–Johns Hopkins Universities study, led by Roger A. Fielding, PhD, found that rapid contractile movements, such as a speedy upstroke on a leg extension, will quickly bring back your thick, powerful "fast-twitch" muscle fibers. These short, bulky fibers, unlike the smoother, longer, more aerobic-oriented "slow-twitch" fibers, will wither substantially by age 50 and can virtually disappear in old age without stimulation. On the bright side, the lack of fast-twitch fibers doesn't hurt you as much in pure endurance activities as in speed-based events, which is why many marathon runners and cyclists have done well into their late 30s—and even 40s. On the flip side, the rapid fall-off in fast-twitch fibers severely impacts reaction time. That's why you're a step slower on the basketball court at 35—and can fall and break your hip while vacuuming at age 70.

continuum, the power loss accelerates. A 50-year-old man may still be able to climb the same hills on his mountain bike about as fast as

Among his test group of 73-year-old women, Fielding found that superfast contractions and regular speed contractions brought similar strength gains, but the superfast contractions stimulated far greater gains in fast-twitch fiber volume and peak power output. "But why wait until 73?" he told *Bike for Life.* "In younger people, they'll come back even faster."

Note: Don't forget to hit the triceps, the muscle on the backside of the upper arm, as it is predominantly (90 percent) composed of fast-twitch fibers, said Michael Bemben, PhD, director of the Neuromuscular Research Lab at the University of Oklahoma. Also, pound calves and forearms, which wither quickly for another reason: They're routinely stressed less than muscles nearer the body's core.

Solution 2b: Spike growth hormone levels with heavy, no-rest training.

Human growth hormone (HGH) is the body's fountain of youth, promoting lean muscle mass, body-fat reduction, youthful skin, thick bones, strong connective tissue, and deeper sleep. Unfortunately, your body's production of HGH tumbles after your mid-20s, some say by as much as 24 percent per decade. Your body produces about 500 micrograms of HGH a day at age 20, 200 at age 40, and 25 at age 80. Beginning in middle age, men lose 5 pounds of muscle per decade. Result: You may weigh the same at 48 as you did at 18, but your body composition is more fat, less muscle.

The US Food and Drug Administration (FDA) approved injections of artificial HGH in 1996, but slowing the slide that way is controversial due to the numerous side effects that HGH in this form can have (see sidebar on "Artificial HGH: High Price for Eternal Youth"). Fortunately, however, you can increase the frequency and amplitude of HGH "spurts" naturally through lifting weights. The method is simple: Perform three sets of 8 to 10 reps to failure (the point at which you can't maintain

form), with no more than a minute's rest between sets.

This intense sequence of lifting may seem difficult, but it is doable by structuring the workout in pairs of non-overlapping exercises, such as push-pull or upper-lower. An example of push-pull is following a bench press, which works the chest, with a complementary, oppositional exercise like a seated row, which works the back. The chest rests as the back is worked, eliminating downtime.

"This method floods your muscles with lactic acid, which cues the pituitary gland to secrete growth hormone," said William Kraemer, PhD, of the University of Connecticut, a leading HGH researcher. "Just cut out the talking and work out for at least 15 minutes to maximize the spurt."

ARTIFICIAL HGH: HIGH PRICE FOR ETERNAL YOUTH

Hoping to reverse the muscle-mass shrinkage and body-fat increases associated with the drop-off in human growth hormone after the teenage years, researchers first harvested HGH from cadavers, then, 20 years ago, began manufacturing a synthetic variety for clinical use. To build strength and recover faster from training, competitors in a variety of sports began to use it instead of anabolic steroids, which do the same thing but are readily detectable in drug tests. Because HGH is produced by the pituitary gland at the base of the brain, it's difficult to prove whether it has been taken artificially. At the 2004 Tour de France, cyclists were not yet being tested for HGH, because the requisite blood test had not yet been given full World Anti-Doping Agency (WADA) approval. Athletes were first tested for artificial HGH (which is banned by WADA) during the 2004 Athens Summer Olympics, and a first "positive" was recorded in North America in 2010.

Today, injecting human growth hormone is a thriving industry in the United States. A
(continues)

Solution 2c: Ease into it and build in recovery.

Ironically, although you need more intensity with age (to produce HGH and fast-twitch fibers), safety requires you to take it easier: Use lighter weight on your first set (to warm up), take more recovery time (rest and sleep) between workouts, and gradually build up to heavier workouts over time. Since muscle fibers need at least 48 hours to recover from a hard workout, don't lift two days in a row. In fact, alternate heavy and light workouts. "If you're 35 or more, make every second workout a 'recovery workout' (below 80 percent of max), and every fifth week an easy week," said Dan Wirth, president of Sierra Fitness Health Clubs of America and a former University of Arizona strength coach.

Solution 2d: Periodize your weight lifting.

To prevent gradual decline, Wirth and many other coaches promote cross-training and "periodization"—working muscles with different weights and reps every couple of months.

Ironically, while the periodization program *Bike for Life* describes in Chapter 2 applies the same principles to aerobic cycling training, Romanian coaching guru Tudor Bompa actually developed the periodization concept for strength training. He noticed that muscles "learn." As you get stronger, a movement that initially took 10 muscle fibers to move soon takes 9 fibers, then 8. To keep firing all the fibers, you need to change your routine. At a macro level, lift heavy weights with low reps for a month, then switch to light weights and higher reps. At a micro level, change technique. Do bicep curls, but change your grip from underhand to overhand. Instead of a military press machine, find a wall and do handstand push-ups. Change brands of machines; the Universal incline-press machine involves slightly different biomechanics than the incline press on an Icarian.

PROBLEM 3: DETERIORATING JOINTS
Solution: Warm up, cool down, avoid risks, build up weak spots.

Muscles can be rebuilt, but joints aren't so lucky. Micro-thin synovial membrane, already a tissue-thin lining that covers bone ends with lubrication slicker than wet ice, gets thinner and more worn with age. Meniscus cushions in the knees get ripped. The humerus bone dangles precariously from the cavity of the shoulder blades, making the shoulder prone to impingement and rotator-cuff injuries. Blood, barely able to penetrate joints due to lack of capillaries in tendons and ligaments, delivers fewer healing nutrients with age. What to do?

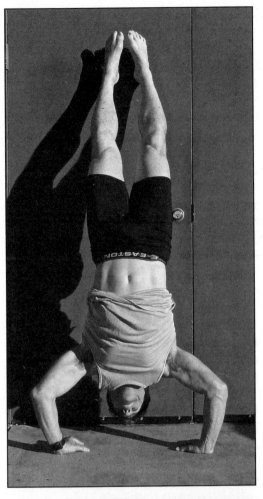

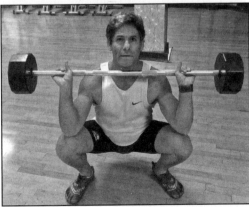

Strength training is essential. Use both body-weight and weighted exercises.

Solution 3a: Do an extensive warm-up.

Do you really have the time to do a 15-minute warm-up?

"The question is, do you have time not to?" asks Rob Bolton, a certified strength and conditioning coach at UC Santa Barbara, who advocates "functional" fitness, the popular movement advanced by Vern Gambetta, the New York Mets director of athletic development, who sees muscles as links in a "kinetic chain" that must be worked out together, not in isolation. "No matter if you're young or old—but especially if you're old—you need that long to gradually increase your heart rate, get synovial fluid lubricating knees, elbows, and shoulders, and work up a light sweat, indicating your body is ready for action," Bolton says. "Don't lift or run or ride without lubing the joints."

Bolton's warm-up includes body-only moves and light weights. It starts with five minutes of jumping jacks, then systematically hits all joints from top to bottom: neck rolls, shoulder shrugs, alternating arm circles, hip circles, trunk rotations (hands on hips, rotating in circles), leg swings (side-to-side like windshield wipers, and forward and back, like kicking a soccer ball), knee bends (put hands on quads, to avoid overloading them), and "old-school" knee circles.

Next up are core-focused single-leg balance exercises. Reach forward, back, sideways, and to a 45-degree angle with one leg while balancing on the opposite foot, then do the same thing with arms extended straight up. Follow that with five minutes on the Lifecycle or elliptical, and quick stretching to avoid cooling down. Then proceed to a regular weight-training program.

Solution 3b: Strengthen two high-risk areas: Rotator cuff and lower back.

Rotator-cuff exercises: Since injuries to the shoulder are the most common injuries in sports, strengthening the four rotator-cuff muscles that stabilize it is critical. "Unfortunately, it's not so easy," said physical therapist Robert Forster.

"The cuff gets little blood flow, and is invisible to the naked eye, so it's ignored, understrengthened compared to the glamour muscles, and subject to tears."

Three exercises in particular strengthen the rotator cuff. Starting with 2- or 3-pound weights in each hand, do three sets of 10 to 15 reps, twice a week.

To work the supraspinatus, which helps the deltoid raise the arm to the side, raise both your arms straight out. Hit the infraspinatus and teres minor, which pull the arms downward (as in a pull-up), by lying on your side with your elbow on your hip, then pivoting your arm upward. To work the subscapularis, which assists with inward arm rotation, pull surgical tubes sideways across your body, like windshield wipers.

Lower back and transverse abs: A lifetime of sitting tightens the lower back's spinal erector muscles and weakens the transverse abdominus, the deep abdominal muscles that draw the belly button to the spine. Strengthening and stretching both can improve posture and eliminate back pain. Three exercises do this:

Back extension: lie belly down with your arms at your sides and raise your head and upper back to work the spinal erectors.

Dying-bug: To work the core from both sides, lie face-up with your arms at your sides and your legs stretched out straight, press the small of your back to the mat, and tighten your core by making a "pssst" sound. Then raise and lower your opposite legs and arms at the same time without moving your spine. Then reverse.

Transverse abdominus (TA): stand up, holding light dumbbells at chest level with arms either bent or straight (depending on your preference), and twist side-to-side as you draw a sideways figure eight. Then do cross-crunches: Lying on your back with your legs raised and your knees bent, fold your left leg over your right knee and cross over the midline of your body with your elbows

in a slow, controlled motion. That hits your TA muscles, intercostals, and obliques.

Solution 3c: Avoid extreme ranges of motion in at-risk joints.

Many trainers and therapists nowadays warn against extreme ranges of motion for all weight-training exercises, regardless of age, due to potential joint injuries and lack of functional benefit. At extreme ranges, dips, push-ups, and flys can jeopardize the humerus/shoulder joint, which is supported only by tendons and ligaments. General rule: To avoid rotator-cuff injuries, keep your elbows visible in front of the body. Many trainers have banned the military press for its injury risk and lack of function. If you have knee pain, avoid deep squats that take your butt lower than your knees.

Rob Bolton even warns against the apple pie of the weight room, the bench press. "You can't avoid pinching your shoulder joint on the bench press because it inhibits the scapula [shoulder blades]," he said. "The scapula is pinned between the bar and the bench, causing the humerus [upper arm bone] to grind into and overload the glenohumeral joint. Besides that, it doesn't train you for anything in real life." He favors pulling exercises in general and replacing the bench with a standing cable-machine press, which frees the scapula and uses the hips, stomach, and lower back to stabilize the body.

Solution 3d: Cool down with a recovery spin and stretching.

"After lifting, your capillaries are dilated and pooling with lactic acid," said Bolton, "so jump on an easy cardio machine to pump it out. The bike allows you to slowly take your heart rate down to 90 bpm."

Elasticity of tissues drops with age; instead of bending and stretching, they break. "So stretch more and avoid injuries that are hard on these tissues," adds Forster.

Solution 3e: Baby your knees by changing your running form.

Running is a fantastic cross-training activity for cyclists, a quick and convenient way to maintain and even ramp up your cardiovascular fitness between rides that can be very important for preventing osteoporosis (see Chapter 9) and restoring good posture. But it can also injure knees and ankles—when done incorrectly. That's due to the harsh impact of a heel-strike landing, which, ironically, is made possible by thickly cushioned running shoes. The solution: Try a more minimalist shoe and an injury-reducing "soft" running form that lands you on your forefoot with a bent knee, not on your heel with a straight leg. A shorter stride, with touchdown directly under your body (not out ahead), and a faster cadence keeps you off your heels.

Over the past decade, there has been a strong emphasis on this soft running form, which is how ancient man ran in moccasins or when barefoot. I believe in the concept, wrote the first big national story about soft running for *Runner's World* magazine ("I Will Learn to Run Better," October 2004), run barefoot myself and followed *Bike for Life* with several running books, including *Run for Life*, *Barefoot Running Step by Step*, and *Healthy Running Step by Step,* that advocated a soft landing. It works, turning running into a fun skill-based activity that can improve performance and virtually eliminate injuries—if you *gradually* adapt to the new form and learn to match shorter strides with faster turnover.

I put "gradually" in italics because I can't emphasize it enough: Many newbie barefooters and minimalist toe-shoe wearers tend to do too much too soon, and end up straining their calves and Achilles tendons. You see, while soft running restores natural biomechanics and is much easier on your knees, it is new for calves and Achilles foreshortened by decades of wearing high heels and running

shoes with lots of heel cushioning. In 2014, the Vibram company, makers of the FiveFingers "barefoot" toe shoe, settled a large class-action lawsuit because it claimed that injuries would disappear with their shoes. What they forgot to mention is that you need to start slowly. Start with 5 minutes of the new form and slowly work up to 20 minutes over the period of a month to give your legs time to adapt. If you do, you may be able to run to mile 100 as well as ride to age 100. Add swimming, and you're looking at doing a triathlon at 100.

PROBLEM 4: LOSS OF FLEXIBILITY
Solution: Stretch a lot.

If you wonder "*Why stretch?*" you may need a different perspective. "The real question," said Bob Anderson, is "*Why get old?*"

Anderson is the author of *Stretching*, widely known as the bible of flexibility. "Stiffness really has nothing to do with age," he said. "If you keep stretched, and keep active, you feel young—no matter what it says on your driver's license." Anderson lives his words. On the day I caught up with him, he had just returned from a "typical once-a-week" mountain bike ride of 5.5 hours, 52 miles, and 6,500 feet of climbing. He said he rides 25 to 30 hours a week in Pike National Forest trails near his Colorado home. He packs 138 pounds of "pure muscle" on his 5-foot-9 frame, looks and feels far younger than his 67 years (as of 2014), and has a resting heart rate in the 40s. "Most of all," he said, "I try not to whine, because no one listens."

The world has listened, though, as Anderson has spread the stretching gospel. Two key points to remember: Tightness is the rare malady of aging that anyone—athlete or couch potato—can completely reverse. And for cyclists and other athletes, the immediate benefits of stretching, and ridding yourself of this tightness, are too good to pass up:

1. Faster speed, due to more efficient biomechanics

2. More force, due to the increased leverage of lengthened muscles

3. Faster post-ride recovery, due to speedier outflow of waste products and correct muscle shaping

For an example of flexibility's benefits, look at one pair of muscles: the hamstrings. Flexible hams yield more power by (1) allowing further extension of the quads, and (2) allowing a dropped-heel pedaling position, which allows for fuller use of the powerful glutes.

The Connective-Tissue Skeleton

Flexibility is defined as the ability to move joints freely through a wide range of motion, according the American College of Sports Medicine. It may be best illustrated by those who don't have it: the elderly. "They walk like they are old—totally stiff," said Anderson.

That's because their connective tissue—the white, glistening sheaths of collagen that surround and shape bundles of muscles and, when condensed, become tendons—is tight, which makes their muscles tight. For that reason, the real focus of stretching is not the muscle itself, but what Bob Forster calls "the connective-tissue skeleton" that gives shape to our bodies.

"You stress this 'soft skeleton' every time you work out, and your body then lays down more connective tissue haphazardly, making you tight and imbalanced," Forster said. "So the goal of stretching is to remodel it into a functional pattern—to remodel your infrastructure."

Cycling, given its unnatural position, lays down connective tissue in such a way as to leave your biomechanics inherently imbalanced, according to Forster. The bent-over riding position shortens the hip flexors. The abductors become weak because of the lack of lateral movement— what you'd get from playing tennis or basketball. The quads and hamstrings get short, squat, pumped, and tight from working so much. The

neck muscles get tight from holding up the head at an unnatural angle.

"Chronically tight muscles, left unstretched, will adapt to this position," said Forster. "That will alter joint mechanics and increase the potential for injury." To lengthen, relax, and ultimately strengthen the muscles and correct the body's biomechanical imbalances, you must stretch them.

Stretching Rules

If possible, stretch "passively"—while lying down on the floor. Generally, it's harder to relax a muscle while stretching under tension.

1. Easy in, easy out: Be in a position where you can breathe properly.

2. Use the "subsiding tension principle": Move slowly into the stretch and allow for tension to register before adjusting the intensity.

3. Never reach over to touch your toes from a standing position: The lower back is concave; this move makes it convex. "Your back ligaments are already stretched out by cycling, and they don't need to be stretched more," said Forster. "A guy with a discectomy isn't finding enlightenment."

4. Go slow: Rapid stretching can stimulate the muscle to tighten up.

When to Stretch

1. Before: As part of your warm-up—within 45 minutes of a workout or race. Use a five-second "release" to prepare the muscle to perform in its normal range of motion. Don't hold it any longer. You do not need permanent elongation at this time.

2. After: Within 45 minutes after a workout, while warm. At minimum, do a release. A longer session aids circulation and recovery, flushes lactic acid out of the system, corrects gross imbalances and contracture, and effects permanent architecture changes.

3. Nighttime: Before bed, to promote a functional remodeling of connective tissue to create a stronger infrastructure.

Bob Anderson's Top 10 Stretches for Longevity

The latest edition of Bob Anderson's *Stretching* is 223 pages long and filled with drawings of nearly 1,000 stretches. The author recommends that you find 4 or 5 that "really help you" and do them several times a day, including before bed. *Bike for Life* asked him to recommend 10 basic stretches to start with that will help maintain range of motion from toe to head. Here goes:

1. Ankle Rotation

The ankle is important for overall flexibility. "Nothing says 'old' like a stiff-ankled walk," said Anderson. To keep it loose, sit on the floor with legs spread, then grab one ankle with both hands and rotate it clockwise and counterclockwise through a complete range of motion with slight resistance provided. Rotary motion of the ankle helps to gently stretch tight ligaments and improve circulation. Repeat up to 20 times in each direction. Do both ankles.

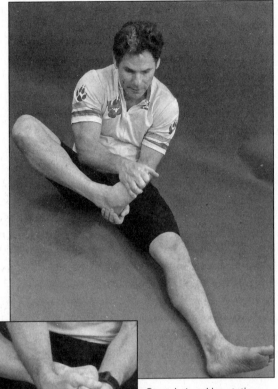

Stretch 1: ankle rotation
Stretch 1: ankle out

2. Sitting Calf and Hamstring Stretch

This movement stretches the lower leg's rear muscles and the area behind the knee.

Sit upright with one leg straight ahead and the other leg bent at the knee, with the bottom of the foot flat against the other leg's inner thigh. If you are not very flexible, point the toes toward your body and lean at the waist toward the extended foot until you feel a stretch in the back of the knee. Hold this position for 10 to 15 seconds.

If you are flexible, assume the same position but reach out with the same-side hand, grab the back of the toes, and pull them toward you. Keep the head up and back as straight as possible.

"People say, 'Oh God, I can feel that one!'" said Anderson. "They're surprised that they feel that tight."

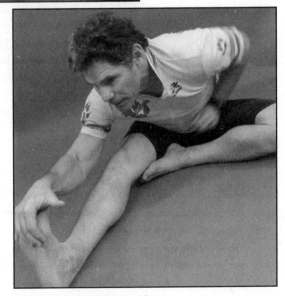

Stretch 2: calf and hamstring

3. Opposite-Hand/Opposite-Foot Quad Stretch

Lying on your side, hold the top of your right foot with your left hand and gently pull your heel toward your buttocks. The knee bends at a natural angle when you hold your foot with the opposite hand. This is good to use in knee rehabilitation and by those with problem knees. Hold for 30 seconds, each leg.

4. Spinal Twist: Lower Back and Hamstrings

Although Anderson warns that this stretch is difficult for the average person to do, it is highly beneficial for cyclists' backs, which are subject to very little movement.

Sit on the floor with your right leg straight ahead. Bend your left leg and cross your left foot over to the outside of your upper right thigh, just above the knee. During this stretch use the elbow to keep the left leg stationary with controlled pressure to the inside. With your left hand resting behind you, slowly turn your head to look over your left shoulder, and at the same time rotate your upper body toward your left hand and arm. This should stretch your lower back and the side of the hip. Hold for 15 seconds. Do both sides.

5. Groin and Back Stretch

This comfortable stretch is an easy, safe way to stretch an area that is often tight and hard to relax: the groin. It also flattens your lower back, helping to counteract a hump. Lie on your back with knees bent, soles of the feet together, and hands resting at your sides. Let the knees hang down toward the floor so that the pull of gravity will be stretching your groin. By contrast, people often sit up and perform a groin stretch by leaning forward with a rounded-back torso that is hard on the back ligaments.

6. "Secretary Stretch" for Lower Back and Hips

Great for cyclists and people with sciatic pain, this stretch begins with you lying on your back with your knees up in a sit-up position. Interlace your fingers behind your head and lift the left leg over the right leg. From here, pivot your left leg to the right, pulling your right leg toward the floor until you feel a good stretch along the side of your hip and lower back. Stretch and relax. Keep the upper back, shoulders, and elbows flat on the floor. Hold for 20 to 30 seconds. Repeat on the other side.

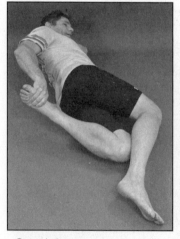

Stretch 3: quad stretch

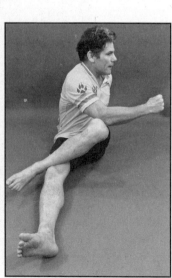

Stretch 4: spinal twist

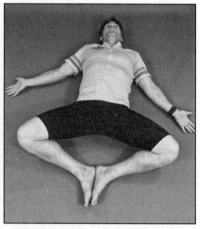

Stretch 5: groin and back

7. The "Saigon Squat"

"If I had one stretch to do, this would be it for keeping overall muscle and joint flexibility," said Anderson. "It's the most natural position in human history—squatting to relieve yourself in a floor-pit toilet." The squat stretches everything from the midsection down, including the ankles, Achilles tendons, groin, lower back, and hips. Anderson is fond of pointing out that it taxes humans much more than the seated position Western toilet, which is why countrified Asians often have better postures and livelier steps than their occidental counterparts.

The squat is simple to perform: With your feet shoulder-width apart and pointed out to about a 15-degree angle, heels on the ground, bend your knees and squat down. Hold for 30 seconds. If you have ultra-tight Achilles tendons, can't balance with flat feet, and generally have trouble staying in this position, hold onto something for support. If you have knee problems, discontinue at the first sign of pain.

8. Williams' Flexion Hamstring Stretch

Considered very relaxing and safe after a ride or a run, this easy stretch is great for pelvic flexibility, the hip flexors, the back, and the circulation (since it gets the foot above the heart).

Lie on your back, keeping your back flat, and draw one knee into your chest by pulling it in from the back of the knee. Repeat with the other leg. For variation, pull the knee toward the opposite shoulder.

9. Elongation Stretch/Total Body Relaxer

This nearly flawless post-exercise stretch feels good, stretches many muscles—abdominals, intercostals, top of the foot and ankle, back, and more—and is particularly good for cyclists because of the way the sport bends them over. "No one's ever criticized it," said Anderson.

Lying down flat on your back, make yourself as "tall" as possible, straightening your arms and legs in opposite directions, pointing your toes, and extending your fingers. Stretch and then relax.

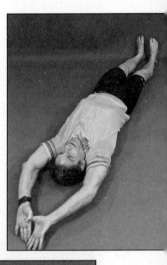

Stretch 9: elongation

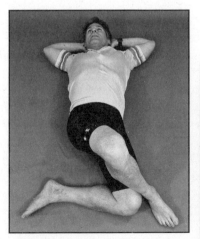

Stretch 6: secretary stretch

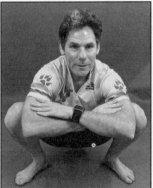

Stretch 8: Williams' flexion

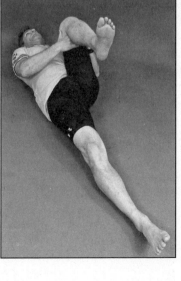

Stretch 7: Saigon squat

Hold for five seconds. For variety, stretch diagonally, extending your opposite arm and leg, then repeat, stretching the opposite sides.

10. Triceps and Tops of Shoulders

Anderson calls the upper body "a storehouse of mental and physical tension." The tension can be caused by cycling as well as non-athletic pressures, such as getting yelled at by the boss at work.

In a seated or standing position with your arms overhead, hold the elbow of one arm with the hand of the other arm, then gently pull the elbow behind the head and push it down, creating a stretch. Do it slowly. Hold for 15 seconds. Do not use drastic force to limber up. Stretch both sides. You can also do this stretch while walking.

Anderson suggests that cyclists take the stretch further by placing the back of the head against the bent elbow and bending to the opposite side. "This counteracts the cycling position and keeps cyclists standing straight up as they age," he said. "It's especially helpful for men, as we tend to get tighter with age than women."

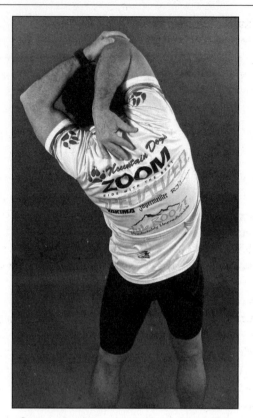

Stretch 10: triceps

PROBLEM 5: SLUMPING POSTURE
Solution: Straighten yourself out before you ride or lift weights.

Let's pull no punches here: Cycling is simply not good for your posture, morphing your back from concave to convex as it freezes you in an unnatural, crunched-up, bent-over position for hours at a time. Frozen in an imbalanced, crab-like position off the bike, you'll be compromised and injury-prone in normal life and other athletic activities designed to complement the sport, such as strength training. That's why postural therapist Patrick Mummy, founder and CEO of the Symmetry pain relief clinic in San Diego and Sacramento and the designer of the back-straightening exercises described in the "Biker's Back" section of Chapter 8, says that lifting weights with bad

posture is "like building a Ferrari on a bent chassis." His 12-exercise routine (starting on page 186) is an antidote to the slumping, hunching posture that he said is often first apparent by age 35. The exercises will stretch the hip flexors to restore the correct pelvic tilt, reposition the shoulders, and equalize the hips to restore bilateral symmetry.

"Step One of any anti-aging maintenance program, by definition, must be posture," Mummy said. "Otherwise, everything you are doing to build yourself up is reinforcing the problem." Perform the exercises twice daily in order, especially before doing any weight training or aerobic exercise. At 1 to 2 minutes each, the exercises should take 10 to 15 minutes total.

PROFILE: VIC COPELAND AND THE FOUNTAIN OF YOUTH

THE SECRETS OF THE WORLD'S GREATEST OVER-55 BIKE RACER

When the first edition of this book was published, then-62-year-old Vic Copeland, an optometrist from Rancho Santa Fe, California, was officially the world's greatest old track cyclist, with a treasure trove of age-group time-trial records. From 40-plus to 50-plus, in distances ranging from 200 meters to 3 kilometers, he was the US record holder. His victories included a world's best 500-meter in the 60–64 age group (35.654 seconds, set in 2004). At the 2003 world track championships in Manchester, England, when he won the 500, the 2K, the points race, and the match sprint (the same four events he had swept six years earlier with *slower* times), the Union Cycliste Internationale (UCI, cycling's governing body) named him "Outstanding rider in the world over age 35"—at age *60*.

Well, over a decade later, nothing's changed. He added more world records in the 500 in the 65–69 age group (37.034, in 2007), and the 70-plus age group (37.855, in 2012).

What's his secret? Good genes, good training, and an off-the-charts will to win, according to his coach, Eddie Borysewicz. "He could have been another Greg LeMond if he had started the sport in his teens," says Eddie B (profiled in an interview starting on page 212), who also coached the three-time Tour de France winner. That's a pretty good comparison for a guy who only got into cycling because it was easier than doing triathlons.

A natural athlete, Copeland had excelled in football, basketball, and track in school and proved to be a fast learner in triathlon. In 1982, as a recreational runner who rode his wife's clunker bike and dog-paddled on the swim ("I grew up in Kansas," he explains), he finished dead last in his first tri, the United States Triathlon Series (USTS) San Diego race in Torrey Pines. Two years later, he won his age group. But after doing five Hawaii Ironman triathlons from 1983 through 1987, including setting a personal record (PR) of 11:00:09 in 1986 at age 42, Copeland walked away from the sport he loved. In 1988, with his kids entering their teens, he and his wife, Joyce, concluded that triathlon training was taking too much time away from the family.

"I had to get into something less all-encompassing," he said. "I thought cycling was something I could do to keep in shape." Talk about an understatement.

One day, while Copeland was riding with the same bike club he'd trained with during his triathlon years, they challenged him to do a cycling race. He finished fourth . . . and the rest is history. He hired Eddie B when the legendary coach moved to nearby Ramona. At the 1988 Masters nationals, he won the criterium and took two second places and a third place on the track. By the mid-1990s, Copeland was known as the Mark Spitz of age-group cycling, scorching the record book with 14 national records in events ranging from the kilo to the road race. At age 49, going against 20-year-olds, he placed eighth overall in the kilo at the Olympic trials. At 50, he set a record for the 35-year-old age group.

How does he explain his success on the bike?

"Besides good genes, the Ironman," he says. A naturally fast sprinter, Copeland believes his long-distance Ironman training taught him how to hold his sprint speed longer than most—a theory he says is borne out by the exceptional performances of Australian track sprinters, who do a lot of long-distance work earlier in the season.

The result? "The younger guys would be ahead of me in the first half of the kilo, but their speeds would drop off the second half," he said. "My speed stayed the same, so I'd win in the last half." Records that Copeland set range from the shortest to the longest: the flying-start 200-meter time trial (11.5 seconds) in 1995; the standing-start kilo (1:07) and flying-start kilo (1:02), both in 1993; the standing-start 3K (3:38), and the tandem 40K (48:18), both in 1996.

(continues)

Initially, winning against younger men got Copeland a lot of attention, but that soon was a non-issue to his opponents. "Occasionally, somebody would come up and joke, 'Hey, I've got 20 more years to get as good as you.'"

Cycling success became a family affair for the Copelands. Son Zack won a national junior championship on the track one year and was on the national team; father and son both competed for match-sprint slots at the 1992 Olympic trials, but never met head-to-head because Vic didn't survive his qualifying round. (Zack barely missed the Olympics, finishing fourth). Daughter Joannie, then 16, set a world junior record in the 1K in 1992 and won the junior criterium nationals the next year; she finished high school in Colorado Springs because she was a member of the US national junior team. Both gave up cycling in college and haven't looked back.

Told that Eddie B said he was born with as much talent as LeMond, Copeland said he has never dwelled on what might have been. But it might have been impressive: His record 1K time in 1992 (though done on a smooth indoor velodrome with high-tech equipment not available 30 years earlier) would have won him the Olympic gold medal in Tokyo in 1964. "If I did it at age 49, certainly I could have done it age 21," he says.

Copeland's greatest challenge was a scare that came after the US national championships in Colorado Springs in August 2004, when he won four gold medals and set two world records in the 60–64 age group. At the US road nationals, he got faint as he went into atrial fibrillation, a rapid-heartbeat condition that prevents blood from circulating through the upper chamber of the heart.

"It was caused by my training—and is triggered by riding hard," he said. "I can go to 87 percent of my maximum heart rate of 160, but can't go anaerobic. At 90 percent or above, which is what you have to do to win races on the track, that will be trouble." For several years, he kept his efforts down to 85 percent, but that couldn't hold him back. He won the 70-plus category again at the 500 meters at the worlds in 2013, and has no plans to slow down.

TRAINING TIPS: HOW COPELAND DID IT

1. Hammer and recover: Coach Eddie B only lets Copeland do two days of intensity a week. "Eddie holds me back," he said. "He says that high intensity raises the acid level in the blood, and that you need longer, slower rides to renormalize." Copeland rides two hours a day, indoors on a trainer and outdoors at the track at San Diego's Balboa Park.

2. No mega miles: "It becomes comfortable to take long, slow rides—but that only trains you to go long and slow," he said. "And they leave you too tired to go fast." During his triathlon days, while his competitors were biking 500-mile weeks, Copeland logged only 150 miles.

3. Specificity: "I break an event down into each segment. If a bike course is hilly, I'll train by doing hill repeats over and over and over."

4. Visualization: Psychologically, Copeland begins his preparation the day before the race. "I try to act as if I've already won the race, in the way I talk to people and act. It creates a winning attitude." Additionally, he visualizes important moments of the race itself, so that his race reactions and strategy will be automatic.

5. Resistance training: Copeland does not lift weights, but for two years has used a one-of-a-kind bike trainer invented by his son in which the pedals turn backward with resistance. "It increases the stress on my muscles in a cycling-specific motion, yet doesn't stress me cardiovascularly."

6. Mind of a champion: "I always had confidence, and Eddie B liked that," he said. "Eddie is not interested in you as a rider unless you're highly motivated already. I've never seen Eddie once push people to ride harder. He wants a mental champion who he can mold." So regardless of your level of talent, think of yourself as a champion. Every day, every ride, can be a race against yourself that you can win.

John Howard

THE MAN WHO CAN DO ANYTHING

Many people have called John Howard "Greg LeMond before there was a Greg LeMond," but that characterization is far too limiting. A monster talent who blew out of the backwoods of Missouri at a time when few Americans raced a bike and even fewer had tried their luck in Europe in decades,[*] Howard has pushed the envelope in every imaginable sphere of cycling. He won a national championship (in 1968) before he could vote, added three more in the 1970s, and so stunned the US Olympic Committee with his 200K win at the 1971 Pan Am Games that it restored financing to a sport it had planned to let expire. The three-time Olympian saw Black Power fists raised in Mexico City in 1968, heard terrorist bullets in Munich in 1972, and competed again in Montreal in 1976. He was still America's top road cyclist in 1979, when he was unceremoniously booted off the US Pan Am team for, as he remembers it, not being a "team player."

Seeking new challenges outside mainstream cycling, Howard won the Hawaii Ironman Triathlon in 1981, finished the first Race Across America in 1982, and risked his life in 1985 in setting an astounding bicycle speed record of 152.2 mph behind a custom-built land rocket. Since then, he's built and sold pedal-powered water bikes; accumulated scores of Masters road- and mountain-bike championships; broken dozens of bones; authored hundreds of articles about form, training, and bike fit; acquired a taste for antique cars; and, of course, been inducted into the US Bicycling Hall of Fame (in 1989).

Infinitely curious and open-minded about unorthodox technologies and fitness regimens (don't get him started about lung trainers and belly breathing), Howard lives in a house in North San Diego County that includes a self-designed indoor-cycling studio and a cycling museum. He runs one of cycling's best-regarded coaching clinics, the John Howard School of Champions and the John Howard Performance Sports FiTTE Clinics. And, by the way, as he mentioned during his Bike for Life interviews in March 2004 and October 2013, he claims to have ridden 800,000 miles. That's about 31 times around the circumference of the Earth.

A COMIC BOOK changed my life. When I was 16, I saw Schwinn Bike Thrills at the local Schwinn shop in my hometown of Springfield, Missouri. I was fascinated. It told the story of Alfred Letourneur's world record—108.92 mph on a Schwinn Paramount drafting a racecar in 1941. Letourneur, known as "the Red Devil," was the most famous six-day bicycle racer in French history and one of the most famous in the world. I thought, God! I've got to do this.

---

[*] Note: Joseph Magnani from Illinois competed in Europe during the 1930s and '40s, and even raced the Giro d'Italia and world professional road championship in 1947.

I went to the library and found a book called *The Big Loop*, a story about the Tour de France. I thought, God! What a wonderful sport. So I went back to the bike shop and bought the first ten-speed in Springfield, Missouri—a Schwinn Continental, a high-end race bike.

Trouble was, nobody in Springfield knew anything about bike racing. The closest I could find was the AYH—American Youth Hostels. They're into touring—the kind with panniers. I wanted some organization, to ride with a group, to find a connection. But after I rode with them, I realized quickly that they were way below my level. Some were serious, but not many. I was just this young stud....

I was a good intramural athlete in baseball, football, and basketball, but the only varsity thing I did was running. I did the mile and would call myself mediocre, even though I won the Ozark Conference mile-championship race. But from the beginning, cycling was my forte. I always seemed to be able to outdistance the rest of the kids in the neighborhood. And I was always into the lightweight equipment; got a three-speed at 12 or 13, a big step up from the cruiser bikes. Then came the move up to the Continental with its derailleur gears—pretty hot stuff back in 1963. My brother and I prided ourselves on being on the cutting edge. He's about a year younger than me—my competitor and best friend.

I always rode more than he did. I loved the blue sky and fresh air. Even on my three-speed, I was traversing hills in the Ozark Mountains—some of the toughest little climbs anywhere to be found in the country. As soon as I got the Continental, I would take that thing down to the Lake Country, a 70-, 80-, 90-mile ride, alone. There was nobody else who would do it. Why'd I do it? [Long pause.] Because it was there. Because I saw the potential. Everyone wants to be good at something. In my case it was covering ground.

I had good cardiovascular, but cycling was different. With a bike I could make progress more rapidly, because the sport itself was on

such an infantile level back then. The true competition in the United States in the '60s was in the velodrome. And right away, I found that it didn't take much to get to the top of the sport. By the time I was 19, I was there.

I would literally ride away from the field and cover 50 miles on hilly courses under two hours, which was unheard of. So I knew this is what I am good at. This is what I can do. At 19, I won the 1968 national championships. The top guys—Parsons, Hiltner, Butler, Van Boven. I beat all of them.

Religion, RAAM, and 152 MPH

PEOPLE DON'T LET me forget that I once called my bike my "Iron Mistress." Metaphorically, it means it was a tool. I won't say that I hadn't discovered girls, but the girlfriends I had were short-term. I can't believe I was ever this way. But back then, I was more focused on the bike. It gave me much more than another person could—particularly a spirituality.

I found myself practicing a very profound, personal form of worship when I turned those pedals. On a bike, passively covering ground for two or three hours, I would experience a wonderful sense of self-discovery, of being a part of a universe that was much more powerful than myself. I say passive for a reason. I can remember covering 20 to 30 miles and having no recollection of being anything but in a complete form of perfect bliss.

Growing up, I was religious—did go to church quite a bit. Being of the Bible Belt, my parents were fairly religious Presbyterians. It was what I did, who I was. But the bike replaced that. It brought me into a whole different landscape. The spirituality of the bicycle was a self-discovery that went much deeper than the four walls of a church. The feeling of being in control of my own destiny, as opposed to having it scripted through the organization of religious doctrine.

To go there by myself, with no training partners, these journeys into the spiritual world, into a separate universe, were powerful motivators.

The spiritual focus changed as the world became more complex and competition came into the mix. But it came back as I got older.

Today, I practice kind of a mix of optimism, Taoism. I believe we are what we practice. I really put more emphasis on the positive nature of things. I feel like that's really the essence of it— coming back to just feeling good about yourself and practicing exactly that. I meditate on this; meditation has been a profound step. I learned to do this during the Race Across America.

For me, the Taoist view of life was extremely profound during RAAM. In 1982, John Marino, Lon Haldeman, Mike Shermer, and I did the first RAAM, the true cycling ultra-event: L.A. at the Santa Monica Pier all the way to the Empire State Building in New York City. It took me 10 days, 10 hours. Tough ride. Headwinds all the way from Kansas through Illinois clear into West Virginia. It was a tough, tough ride.

The sleep deprivation had an impact on me. Going into a trance state, some of my visualizations were extremely powerful. I really didn't associate them at the time with what reality was or should be, but over time I could see that it was an experience that shaped me as an individual. I really understood a lot more about my limitations. My inflexibilities. My temper. All the things I didn't like about myself, I had to come to grips with. In a real, powerful way, I realized what I needed to discard and what I needed to work on and where I needed to go with my life. I would never do RAAM again for anything—it was so grueling. Yet it was a unique time for me—a self-analysis that lasted 10 days; I saw myself at my best and I saw myself at my worst. Where do you have an opportunity to do that?

Since RAAM, I've been better able to control my anger and channel that into more positive progressive experiences. I've been able to use those experiences to understand what I need to do to advance in business, to make a living— what works, what doesn't, what to discard, what to keep. I realize that a lot of the anger that was directed at my crew was really a reflection of my own insecurity problems. I'm still working on it, but I think I've come a long way since 1982.

I clearly see one of my [RAAM] visualizations even today. I was standing by the motor home, waiting for the fog to clear so we could get back on the bikes. Freezing cold. It was in West Virginia, probably less than two days out of New York. Three in the morning and no traffic. Appalachian Mountains. It was so foggy on the descent, it was actually dangerous. I so badly needed sleep. I didn't want to take a risk. While somebody was gathering up something—I don't remember if it was food or what—I was leaning against the motor home. Then this black Lab came up from out of the ditch and started nuzzling me. I remember the cold snout of his nose against my warm palms. And I thought that was great. I played with that dog for a while. Then it was like my eyes were like shutters on a camera. I clicked and the dog was lying down at my feet. Here I am, so tired. I looked around. And when I looked back down a second later, the dog was a pile of bones. Road kill.

I could feel that warm snout. I can feel it— even today. But that experience, God, I get cold chills every time I think about it.

I'm not sure I can apply any meaning to it. Maybe I just chose not to. But there were four or five experiences like that that happened en route at various times during the ride. Through sleep deprivation and lack of good, consistent diet, I just put myself over the edge. But I look back and, like I said, I'd never change anything. But I'd never want 'em repeated.

Although I didn't win, RAAM was the hardest thing I'd ever done, much harder than winning the Hawaii Ironman Triathlon the year before. Then I had to face something even harder: the third act in my four-year post-bike-racer plan, the new bicycle world speed record.

By 1985, I wasn't at my peak anymore—nearly 40 years old, I had been spiraling down since 35. So I had to develop something else: mental fortitude. I was heavily into meditation then, and that was my key to getting over the incredible pressure of the speed record, a confluence of stress I'd never experienced. There was training stress, the monetary stress, the stress of organizing everything—building the supercar, building the superbike, hiring all the people, getting the *Sports Illustrated* article, the sponsorship deal with Pepsi and Wendy's and Specialized, the training, the worrying about the weather conditions on the Bonneville Salt Flats, the fear of death—a very real fear at the speed I'd be going. I didn't want to push the safety envelope, but I had to push it to get the ink we needed to pay off the sponsors, to sell the show to *That's Incredible*. Total pressure—far more than anything I'd ever done. More than winning the Tour of Baja [the first win ever of a big international stage race by an American], scoring high in the Milk Race [the Tour of Britain], taking third in the Tour of Ireland [then the best-ever placing by an American in Europe], winning the Ironman, and doing RAAM.

This speed record was half terror, half exhilaration. I badly needed an edge. It would either bring me to a new realm of self-discovery—or a nightmare that could leave me permanently broken. So as I meditated, I came to my method of dealing with the pressure: visualization. It's the deepest I've ever gone. The image replays like a video camera in my brain. I visualized it—streaking above the vast, endless ribbon of salt flats, a mirage on top of a mirage, the image above me flashing in giant red numbers in the sky: 152. I saw it before it took place. And that day, it was 105°F. I'm covered in my leather suit. Three years of putting this all together—for five minutes of action. No mistakes possible. No do-overs. And when it was over. I looked at the number: 152.2 mph. Didn't just beat the old record (140 mph), but did what we said I'd do: Shatter it.

Fitness, Aging, and Wives' Tales

IN THE EARLY '70s, I had a VO$_2$ max of 82 milliliters per kilogram, up there with all the best pros today. Now, 30 years later, I'm 18 percent lower. I've done my best to counter it, and think I have done quite well.

There is a popular belief that decline is bullshit and we don't deteriorate. But it is very much a genetic issue and it can happen to the best of athletes anytime. We all reach a point where we diminish in terms of vital capacity. You can accept it or just deny it.

I've tried to fight it. One way is that I've vastly improved my range of motion, using specific stretches to gain maximum utilization of my lung capacity. Some of it is Pilates-based. Some of it is yoga. I've used a number of sources to create a program that is the nucleus of our training school. Because I feel like my career has been a guiding point for us and I've used that to help other athletes. I'm very proud of the fact that we've had over 130 national championships won by people I've worked with.

Much of coaching in cycling is steeped in tradition. Old-school stuff. And some of it's good, most of it isn't good. We really believe in following technology as much as possible. Without naming names, let me say that the old way of bike fitting that the French taught us 25 years ago is backward. It doesn't take into consideration the biomechanics, much less the aerodynamics. Christ, I back-test everything I do using the most sophisticated programs available anywhere in the world. We have access to the Allied Aerospace wind tunnel, the most sophisticated low-speed wind tunnel in the world. What the hell. I love [name withheld by request] like a brother. But the bottom line is he's not a coach and all he knows is what the French told him 25 years ago.

It's frustrating to be so clear on the way to improve performance and yet this kind of bogus crap is being pitched out there in [cycling publications]. Old wives' tales. That is exactly what it is. There is very little scientific documentation. On the other hand, my coaches have done a thousand fits a year, and we have an understanding of the way it should be done. We have the electronics to back up what we do. To see it done so wrong is kinda frustrating.

Example: The age-old formulas for saddle height don't take into consideration a lot of important factors. Overall, the traditional bike-fit seems to have absolutely no scientific basis whatsoever.

Everybody should be different with regard to saddle height. It's based on trochanteric leg length. It's based on hamstring flexibility. It's based on the tilt of the saddle. It's based on the amount of hip rotation you have. It's based on how the IT [iliotibial band, the tough muscle sheath on the outside of the thigh running from hip to knee] is lined up. It's based on bone configuration. All of which can be systematically tested. Our work we do is like dyno-testing a racecar. We can show minute changes in performance in terms of torque and wattage. The average guy just can't do it on his own. But we can use our principles to show the simple way to do it—to make somebody comfortable and fast.

People typically have their saddles too low and too far back. You can change the pivot point of the cleat and change torque and watt output for optimal performance. In many cases, the cleat is jammed all the way forward—or too far back. You should be on the ball of your foot, absolutely, for optimal power.

There's an optimal way to do everything—even falling. I've gotten hurt way more mountain biking than road biking. But you can minimize breakage by developing a strategy for going over the bars—essentially a tuck and roll. Very difficult to do, but effective. It needs to be second nature, which means you need to practice it. Throw your shoulders back and try to stay off the collarbone. Stay off the shoulder. Or let the bike absorb the crash. Don't put your hands straight out to break the fall—that breaks the collarbone. I dunno one in a hundred people who'll practice that sort of thing. But if you have the presence of mind to tuck and roll, you're always going to come out of it better. You may lose a lot of skin

on your back and shoulders. But believe me, that grows back a lot faster than a collarbone.

My diet hasn't changed appreciably over the years. I eat a lot of vegetables. A lot of good solid protein. Basic food groups. The essence of it is to try to get the macro levels to supply as much of the nutrients as possible. Failing that, or to supplement that at harder levels, you need some micronutrients. Generally, as you age, think about prevention issues. In males, think prevent prostate cancer. Eat roughage. Leafy vegetables.

On the bike, I still try to put in the miles and do the training—100 to 160 miles per week. But it's smart training. It's what I can do to stay at the top of my game without being competitive. My emphasis has changed. After a life of competition, I no longer compete. Riding for me now is therapeutic. It's beautiful. I go out and experience the bicycle the way it should be. I don't see that [feeling] with retired European pros—they sit back, get fat. Not all of them, of course. But generally, they don't see the bike as I see it: a life tool.

More Than a Wheelman

YET A BIKE'S not the only tool. Even though people may raise their eyebrows at this, I resent being labeled a "cyclist." I think in the human body there are generative vital spirit energies; while cycling brings those out, the ultimate manifestation of energy is not to be tied down to one medium or one source—that is risky. For example, cyclists tend to be stoop-shouldered as they get older, because they are not balanced.

The last thing I would want for somebody to say is, "Oh, there's a cyclist." I don't want to be labeled that way. I want to have balance. To me, that balance is more than physical. It's mental as well. And I look now at the Masters cyclists who are really the ultimate manifestation of what I do, and I think, you know, I don't need that racing anymore. Racing doesn't do it anymore. I don't need to prove that. I've been there. Done that. I have all the titles I'll ever need. And I don't want the degenerative break in what is important physically, you know? I want to have good muscle control. I don't want my low back to be compromised by sitting in the saddle for hours and hours. I came to a conclusion that sort of relates to one of the most important things I learned from the RAAM—that all of us are geared for x-number of miles at effort. When you use that up, it's probably going to be gone and you're going to have to find something else to do.

I really believe in it. I've tempered my whole life with the idea that I don't want to use this energy up. Now I understand that there's a yin and a yang. But I choose on my own now not to race; to me, that's wasteful dissipation of the energy. I'm not saying I'll never race again. But I see it better spent in using it to prolong my feel for life and just enjoying the body shell until it eventually wears out and dies and it will be gone.

I've reached a point where I know that there is no immortality. What's important for me is to prolong, elongate the process of life and to experience it on a positive, blissful level. Play with it. Use the pattern that is set up in a positive way. Move out of this belief that we have to express it in a competitive realm. Because to win something, to win a race, means to make other people lose; in and of itself, that is a hypocritical way of looking at things. I really feel I have evolved beyond the point where I have to compete anymore. It's not the same. It's not international competition. Where are we getting? We don't get on TV anymore. Why do we need to express it that way? I just feel like there is so much more I can impart in terms of coaching, from all of the millions of things I've learned. That, to me, is the real importance of what I do and where I'm going. I want to be the best coach in the world. I want my other coaches to experience what I know so that we collectively can be the best at what we do.

One of my campers said something that really clicked. He'd been to the Carmichael program, and said it pampers you. It lets you experience just what it's like to be a pro cyclist. "But you guys," he said, "you show us how to be a pro cyclist." To me, that was the ultimate compliment. It told me that after all these years, I've learned how to do my job right.

Update

BIKE FOR LIFE checked back with John Howard in October 2013. At age 66, still sprinting at 30 mph on group rides with young "hard-core unemployables" (as he calls them), and competing in events like the El Tour de Tucson (where he typically finishes in the top 15, and suffered a horrible crash in a 40-mph sprint finish in November 2012 that tore half his face off and required major plastic surgery), he reports that his VO2 max is down 22 percent from his prime.

"I might have lost a little snap—my explosive sprint—but I am *not* slower," he asserted. "I can stay in my 53x12 and hang with guys in their early 40s. I just have to work damn hard to do it. When you lose 22 percent of your oxygen-carrying capacity, you have to search for other areas to make up the gap."

For Howard, that includes lots of stretching and strength training, particularly for problem areas like the external rotators, tensor fascia latae (TFL), the IT band, and the lower back stabilizers. He focuses especially on three areas: the glutes, the core, and the upper body. "If the glutes are weak and have poor range of motion, you can't generate force," he said. He does lots of pull-ups and push-ups, which allow him to stand out of the saddle and leverage the bike better by pulling up on the climbs more than he used to.

"I'm stronger than I was at 35—because I need to be," he said.

Howard is dead-set against long, slow, distance (LSD) training. "Going out and logging big miles is a mistake," he said. "An older cyclist will just get slower and slower by focusing on longer events. It's better to go shorter and faster. Limited time is not limited progress. It's more fun riding fast, anyway. Find younger friends—and push it hard."

2

TRAINING

Building a better engine through goal-setting,
periodization, strength training, cycling-specific yoga, recovery,
and staying out of the Black Hole

"Larry! LARRY!! Wake up! WAKE UP! YOU ARE GOING TO DIE!"

I wasn't exaggerating. At 1 a.m., deep in California's High Sierra after 27 straight hours of riding, my friend Larry Lawson and I and 60 others were rolling down a 10,000-foot mountain at 45 mph, and he was nodding off. So I kept us both awake by screaming at him all the way down to the little town of Susanville, where we'd finally get some sleep before riding back to our car, 310 miles west and south in Davis, near Sacramento. It was June 1991, and this was the final qualifier for the mother of all bike rides, the Paris-Brest-Paris randonnée, to be held the next month in France. I was inches from a 1,000-foot drop-off, every fiber of my being consumed by the most monumental challenge of my athletic life. But it didn't dawn on me at the time that I was simply about halfway done with a training ride. A 620-mile training ride!

That was a pretty extreme distance for a guy who, four months earlier, had rarely ridden over a century in any one day, and had never formally "trained" a day in his life on a bicycle.

During the 1980s, I ran for fitness and biked for adventure, only yanking my trusty Univega touring bike out of the garage the day before a two-week or two-month bike tour. I gave no thought to doing any

organized death march, much less training for it. I paid the price occasionally—one time bailing out of a five-day ride from San Francisco to Los Angeles on Day 3 at the San Luis Obispo Greyhound bus depot because I hurt so bad I could no longer walk—but on most slower-paced trips I'd just pedal into shape. Train? What for? Then Larry, who had toured the length of the Mississippi River with me in 1989, suggested we do Paris-Brest-Paris.

Say what you will about the French, but they have a strikingly beautiful country that is heaven to bike-touring, a deep love for cycling, and an uncompromising knowledge of training. If you wanted to do their beloved, quadrennial 1,200-kilometer (746-mile) ride from the capital to the Atlantic coast town of Brest and back, a tradition that began in 1891, you were required to survive a butt-numbing series of progressively longer, time-limited qualifiers called "brevets": a 200K, 300K, 400K, and 600K. For me, each brevet, spaced about three weeks apart, was a new landmark of distance and agony...and revelation.

As I pushed myself further and harder than ever before, then collapsed back home in an orgy of relief, rest, and healing, I was amazed again and again to find my body emerging remarkably stronger and more powerful at the next brevet. Before my very eyes, I was transforming every 21 days, mutating like the Incredible Hulk, ramping up to a new PR, a new level of cycling insanity—186 miles, 248 miles, 372 miles. When we survived the final 1,000K (621-mile) brevet from Davis to Susanville and back—a special requirement the French imposed solely on US riders in response to our exceedingly high drop-out rate at the '87 P-B-P—I crossed the line wasted, moaning with every pedal stroke, barely able to walk, hating the very sight of that vile pain machine. In fact, I wouldn't touch my bike again for a week. But I wasn't worried a bit.

I knew by then that this amazing, stair-step training effect of "kill-yourself-and-rest"—an extreme example of the "periodization" program outlined in this chapter—would morph me into a cycling cyborg by the next month in France. Despite numerous mechanical problems and major time off the bike, I finished P-B-P in 88 hours, 55 minutes—an hour under the 90-hour cutoff. Americans as a whole that year had the highest finishing percentage of all nationalities among the 5,000 participants.

This experience changed me; now, I crave the hard challenges and the training they demand. Yes, I still love the freedom of touring, of randomly exploring, of going out with no goal other than to be as free as a bird to see what I can see. The bike allows that like nothing else in this world. But discovering that you are in possession of a strange, wonderful, self-improving machine—your own body—that in a few months can be molded and transformed through training into a high-performance being that can survive P-B-P or La Ruta or the Furnace Creek 508 or a double century or that 10-mile hill climb in your local mountains, brings about a different, empowering kind of freedom that can be even more satisfying.

Situation: A friend—say, someone you haven't seen in five years, since he moved to Singapore—calls up one day and says, "Hey, I'm flying into town tomorrow for a business meeting. How

about on Tuesday we get together and do our old four-hour mountain bike loop up Silverado Canyon?"

You freeze. You haven't done anything athletic in weeks—months, if dog walking doesn't count. If you say yes, you know what to expect: lung-wheezing, leg-burning, back-aching pain, followed by a week of limping on sore knees and frayed tendons. Maybe a doctor visit, too. "Yeahhh, ughh, okay," you stammer, too embarrassed to say no, all the while wondering how you managed to get so out of shape.

The answer might be that you're lazy or too busy. But it's more likely that you simply don't have a training plan.

Fact: People tend to respond to plans—and slack off in the absence of them. On the job, you follow a business plan—1-year, 5-year, 10-year. You plan for your retirement with a 401(k), an IRA, and income property. By the same token, if you want to ride the way you did at 30 when you're 50, or do the Furnace Creek 508 race at 71, like Berkeley's Gerd Rosenblatt did (see his story in Chapter 10), or generally be confident enough to take on an unexpected ride at any age, you can't just wing it. You need a plan. Cycling, which, with its huge menu of highly motivating events and exhilarating biomechanical efficiency, encourages long, fun hours of exercise, is the ideal sport to build an athletic training plan around.

The word "training" may seem scary to some, because it sounds like—and is—hard work. But if you understand that training should not be a daily hammerfest but a structured process that encompasses a logical series of easy and hard, long and short, on- and off-the-bike workouts, the hard work won't seem so daunting. In fact, given training's benefits—a regular endorphin rush; almost-instant feedback, in the form of identifiable, enhanced fitness and a more youthful appearance; and the Superman-like pleasure of knowing you can perform feats younger people can't—you may come to look forward to, and even love, the hard work of training. Yet, in the same way that you can't truly love a person unless you understand him or her, you can't love training and feel compelled to do it often unless you understand its logic.

Training for both competition and healthy longevity must include the three-legged stool of fitness described in chapter 1: aerobics, strength, and flexibility. These three elements are addressed in this chapter by two different training strategies: *Periodization*, a classic race-preparation buildup plan; and *The Blend*, an unconventional, nonspecific default mode designed for all-around fitness and longevity. Here are summaries of each with details following.

1. Periodization—Used by the world's greatest athletes for decades, this classic training plan slowly ramps up and peaks your fitness for a long-distance endurance event through five training phases, or periods. It starts with the all-important "base phase," an eight-week period of low-heart-rate aerobics that keeps you out of a deleterious, too-fast "Black Hole" pace (more on this later) as it converts your body into a "fat-burning machine" that can ride all day on your unlimited stores of body fat. After that, it adds strength and speedwork phases that bring you to top form on race day. Developed in the 1950s in Eastern Europe, codified in the 1960s by Romanian coach Tudor Bompa, and a mainstay in the West since the late 1970s, periodization is the foundation of all modern training for a simple reason: It works—if you have the patience to stick with it. Leaving nothing to chance, it is a virtually foolproof training regimen.

2. The Blend—A general-purpose, all-around mix of aerobic and strength work, The Blend will keep you ready for anything, from century rides to triathlons to mud runs to snow shoveling. Incorporating a broad mix of cross-training, heavy weight training (a unique and effective strength program called "Maximum Overload," which is debuting in this new edition of *Bike for Life*), intervals, and low-heart-rate LSD (long, slow, distance) rides, The Blend is the default workout strategy for the rest of your life whenever you are not training for a specific race. It works on a simple principle: *Follow a hard day with an easy day.* The hard challenge gives your body the stress that motivates it to adapt and get stronger, while the easy, low-heart-rate day gives it the recovery time it needs to consolidate the improvement. This simple hard-easy paradigm at the heart of all good training plans (including periodization) will keep you physically and mentally fresh and provide built-in flexibility, fun, and do-ability. No matter where you are and what workout facilities are available, you can create a hard workout and an easy workout. The Blend is not ideal for longer endurance events, which require more sport specificity and the fat-burning efficiency of a strict periodization plan, but it will allow you to start any periodization training from a high base of fitness.

Think of periodization as the template for optimal race performance, and The Blend what you do all other times for all-around fitness. Used as prescribed, the two methods will reduce overtraining-borne injuries and illness, raise your speed, slow age-related decline, and provide the blueprint for superfit longevity.

But before they are discussed further, you need a focus that gives you the motivation to train in the first place. That's why Step 1 of any training program is setting goals.

STEP 1: SETTING GOALS
Make Your Life a Non-Stop Event

At 45, Rich MacInnes wanted to be a top-level competitor, just like he was back in college. Dan Crain, 60, wanted to set an untouchable record. When he hit 50, mountain bike superstar Tinker Juarez decided to keep racing—and winning—against competitors half his age. All three, profiled in this chapter, succeeded because they decided to give themselves an extremely important gift: a goal.

Goals give you a reason to get on the bike. They give your training purpose, urgency, and excitement. And, maybe most important, they put the fear into you. I've often thought to myself, "If I don't climb the hills today, don't lift the weights, I won't survive La Ruta . . . or the BC Bike Race . . . or the Beverly Hills Gran Fondo"—which inevitably forces me to work out on days I probably wouldn't have otherwise.

Big ones, small ones—you need a whole series of goals to reinforce one another: lifelong goals (e.g., ride a century at age 100), decade-by-decade goals (e.g., climb Maui's 10,000-foot Mt. Haleakala faster at age 50 than you did at age 40), annual goals (e.g., earn a California Triple Crown T-shirt by doing three double-centuries), and monthly goals (e.g., do at least one four-hour bike ride with your friends). Mix the goals up every year to stay fresh. Write all your long- and short-term goals down in your appointment book, just as you would business deadlines.

It's easy to get motivated to train for a challenging event a couple of months down the road. That's near enough to keep you focused for a while. But I think training to maintain a fitness lifestyle that keeps you strong enough to hammer at 50 or 60 or 80 requires at least one major challenge per season, plus several smaller "booster shots" to keep you on track. Cycling offers a vast variety of activities to keep your interest high: multiday cross-state rides, charity benefit rides, hill-climb challenges, weeklong mountain bike stage races, and epic one-day events (see Chapters 11 and 14 for ideas). To keep the training fever hot, also take advantage of the age-group format of Masters racing and triathlons; thousands of cyclists actually look forward to "aging up" to, say, the 55–59 age group, where they'll be the young studs for a couple of years.

Beyond keeping you focused, goals provide definable memory markers that are often missing in adult life, when one year of fighting traffic and paying bills can seamlessly blend into another. Kids instantly identify years with grades, teachers, proms, and soccer championships. But after college, life can fade into a fuzzy morass of adult responsibilities. Yet there's one easy way to prevent the decades from slipping by unannounced: Mark the years with memorable fitness benchmarks.

"2020? What a year!" you'll tell your great-grandchildren 50 years from now. "That's the year I turned 50 and did the TransAlp Challenge." They'll look at themselves and wonder: How did the old codger do something that crazy at 50? And how does he remember all that stuff a half-century later? Answer: It was something worth remembering—and training for it kept you in shape and excited all year. Heck, even if your memory frays, you'll have the photo albums and finisher's medals to jog it.

However you do it, the ultimate objective of setting goals is to turn your life into a non-stop event—which, by definition, requires non-stop training. Goals make you afraid to get out of shape, afraid to grab the Cheetos and ride the couch. When that happens, training may become an end unto itself, the chicken *and* the egg, a necessary and enjoyable part of life that you look forward to, much like eating, sleeping, and brushing your teeth.

STEP 2: BUILDING THE AEROBIC ENGINE WITH PERIODIZATION & THE BLEND
Training Option A: Periodization: Perfect Prep for a Race

The Einstein of athletic training is Tudor O. Bompa, who outlined the framework on which most modern training today is based. In 1963, the Romanian coach developed his own "unified theory" of fitness: "periodization," a relatively simple series of stair-step training schedules that were first used successfully by athletes in Soviet-bloc countries. Bompa originally developed periodization for weight lifters, but the method is now used by the world's best athletes in every sport—from cycling to running to swimming—and virtually ensures success when followed. Periodization develops remarkably high fitness by making every workout count.

In a nutshell, periodization is a series of methodical, progressive physical challenges that are peppered with variety and punctuated with rest. It starts with a goal and plans a workout schedule aimed at reaching it, breaking the training year up into five "periods," training phases that vary the volume, timing, and intensity of workouts. Many call it "planned variation."

Why the need for variation? Researchers predating Bompa found that doing the same thing over and over eventually causes the body to stop improving, a process known as the "general adaptation syndrome." It turns out that the body is a very efficient adaptive learning machine: It improves in response to incrementally increasing stress—for a while; at a certain point, it will adapt and plateau. Over time, your body actually "learns" how to ride your favorite 20-mile loop (or bench press that same 150 pounds at the gym) more efficiently—but then your muscles cease to get stronger. What they get is more efficient—because you are building neural pathways that let you do that same work with less muscle. So, ironically, you can actually *lose* some of your former strength since you lose what you don't need to accomplish that particular task.

The solution is to stress your body, rest it, then stress it again even more. That's periodization. By altering your workouts (adding more hills to your bike route, or using a different hand position when doing a bench press), you force your muscles to grow in new ways, recruiting new fibers in a different order and adding to overall strength.

In periodization, deliberate rest and recovery times are also planned. That's because your body actually consolidates the gains of your workouts during downtime. Hard workouts, in particular, must be followed by rest and easy "recovery" workouts. Technically, the body doesn't get stronger during a workout; it gets broken down. It is during the rest phase that it repairs, rebuilding itself to be stronger than before.

What exactly gets stronger? Periodization simultaneously develops two types of fitness: *aerobic* and *structural*. Aerobic, or metabolic, fitness builds your cardiovascular system (heart, veins, and capillaries), pulmonary system (the lungs), endocrine system (hormones), and nervous system as well as the energy production in the muscles themselves. Structural fitness includes strengthening muscles, tendons, ligaments, and bones.

Summary: If you ride the same miles at the same speed all the time, you'll plateau. Your body responds to periodization's escalating variety of challenges and subsequent rest by getting fitter and better able to handle hard work and by safely and gradually making gains in strength, speed, power, and endurance. The changing variation also alters motor coordination and gives muscles balanced shape and size. On the other hand, "variation" doesn't mean chaos. While random workouts will aid overall fitness, they won't help you reach a sport-specific goal as effectively as periodization will.

Five Periodization Phases: Base, Strength, Power, Peak, and Taper

Periodization uses five periods, or phases, to prepare you for your goal. Each phase has a specific conditioning purpose and can last anywhere from a few weeks to several months, depending on your objective, whether it be riding a seven-hour century in June; mountain biking across Costa Rica in November; or keeping up with your 11-year-old grandson on the bike path by Christmas. In periodization, every workout is performed with your specific objective in mind.

Sample goal: Let's say it's February, you've spent most of the snowy winter swimming or cross-country skiing, and you want to do a moderate hilly century ride in June. Here's your plan:

Phase 1: Base Training

Duration: Eight weeks

Workout plan: Long, slow rides at sub-threshold heart rate, with an extra-long weekend ride.

Base training is the key to periodization, so don't rush it. The phases that follow will make you faster and stronger, but your base is crucial because it's what allows you to go the distance. It takes about eight weeks for the human body to make the improvements in its structure, muscle power, and fuel-burning ability that will allow you to ride comfortably all day. The base uses a gradual mileage ramp-up with low-intensity, low-heart-rate workouts. It includes long weekend rides as well as recovery days. Base training forces the body to make adaptations that will safely improve your endurance in several ways:

1. Turns you into a "fat-burning machine." Your fueling system converts to rely mainly on fat, of which all bodies have a near unlimited supply. Fat also packs a lot of bang for the buck: 9 calories per gram versus 4 calories for carbs (glycogen). So, once you learn to burn it efficiently, you can ride all day on fat—saving your limited stores of carbs for your brain.

2. Builds up your metabolic and structural foundation. The physical stress of training improves your cardiovascular infrastructure (lungs, heart, veins, capillaries) and hardens your body's bones, muscles, and connective tissue for the tougher workouts to come.

3. Increases mitochondria. These tiny production factories within the muscle cells, which create energy, are stimulated by ever-longer low-intensity rides. The body meets the demand for more energy by packing each cell with more mitochondria. Think of them as cylinders in a car engine (except that fats and oxygen are mixed and ignited, instead of gasoline and

oxygen). When you follow the classic slow build-up of your base, you are essentially turning your four-cylinder metabolism into a supercharged V-8. To provide more fuel to this bigger engine, more capillaries (see No. 2) arise.

4. Increases glycogen storage. The weekend LSD workouts not only will improve your fat-burning engine, but train your body to store more glycogen (carbs). By depleting it, in a process called "supercompensation," you teach your muscles and liver to store even more glycogen—from maybe 1,500 to 1,800, 2,100, or 2,500. (But remember, that's still only enough to ride a couple of hours on, max.)

5. Prevents overtraining. A regimented plan of stair-step increases and built-in recovery days prevents the classic signs of overtraining: feeling burned out, getting sick and injured, and poor performance.

To help the cause, you'll also train with light weights, which will help isolate and strengthen all the little "helper" muscles that act to stabilize each joint and perfect your cycling mechanics.

The base phase contains two four-week subphases in which training hours slowly increase to prevent overtraining. The second subphase starts at a lower level than where the first ended.

Again, the key to base training is to go slow. Ramp up the miles and pace by no more than 10 percent per week. Be patient. Hold back. Fight the urge to surge. Base training is all about low-intensity workouts at maximum volume— long, slow, distance rides (LSD). The "S" in LSD could be "slow" or "steady." Either way, it means keeping it challenging without pushing it over the limit.

The limit is a specific heart-rate level called "threshold," the point at which you begin to convert from aerobic to anaerobic metabolism. (To help you identify this point, read "Take the Talk Test" on page 36.)

The importance of staying aerobic for at least eight weeks can't be overemphasized. "That's how long it takes to optimize your fat-burning metabolism," says physical therapist Robert Forster, a trainer of Olympic athletes, owner of the Phase IV high-performance training center in Santa Monica, California, and a longtime participant in mountain- and road-bike stage races such as the TransAlp Challenge. "Push it too hard before base building is done and your muscles will reach for [faster-burning] carbs, compromising the building of your fat pathways." Those pathways include miles of new capillaries, the tiny vascular pipes that deliver O_2 to the ever-denser mitochondria. One problem: capillaries respond much slower to stimuli than muscles and lungs. You must build the base slowly.

Remember that the goal in burning a higher percentage of fat for fuel is to spare glycogen, an essential brain fuel which will only last a couple of hours. Fat can fuel you all day if you teach your body to tap it.

By the end of the two-month base-training period, a prospective century rider should have built his or her body and fat-burning engine up to the point where it can survive a 75- to 80-mile ride without body aches and bonking. Now it's time for Phase 2, when you add the strength and speed that will allow you to survive—and thrive—at a fast, hilly 100-miler (Note: Please read the Talk Test sidebar before moving on to Phase 2. It describes the ideal pace for fat burning and how to stay out of the indidious "Black Hole," an alluring but detrimental effort level.)

Phase 2: Strength Development

Duration: Four weeks

Workout plan: Shorter, faster rides with more hills (just under threshold); five-minute cruise intervals; heavier weight-lifting; and a long ride every two weeks

This higher-intensity training cycle utilizes hill climbs and heavier weight-lifting to increase the strength of the tendons, bones, and bigger muscles that propel you forward. Do 10 to 12 reps of weight

exercises, but not to failure. Since mileage is inversely related to intensity in periodization, reduce your mileage.

Now that you've built your metabolic and structural base in Phase 1, you'll try to raise your ability to do hard work—to, say, climb several miles without significantly slowing down. Technically, in Phase 2 you are trying to raise your threshold. If you do, you'll stay aerobic at a higher heart rate, keep burning a high-fat/low-carb fuel mix, delay the production of lactic acid, and keep out of the Black Hole, which is being pushed up into a higher bpm range.

Your tools to accomplish this will include low-heart-rate hill climbing, sustained long intervals ("cruise" intervals), and training sessions with moderately higher intensities than those encountered in Phase 1. Since what isn't trained gets de-trained, long efforts are still part of this phase. Every second week, you will ride a distance close to your longest day of base training and follow it with a recovery day to prevent overtraining.

Bottom line: If you raise your threshold, you'll be able to ride faster for a longer time without breathing heavy and feeling your muscles burn. You'll delay going anaerobic—and keep burning all that wonderful, high-calorie fat.

Phase 3: Power Conversion

Duration: Four weeks

Workout plan: Shorter mileages; short, intense intervals; hill repeats; and short, heavy weight workouts with basic power exercises at 6 to 8 reps to failure; along with maintaining the LSD ride every other week

Intensity: Intervals

Food note: Although you're now a fat-burning machine, able to incinerate fats at higher intensities, you'll need to add more carbs (healthy ones, of course) for the harder, more anaerobic workouts in this phase.

Weights: Two times per week. Aim for faster

TAKE THE TALK TEST
IT'LL KEEP YOU BURNING FAT AND OUT OF THE BLACK HOLE

Since you need to optimize your body to burn your fat as fuel, the Base Training period, you must make sure it gets all the oxygen it needs to do so. You do this by keeping your effort—and heartrate—low.

But how low? Where exactly does a too-high heart rate begin?

The line between low and high heart rate, aerobic and anaerobic metabolism, is technically known as *threshold*. Threshold will be different for everyone based on heredity, age, and fitness. How do you find it? The easiest and cheapest way is the "talk test."

The talk test simply involves saying the Pledge of Allegiance while you ride. Start at a low speed that allows you to speak the words continuously without getting out of breath. Then, increase your speed by 1 mph every two minutes. As you settle in to that pace, repeat the Pledge again and note the ease or difficulty of your breathing. Finally, when you reach a speed at which you cannot say the Pledge straight through without gasping for breath, check your heart-rate monitor: That is your threshold heart rate.

If you've got the time and money, you can get a more exact threshold number by going to a lab, hopping on a stationary bike, and taking an LT test—lactate threshold. This involves someone pricking your fingers and drawing blood samples (instead of you reciting the Pledge) while you are riding at different speeds. The blood is then analyzed and graphed for the presence of lactate, a waste product produced during the burning of carbohydrate, which rises as you go more anaerobic. When the graph shows an abrupt rise in lactate concentration, that is your threshold heart rate.

At all times, you burn a combination of fat and carbs for fuel. To develop a metabolism that runs on the highest possible ratio of fat to carbs, you must stay below threshold. That is the overriding goal of the base training phase.

Unfortunately, most people routinely exceed their threshold heart rate, unwittingly training in a harmful and insidious heart-rate zone just above it. This zone is known as the Black Hole.

The Black Hole is harmful because it can really mess up your recovery. And it's insidious because you can slip into it without knowing.

The Black Hole is located in a narrow heart-rate range just above pure aerobic range—from 100 percent to 105 percent of your threshold. Therefore, if your threshold is 150 beats per minute (bpm), your Black Hole will be 150 to 157.5 bpm. The trouble with this effort is that it is sort of hard and satisfying to stay in, but not *that* hard. Stuck in the no-man's land in the middle of easy and hard, the Black Hole pace is double trouble: not as hard or painful as sprint/interval training, but harder than staying strictly aerobic with LSD workouts. It's not hard enough to make you stronger, but it's too hard to allow for recovery. So staying there leaves you slightly fatigued. Stay in the Black Hole for weeks at a time, as most people seem to do on their daily rides, and you will inevitably get sick, increase your injury risk, and end up slower than you ought to be.

Because anything over threshold spikes your lactate, the Black Hole slows your body's use of fat as a fuel and drains your carb stores. Yet the pace feels so good to ride in that some people stay in the Black Hole for years, not realizing that it's holding them back.

Do you know people who ride and run the same route year after year, and never improve? They're stuck in the Black Hole.

The Black Hole was discovered in 2006–2007 by an international team of sports researchers led by Jonathan-Esteve Lanos of Spain, Carl Foster of the University of Wisconsin at La Crosse, and Stephen Seiler, an American who teaches at Agder University in Kristiansund, Norway. Their survey of endurance athletes, "Impact of Training Intensity Distribution on Performance in Endurance Athletes," published in a 2007 issue of the *Journal of Strength and Conditioning Research*, found that

(continues)

those who minimized their time in the Black Hole and expanded their time in the sub-threshold LSD recovery zone got faster. Those who spent more time in the Black did not—and suffered more training injuries. The findings, which I wrote about in a 2010 issue of *Outside* magazine, were clear: *Better recovery, not additional hard efforts, led to better performance.*

Seiler, an astronomy buff, named this poisonous middle zone the Black Hole because, like a Black Hole in space, it "sucks everything in." It sucks slow bikers into going too fast, and sucks fast bikers into going too slow.

Most of your improvement in speed, endurance, and fat-burning capability will come from riding close to, but just under, your threshold. Wear a heart-rate monitor and resist the urge to slip into the Black Hole. If all you have training time for is Phase 1, no problem. You can make huge gains by staying under threshold and out of the Black.

Mark Allen is proof of that. The six-time Hawaii Ironman triathlon winner, widely acknowledged as the best triathlete in history, was a pioneer in using low-heart-rate training to build a fat-burning engine. His coach, Phil Maffetone, had Allen keep his heart rate below his threshold of 150 bpm, which was so low that at first he had to walk to keep from exceeding it. As Allen got fitter—meaning that he was burning fat at higher speeds—he could ride 25 mph for 112 miles and run sub-six-minute miles over a marathon distance at 150 bpm.

So the rule is simple: Don't exceed your threshold heart rate during the Base Training phase. "I've seen athletes train a couple beats too high, and they're overtrained," said Maffetone. Allen only started doing intervals and speedwork after his base was built and his well tuned fat-burning engine was in place. If you stick to the time-tested periodization plan, you'll get one, too.

KEEP THE RECOVERY DAY PURE

The importance of recovery cannot be overemphasized. You must get recovery after any hard workout, no matter the week or the phase. And if you feel tired after a recovery day, take another one. Base training even builds in a recovery week at the end of each four-week phase. Recovery refreshes your mind and body and lets the effect of your hard-training days sink in, so you come back stronger. A recovery workout must not produce stress; its low intensity is rejuvenating—like a massage. Recovery permits your body (and your mind) to test the limits of athletic potential without falling over the edge into overtraining/under-recovery. Over time, if you don't honor your scheduled recovery days and weeks, exhaustion and mediocre results will follow.

Recovery can mean a lot of things: doing shorter, lower-intensity rides, cross-training, or even just sitting on the couch if you need it.

Cross-training—swimming, skating, running, hiking, doing the elliptical machine, or playing tennis—can be very handy. It helps build a more well-rounded body, and it can be more convenient to do than cycling, especially on weekdays. As always, the goal is to stay aerobically active, but lower the burners.

As you do, resist the urge to throw in even one or two hard efforts. That's because it appears that even a small, short burst of high intensity (or even moderate intensity) can wreck a recovery day. "We think there's a physiological tripwire," said Carl Foster. "Slip into the Black Hole for a few minutes—or do an interval or two—and the body reads the whole workout as hard. It cancels the easy day's recovery effect."

So don't forget: "The Black Hole is poison," said Foster. "It won't get you as strong as intervals, but will leave you just as fatigued. Keep the recovery day pure."

contractions and use the same multijoint exercises as in Phase 2, but reduce the load to 60 percent of your new one-rep max for each exercise and increase your movement speed. This new power will get you over hills faster.

Your goal in this phase is to convert your newfound strength (from Phase 2) into power, an essential ingredient of speed. Power puts a time element into strength—the ability to develop and deliver force quickly through faster muscle contraction. Your tools will be shorter, higher-intensity intervals and short hill repeats.

As you go anaerobic during super-hard 30- to 60-second intervals, your body will burn carbohydrates and leave behind lactic acid as a waste product, which your system will learn to clear or use as fuel via the on-again/off-again nature of the intervals. To teach your body how to do that, you can't just do one or two of them. Aim for eight intervals, a good challenge that makes for a compact 20-minute workout if you rest for 90 seconds after each one. Utilize a bike trainer, stationary bike, or bike hill climbs for the intervals.

Since intervals beat you up, be sure to get recovery the next day, including good sleep, stretching or yoga, an easy swim, and a generous warm-up and cool-down. This will limit the amount of cellular damage from each session and let you come back strong in a couple of days.

Phase 4: Speed or Strength Endurance

Duration: Four weeks

Workout plan: Decreased mileage and increased intensity, with all-out sprints; maintenance of the long weekend ride; and weight lifting once a week at very high reps (30 to 50) and light loads (20 percent of one-rep max) to raise muscle endurance without tightness

Food note: Eat a lot on hard days, but less on recovery days, to avoid weight gain as you reduce overall mileage. Add healthy carbs the night before and after intervals. Your regular meals should maintain healthy fats and protein sources.

The goal in Phase 4 is to eke out a little more speed and fatigue-resistance through holding good form. Your tools are 5-mile repeats, with the focus more on holding form than on absolute leg speed. The idea is train yourself to keep up good cycling mechanics in a fatigued state.

Phase 5: Peak and Taper

Duration: One week

Workout plan: A couple of fast, short rides, three days apart

Relax—but only a little. Now you're at peak fitness (which you can hold for 3 to 4 weeks), but not well rested. For that, you must "taper"—back off on the volume. But this isn't just about rest, as you must work out just enough to stay sharp—two short, intense bike days with no strength work—as you gain a deep recovery that will leave you fresh for your goal event. Work out too much and you'll be fatigued on game day. It's a fine line that plenty of elite athletes cross. You can walk the line successfully if you follow two rules:

Rule No. 1: Forget about a last long ride. You can't develop any more fitness, but you can tire yourself out and sabotage the event you've long been training for. The stress levied on your body must now be unloaded for your top-level fitness to show up at the start line.

Rule No. 2: Maintain the high intensity and frequency of your workouts, but cut the distance. Chop your volume by 30 percent on the first workout, then another 30 percent on the next. Shave duration from longer efforts. You may be able to hold a peak for a month, but not much longer, so when targeting several events, keep them close together on the calendar.

Phase 6: Transition

Duration: At least a week, depending on your next event

Workout plan: Easy riding and cross-training

16-WEEK PERIODIZATION TRAINING PLAN FOR A CENTURY (100-MILE) RIDE

PHASE 1: BASE BUILDING. Goal: Train your body to go the distance on very little fuel so you won't bonk. This 8 weeks will develop your aerobic infrastructure and musculoskeletal resiliency, pack more glycogen into the muscles, and train your body to burn a higher percentage of fat as fuel.

	WEEK 1	WEEK 2	WEEK 3	WEEK 4 (recovery)	WEEK 5	WEEK 6	WEEK 7	WEEK 8 (recovery)
Sun.	Off Day/ Tennis or Golf	Off Day/ Hiking or Golf	Off Day/ Tennis or Golf	Off Day/ Hiking or Golf	Off Day/ Tennis or Golf	Off Day/ Hiking or Golf	Off Day/ Tennis or Golf	Off Day/ Hiking or Golf
Mon.	30 min. indoor bike	30 min. indoor bike	45 min. indoor bike	30 min. indoor bike	45 min. indoor bike	50 min. indoor bike	1 hour indoor bike	45 min. indoor bike
Tues.	Strength Day: Light-weight all-body circuit training (3 sets x 10 reps). Warm-up with Symmetry. Cool-down with 10 min. easy run	Strength Day: Light-weight all-body circuit training (5% over Wk 1; 3 sets x 10 reps). Warm-up with Symmetry. Cool-down with 10 min. easy run	Strength Day: Light-weight all-body circuit training (5% over Wk 2; 3 sets x 10 reps). Warm-up with Symmetry. Cool-down with 10 min. easy run	Strength Day: Light-weight all-body circuit training (back to Wk 2 level; 3 sets x 10 reps). Warm-up with Symmetry. Cool-down with 10 min. easy elliptical	Strength Day: Light-weight all-body circuit training (Wk 3 level; 3 sets x 10 reps). Warm-up with Symmetry. Cool-down with 15 min. easy run	Strength Day: Light-weight all-body circuit training (5% over Wk 5; 3 sets x 10 reps). Warm-up with Symmetry. Cool-down with 15 min. easy run	Strength Day: Light-weight all-body circuit training (5% over Wk 6; 3 sets x 10 reps). Warm-up with Symmetry. Cool-down with 15 min. easy run	Strength Day: Light-weight all-body circuit training (Wk 6 level; 3 sets x 10 reps). Warm-up with Symmetry. Cool-down with 15 min. elliptical
Wed.	Yoga/ Stretching	Yoga/ Stretching	Yoga/ Stretching	Yoga/ Stretching	Yoga/ Stretching	Yoga/ Stretching	Yoga/ Stretching	Yoga/ Stretching
Thur.	30 min. indoor bike	30 min. indoor bike	45 min. indoor bike	30 min. indoor bike	45 min. indoor bike	50 min. indoor bike	1 hour indoor bike	45 min. indoor bike
Fri.	Strength/Butt Day: Light-weight circuit training (3 x 10) + crab walk and lateral butt exercises. Warm-up with Symmetry. Finish with 10 min. swim (or row)	Strength/Butt Day: Light-weight circuit training (3 x 10; Wk 1 level + 5%) + crab walk and lateral butt exercises. Warm-up with Symmetry. Finish with 10 min. swim (or row)	Strength/Butt Day: Light-weight circuit training (3 x 10; Wk 2 + 5%) + crab walk and lateral butt exercises. Warm-up with Symmetry. Finish with 15 min. swim (or row)	Strength/Butt Day: Light-weight circuit training (3 x 10; Wk 2 level) + crab walk and lateral butt exercises. Warm-up with Symmetry. Finish with 10 min. swim (or row)	Strength/Butt Day: Light-weight circuit training (3 x 10; Wk 3) + crab walk and lateral butt exercises. Warm-up with Symmetry. Finish with 15 min. swim (or row)	Strength/Butt Day: Light-weight circuit training (3 x 10; Wk 5 + 5%) + crab walk and lateral butt exercises. Warm-up with Symmetry. Finish with 15 min. swim (or row)	Strength/Butt Day: Light-weight circuit training (3 x 10; Wk 6 + 5%) + crab walk and lateral butt exercises. Warm-up with Symmetry. Finish with 20 min. swim (or row)	Strength/Butt Day: Light-weight circuit training (3 x 10; Wk 6 level) + crab walk and lateral butt exercises. Warm-up with Symmetry. Finish with 15 min. swim (or row)
Sat.	LSD Ride: flat, low-HR 15 miles	LSD Ride: flat, low-HR 20 miles	LSD Ride: flat, low-HR 30 miles	LSD Recovery Ride: flat, low-HR 20 miles	LSD Ride: flat, low-HR 30 miles	LSD Ride: flat, low-HR 40 miles	LSD Ride: flat, low-HR 50 miles	LSD Recovery Ride: flat, low-HR 40 miles

	WEEK 9	WEEK 10	WEEK 11	WEEK 12	WEEK 13	WEEK 14	WEEK 15	WEEK 16
	PHASE 2: STRENGTH Goal: Having built your fat-burning engine in Phase 1, now use heavy weights and slow hill climbs to raise anaerobic threshold and build the muscles that can tolerate higher sustained speed and harder work. Also, continue building LSD miles			**PHASE 3: POWER** Goal: Convert strength into speed, and teach your body to process the lactic acid waste product with intervals, Spinning, and pumping lighter weights with more speed and reps. LSD miles keep building up		**PHASE 4: SPEED** Goal: Reach top-end speed by reducing weight workouts and adding more intervals as LSD peaks		**PHASE 5: PEAK, TAPER & RACE** Goal: Get to start line fully rested but in top shape by eliminating weights and vastly reducing mileage
Sun.	Off Day/ Tennis/Golf	Off Day/ Hiking/Golf	Off Day/ Tennis/Golf	Off Day/ Hiking/Golf	Off Day/ Tennis/Golf	Off Day/ Tennis/Golf	Off Day/ Tennis/Golf	
Mon.	1 hour controlled indoor bike. Raise HR to threshold, but not past it	1 hour indoor bike workout, like last week. Try to push HR a bit higher, but stay at threshold.	1 hour indoor bike workout, like last week. Try to push HR a bit higher, but stay at threshold.	45-minute Spinning class (which includes out of the saddle climbing and intervals)	45-minute Spinning class (which includes out of the saddle climbing and intervals)	1 hour indoor bike, including Spinning class and/or hard intervals	1 hour indoor bike, including Spinning class and/or hard intervals	30 min. indoor bike. Include several hard efforts/intervals
Tues.	Weights: Modified circuit training, heavier 3 x 7 reps to failure of free-weight rows, squats, dead lifts replacing similar machine exercises. Maintain lateral butt exercises. Warm-up with Symmetry. Finish with 15 min. easy run/elliptical	Weights: Same workout as last Tuesday with 5 to 10 pounds heavier weights. Maintain lateral butt exercises. Warm-up with Symmetry. Finish with 20 min. easy run/ elliptical	Weights: Same workout as last Tuesday with 5 to 10 pounds heavier weights. Maintain lateral butt exercises. Warm-up with Symmetry. Finish with 25 min. easy run/elliptical	Weights: Altered workout from last Tuesday by reducing weight to allow 3 sets of 12 reps to failure. Maintain lateral butt exercises. Warm-up with Symmetry. Finish with 25 min. easy run/elliptical	Weights: Same as last week, with 3 sets of 12 reps to failure. Maintain lateral butt exercises. Warm-up with Symmetry. Finish with 25 min. easy run/ elliptical	Weights: Same as last week, with slightly lower weight 3 sets of 12 reps —but NOT to failure. Maintain lateral butt exercises. Warm-up with Symmetry. Finish with 25 min. easy run/ elliptical	Weights: Same as last week, with slightly lower weight 3 sets of 12 reps —but NOT to failure. Maintain lateral butt exercises. Warm-up with Symmetry. Finish with 25 min. easy run/ elliptical	30 min. swim or elliptical. Include several hard efforts/ intervals. (Do not run, as you do not want to risk an injury.)
Wed.	Yoga/Stretching	Yoga/Stretching	Yoga/Stretching	Yoga/Stretching	Yoga/Stretching	Yoga/Stretching	Yoga/Stretching	Yoga/Stretching
Thur.	20 minute slow, steady, bike hill climbs at low-HR to build strength.	30 minute slow, steady bike hill climbs at low-HR to build strength.	40 minute slow, steady bike hill climbs at low-HR to build strength.	20 minute Sprint 8 all-out bike interval session. Warm-up with stretching, squats, and jumping jacks. Finish with stretching	20 minute Sprint 8 all-out bike interval session (push harder than last week). Warm-up with stretching, squats, and jumping jacks. Finish with stretching	20 minute Sprint 8 all-out interval bike session. (Push harder than last week). Warm-up with stretching, squats, and jumping jacks. Finish with stretching	20 minute Sprint 8 all-out interval bike session. Warm-up with stretching, squats, and jumping jacks. Finish with stretching	20 minute Sprint 8 interval bike session (but at only 80% of max effort). Warm-up with stretching, squats, and jumping jacks. Finish with stretching
Fri.	Weights: 3 Sets of maximum pull-ups, push-ups, thrusters, decline situps, and back raises. Do crab walk and lateral butt exercises. Warm-up with Symmetry. Finish with 15 min. swim (or row) at threshold HR	Weights: 3 Sets of maximum pull-ups, push-ups, thrusters, decline sit-ups, and back raises. Do crab walk and lateral butt exercises. Warm-up with Symmetry. Finish with 20 min. swim (or row) at threshold HR	Weights: 3 Sets of maximum pull-ups, push-ups, thrusters, decline situps, and back raises. Do crab walk/lateral butt exercises. Warm-up with Symmetry. Finish with 25 min. swim (or row) at threshold HR	Weights: 5 Sets of 75% of your maximum pull-ups, push-ups, thrusters, decline sit-ups, and back raises from last week. Do crab walk/ lateral butt exercises. Warm-up with Symmetry. Finish with 25 min. swim (or row) at sub-threshold HR.	Weights: 6 sets of the same strength workout as last week. Do crab walk/lateral butt exercises. Warm-up with Symmetry. Finish with 25 min. swim (or row) at sub-threshold HR.	20 minute Sprint 8 interval swim, row or elliptical session (for muscular recovery while keeping metabolic stress). Warm-up with stretching, squats, and jumping jacks. Finish with stretching	20 minute Sprint 8 interval swim, row or elliptical session. Warm-up with stretching, squats, and jumping jacks. Finish with stretching	Yoga/Stretching
Sat.	LSD Ride 60 miles	LSD Ride 70 miles	LSD Recovery Ride 50 miles	LSD Ride 60 miles	LSD Ride 70 miles	LSD Ride 80 miles	Taper: Cut LSD Ride to 60 miles	**THE CENTURY RIDE!**

After the event is over, especially if it was challenging, spend the next week recovering. Swim or row for low-intensity aerobic fitness, or do something totally unstructured; give your mind and legs a break. If another event is planned in a week, go out for a light-effort, low-intensity spin on the bike or a stationary machine a bit on Wednesday and Thursday. If you have an event planned for a month away, recover for a week, build for a week, and recover for two. Above all, stay active.

The six-phase periodization plan is a proven formula that works for all athletes of all abilities for every sport. It also works for the activity for which it was originally designed, weight lifting, which is covered later in this chapter.

Training Option B: The Blend: Time-Efficient Training for a Lifetime of All-Around Fitness

Let's be real here. Who has the time for 8 weeks of Base Training and 16 weeks of periodization? Yes, periodization's been proved for decades. Nothing hones your fat-burning machinery better. But what if you want to ramp it up quicker or just be fit enough to handle any crazy event—cycling or noncycling—that comes along on a moment's notice (which is usually the way it works for me)? Is there a way to shortcut the periodization system—to improve your cycling endurance and ability to ride a century on fewer training miles and hours, and get into good enough shape to handle it in half the time or less?

Enter The Blend.

The Blend generally stays true to periodization in that it maintains an ever-longer LSD weekend ride and shorter LSD cross-training, but it violates the purity of the fat-burning engine-development concept by trying to accelerate the super-compensation adaptation. It does this by sticking to the hard-easy paradigm while combining six workout elements that normally don't get combined:

1. **Interval training (sprints)**
2. **High-intensity strength training**
3. **Maximum Overload (M.O.) heavy strength training**
4. **Yoga/stretching**
5. **LSD endurance**
6. **Cross-training**

The Blend tackles the first three elements with quick workouts that take less than an hour. These sessions build strength, speed, and sustainable power, theoretically replicating much longer training rides on the bike. Yoga gives cyclists the flexibility and postural integrity the sport can harm. A long session of LSD training on the weekends, combined with shorter low-intensity bike and cross-training sessions throughout the week, will build your cycling infrastructure and your fat-burning engine, allow you to progress up to the century mark naturally, and provide the recovery you need from the hard, high-intensity weight and sprint sessions.

Sequence is what allows all these disparate elements to work together—specifically, the familiar mantra that every racer and longevity-focused athlete must live and breathe by: *Follow a hard day with an easy day.* Recovery is built into the Blend, and the benefits of its disparate elements are maximized via the recovery rules.

Purists will scoff at the idea that a blend of different types of aerobic, strength, and cross-training workouts, rather than an all-cycling format, could yield a successful endurance result, but there are precedents. Dave Scott, the great six-time Hawaii Ironman triathlon winner, lifted heavy weights three times a week in his prime. In recent years, I have interviewed many triathletes who were successfully cutting their total workout time while maintaining or improving their race times by using CrossFit Endurance, which combines endurance training with high-intensity CrossFit workouts (although I think CFE mistakenly ignores recovery, which is

THE EVIL SEVENTH STAGE: OVERTRAINING

Is periodization fail-safe? In theory, applying stressor forces to the body in a progressive manner, and breaking it up with rest and variation, will always compel muscles to adapt by getting stronger. But what happens when you apply too severe a stressor for too long? After all, cycling is an addictive sport that tends to encourage hard daily training. And an average load for you one year may be too much the next, when personal circumstances have changed.

Answer: When the body lacks the energy source and/or recovery time to continue adapting, it gets overwhelmed and simply capitulates. This is the dreaded exhaustion stage, most commonly known as "overtraining." For lab rats, overtraining often means death. For humans, it could manifest itself as tendinitis, frequent colds, unexplained edginess—or worse, poor race performance. It behooves you to be aware of its signs, so that you can make adjustments before a crisis occurs.

In his book *Andy Pruitt's Medical Guide for Cyclists*, cowritten with Roadbikerider.com cofounder Fred Matheny, Pruitt identifies four causes and seven symptoms of overtraining:

CAUSES OF OVERTRAINING

1. *Non-stop hammering:* Too much training and racing without adequate rest and recovery.

2. *Runny-nose riding:* Exercising through sickness and injury.

3. *Too much, too soon:* Intense training without a sufficient mileage base.

4. *Empty gas tank:* Poor nutrition, particularly a failure to eat enough carbohydrates and protein soon after a ride to replenish glycogen stores.

SIGNS OF OVERTRAINING

Each of the signs described next are warnings that you need to back off:

1. *Steadily deteriorating performance:* You're getting worse despite—and eventually because of—hard training.

2. *Depression:* "I've never seen an overtrained athlete who wasn't clinically depressed," said Dr. William Morgan, who in the 1970s was one of the first to establish a link between overtraining and depression.

3. *Persistent soreness in muscles and joints:* Since cycling doesn't pound your joints, your muscles shouldn't get excessively sore even after hard rides, said Pruitt.

4. *Abrupt weight loss:* A 5 percent loss of body weight over several days can mean two things, said Pruitt: chronic dehydration, or a lack of glycogen during hard training, in which case the body may begin to devour muscle tissue for fuel.

5. *Diarrhea and constipation:* Chronic fatigue can disrupt the function of the digestive system.

6. *Rise in resting heart rate:* A 7- to 10-beat rise in your normal morning heart rate means your body is tired and your heart is trying to deliver more oxygen and nutrients.

7. *Increased incidence of illness and rise in white blood cell count:* A weak body can't fight off viruses and infections well. Pruitt advises serious cyclists to get a complete blood count four times a year to establish their normal blood-count levels.

so emphasized here). From the academic side, dozens of medical journal articles in the past decade have reported studies showing that simultaneous strength and aerobic benefits can be derived from throwing a bunch of things in a blender and turning it up to purée. In other words, Variety + Intensity = both Speed and Endurance.

As mentioned earlier, strength is a must because it gives endurance athletes the ability to hold power, which prevents deterioration during a race (and during your life). Heavy weights are best because they give your muscles the concentrated "overload" that forces them to improve faster than they could with cycling alone. Overload is taken to a new level with *Maximum Overload*, a radical new strength innovation debuting here in *Bike for Life* (see details on page 57).

Sprints have a similar effect. Very sports-specific and compatible with Maximum Overload strength training, sprints appear only late in a periodized program and are left out of CrossFit Endurance altogether. The Blend uses them right away. *Bike for Life* borrows the proven Sprint 8 program developed by Phil Campbell, an influential coach I've written about over the years. Just 20 minutes long, a Sprint 8 workout is super-simple: eight 30-second sprints separated by 90-second recoveries. Sprints can be done with any aerobic activity (including swimming, skating, rowing, and running), and on both outdoor and indoor bikes.

Additionally, research has shown that the strength and speed effect of sprints can be enhanced by *P.A.P.—Post-Activation Potentiation—* which entails doing the sprints immediately following a weight workout. This protocol also has the effect of being a tremendous time-saver, compressing a weight workout and sprints into 60 minutes.

Throwing a bunch of things in a blender may smack of chaos theory—but if it's done right, there's nothing chaotic or random about The Blend. Again, it adheres religiously to the alternating hard-easy paradigm, where recovery LSD days always follow the strength, sprint, and P.A.P. days.

So how would this translate to training for a century? Here's Week 1 of a seven-week century plan, in the next column.

The Blend week includes six strength and aerobic workouts over five days with two off days, which should be used for yoga and fun physical activities, like hiking, team sports, or tennis (which adds valuable core-twisting motion—see Chapter 8). The five workout days include two aerobic cardio workouts (a long bike ride on Saturday and a shorter cross-training swim, run, or elliptical day on Tuesday); two anaerobic/sprint workouts (one sprint session and one Spinning

THE BLEND: A TYPICAL WEEKLY WORKOUT SCHEDULE

Monday	P.A.P.–M.O. weight training + sprints (40 + 20 minutes)
Tuesday	LSD cross-training recovery day (20-60 minutes swim, elliptical, row or run, always done at sub-threshold heart rate)
Wednesday	Spinning or other intense indoor cycling (40-60 minutes)
Thursday	Maximum Overload strength training (40 minutes)
Friday	Yoga/stretching
Saturday	LSD bike ride (20-80 miles, sub-threshold heart rate)
Sunday	Off/fun day, or tennis, hiking, or other activity

class); and two Maximum Overload strength workouts (if you like, replace one of these with a CrossFit-style, high-intensity workout). The workouts can be collapsed into four days by combining the Spinning day with Friday's strength workout. This combined P.A.P. strength-sprint workout is an hour long, the longest weekday workout, making the weekly total no more than five or six hours initially. Cycling will increase quickly to longer distances and times on Saturday as you tack on another 10 miles per week, topping out at 80 miles, enough to bridge to a century ride the following weekend. This turns century training into an eight-week plan for beginners who start off without a big mileage base. Those with a higher beginning base, who could start Week 1 with, say, a 40-mile Saturday LSD ride, could ramp up to a century in five weeks.

How much does the variety of The Blend compromise the efficiency of the fat-burning engine developed in orthodox periodization? No one knows at this point. But The Blend keeps you in great shape and ready for anything. The carefully sequenced mix of fast-and-slow, long-and-short, cardio-and-strength workouts are complementary. They blast you hard with weights and intensity, then give you the recovery time that lets you rebuild stronger and faster, turning you into a fat-burning machine. Jacques Devore's Maximum Overload strength system gives you the ability to hold form and power in a way that regular strength training and high-intensity programs can't, helping to prevent the dreaded end-of-the-day slowdown. When you make sure all the LSD days (the short one and the long ones) stick to a low-heart-rate intensity that keeps you out of the Black Hole, you assure optimal development of your fat-burning engine, solid recovery that prevents overtraining, and a sustainable, easily understood, and fun fitness plan that I think you can do for a lifetime.

For an average, enthusiastic athlete, the do-ability is the key benefit. Personally, The Blend fits my lifestyle as the default workout plan. When I have a bicycling event, from a stage race like La Ruta to a one-day Gran Fondo, I just substitute in more short, intense cycling during the week and add long rides during the week and/or on the preceding Sunday. If a running event like a Tough Mudder pops up, I switch the cycling days to running. I am no great athlete, but I took 56th out of 212 people on the 6-mile, 2,000-foot King of the Mountains section of the Beverly Hills Gran Fondo in October 2013. Not bad for a 57-year-old whose riding consisted of a weekly three-hour mountain bike ride all summer. I credit the Blend's sprints and Maximum Overload workouts.

At the very least, The Blend isn't boring. It'll keep you excited about working out for the rest of your (extra-long) life.

STEP 3: WEIGHT TRAINING— WHY CYCLISTS MUST PUMP IRON

If you haven't got the idea by now through the periodization and Blend training plans, here it is again, loud and clear: Cyclists need to weight train. It'll help you become a better cyclist—and live longer! Yes, cyclists love the outdoors, and often hate going indoors, unless it's for a Spin class.

BIKE FOR LIFE "THE BLEND" 8-WEEK CENTURY PLAN, OR REST-OF-YOUR-LIFE STRATEGY

	WEEK 1	WEEK 2	WEEK 3	WEEK 4	WEEK 5	WEEK 6	WEEK 7	WEEK 8
Sun.	Off Day/Tennis	Off Day/Hiking	Off Day/Tennis	Off Day/Hiking	Off Day/Tennis	Off Day/Hiking	Off Day/Tennis	Off Day/Hiking
Mon.	P.A.P. – M.O. weights + Bike Intervals*	P.A.P. – M.O. weights + Bike Intervals*	P.A.P. – M.O. weights + Bike Intervals*	P.A.P. – M.O. weights + Bike Intervals*	P.A.P. – M.O. weights + Bike Intervals*	P.A.P. – M.O. weights + Bike Intervals*	P.A.P. – M.O. weights + Bike Intervals*	P.A.P. – M.O. weights + Bike Intervals*
Tues.	LSD cross-training: Swim	LSD cross-training: Elliptical	LSD cross-training: Run	LSD cross-training: Swim	LSD cross-training: Elliptical	LSD cross-training: Run	LSD cross-training: Swim	LSD cross-training: Elliptical
Wed.	Spinning	Spinning	Spinning	Spinning	Spinning	Spinning	Spinning	Spinning
Thur.	M.O. weights*	M.O. weights*	M.O. weights*	M.O. weights*	M.O. weights*	M.O. weights*	M.O.weights*	Yoga
Fri.	Yoga	Yoga	Yoga	Yoga	Yoga	Yoga	Yoga	Off Day
Sat.	LSD Ride 20 miles	LSD Ride 30 miles	LSD Ride 40 miles	LSD Ride 50 miles	LSD Ride 60 miles	LSD Ride 70 miles	LSD Ride 80 miles	CENTURY RIDE !!!

*On all strength days, do a Symmetry warm-up and stretching cool-down.

But get over it. For longevity, quality of life, protection against osteoporosis, riding better, and looking good, you have to hit the gym.

"Many cyclists believe that weight training is unnecessary, given the fitness they derive from riding, but that's wrong," says Christopher Drozd, CSCS, a Los Angeles–based personal trainer, cycling coach, and Ironman triathlete who has developed a weight-training program specifically for cyclists. "Strength training may be *more* important for cyclists than for other athletes. That's because cycling itself is such an incomplete activity." Example: You need glutes [the butt] to cycle effectively and fast, but cycling itself doesn't develop glutes well. You can only really build glutes by some form of weight training.

Weight training provides two important functions for cyclists, says Drozd, one on the bike and the other off the bike: It can reinforce and strengthen cycling movements, helping to make your riding more powerful and stable. And it can correct imbalances caused by cycling, making your off-the-bike life safer, easier, and healthier. Here are the details:

Weight Training's On-the-Bike Benefits

1. Strengthens your core: Ironically, although the core muscles—the abs (i.e., the abdominal muscles), hips, and lower back—are largely ignored by cycling, you need a strong core to ride effectively. "A strong midsection helps you in standing out of the saddle, negotiating obstacles, turning, generally controlling the bike, avoiding falls, even creating a foundation for the legs to push against," Drozd says. "If you're a noodle, you're shifting all over the place, losing energy and power. Use weights to build your core, and you're automatically better on the bike and off the bike in all real-life movements."

2. Improves your power: Weight lifting is an easy way to quickly and thoroughly strengthen cycling-specific muscles, including the quads (i.e., quadriceps), hams (i.e., hamstrings), glutes, and calves. Pulling exercises, such as rows, give your upper body more power when you are pulling up on the handlebars while rocking the bike out of the saddle.

3. Maintains your reaction time and balance: Lifting with fast contractions and heavy weights resuscitates the fast-twitch fibers that can rapidly diminish and lose power and speed over time.

Weight Training's Off-the-Bike Benefits

1. Corrects imbalances caused by cycling: Muscles are stressed through a limited range in cycling, often to the exclusion of others. The quads get worked more than the hamstrings; the vastus lateralis, the outside muscle of the quad, gets worked and built up more than the vastus medialis, the inside of the quad, which is fully flexed only when the leg is completely straightened, which never happens during pedaling. Good balance dictates that agonist and corresponding antagonist muscles (i.e., quads/hams, abs/lower back, biceps/triceps) be of complementary strength. With weight lifting, you can spot-strengthen the under-worked muscles, restoring balance.

2. Adds stability to all your movements: Cycling stresses leg muscles in one direction, but one-dimensional fitness does not give you the resistance you need to handle traumas from all directions. Weight training can provide the omnidirectional stress you need for stability during standing, walking, and lateral-movement sports such as tennis and basketball.

3. Strengthens your unstressed muscles: The cycling position is very static. Many muscle groups—including nearly all of the muscles of the upper body and back—do not see much use during riding.

4. Generally keeps you younger: Need more motivation to hit the iron? Consider that weight lifting also provides great benefits for general

TINKER JUAREZ'S WINNING ANTI-AGING TRAINING PLAN

SCREW PERIODIZATION, WEIGHTS, AND SPRINTS. THE 50-PLUS SUPERSTAR JUST KEEPS RIDING HARD— AND SLEEPS IN A TENT.

"I've been over the hill for a long time. But I can still get over the hills pretty fast."
—Tinker Juarez, then age 46, after winning the 2007 24 Hours of Adrenalin Solo World Mountain Biking Championship

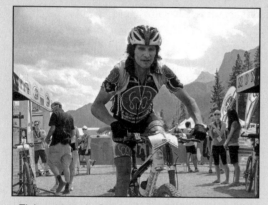

Tinker, 2008, in Canmore, Alberta, at the World Championships. "Weights? I don't do no stinkin' weights."

Nothing seems to have changed since 1986, when David "Tinker" Juarez became a mountain biker at age 25 after a long and successful career as a top BMX rider. The trademark long stringy black dreadlocks hairdo is the same. So is the calm, approachable, low-key personality. And so is the winning—the three-time NORBA national cross-country champion and two-time Olympian won 14 races in 2013, most of them long distance, including his fifth 24-hour national championship. Despite having turned 50 in 2011, he rarely competes in the Masters class, and then only in shorter cross-country events. In long-distance events, which were his forte for decades (he even competed in the 3,000-mile Race Across America in 1996, taking third in 11 days

and 22 hours), Juarez competes against riders young enough to be his kids. He seems timeless.

So is his training.

He does no weight training. No cross-training. No yoga. He doesn't use a power meter, a Strava app, or any other technology. There's no lab. No data. No super-duper diet, and no spiritual guru. "I once got my VO_2 max score—it wasn't that good," Tinker said. "So technology and numbers don't impress me. It's training—pure and simple. If I'm doing my job well, why change? I don't have time to experiment. I know what works for me and I'll stick with it."

An odometer is as techy as Tinker gets on his daily route up and down the bike path on the San Gabriel River near his home in the foothills of Whittier, just east of Los Angeles. Sometimes north to Glendora, sometimes south to Seal Beach—up to 24 hours a week, almost all on his road bike. Hammer and recover, hammer and recover. One day will be a hard day of 75 miles at 21 mph or more. The next day is an easy two-hour recovery day, about 35 miles.

It's hard work, but he has always done it and isn't tired of it yet. "You're doing what you love to do," said Juarez. "I get to ride my bike for a living. If I win, Cannondale keeps sponsoring me." They've been doing that since 1994.

"I don't take anything lightly—nothing for granted," he said. "I know how important sponsorship is. So I keep pushing just like I always have, even though everything is deeper now—the pain, the suffering, the hassle of the traveling."

Yet there is one change lately: Three or four times a week, Juarez sleeps in an oxygen tent. "About four months ago [in the summer of 2013]," he said, "I got talked into it. It was expensive—$2,000. But I always felt good at altitude. And I like it—and have been crushing it hard this year."

There's also the motor home, which he bought in 2006. It makes it easier for him to get away for a couple of days to train—in a very convenient and inexpensive way—if he needs some time in the

(continues)

mountains of Idyllwild or Palm Springs, a couple of hours' drive away.

Juarez does what he can to avoid stress. "And I got lucky," he said. "Never had a big injury, no diseases, not a ton of responsibilities at home. I had a family that let me do what I needed to do. My mom and my wife [they married in 2006] take care of the simple stuff—go to the store, deposit a check, take care of the kid [born in 2007].

"And I've had good timing. When I got into BMX in the '70s, it was all new. When I got into mountain biking in the '80s, it was all new. When I got into 24-hour events after the Sydney Olympics, the same thing. Cannondale was okay with it as they were starting to get big. I decided that the 24-hour scene was more me. I made a big statement to Cannondale when I did well."

One more piece of luck: He hasn't lost his iconic hair, keeping his media-genic dreadlocks intact. "Having a trademark does help," he said. "I grew it for fun and stuck with it because everyone thought it was crazy. I never wanted to be like everyone else, anyway, so it's been good motivation."

Tinker has been riding at high levels since he was a preteen. "I wouldn't have guessed that I'd still be doing this at 50," he said. "In my head, I know I'm 52. But when I ride, I don't feel like an old man. I still have the hunger.

"I've never had a post-biking plan. I never had a strategy—my life is training and racing. I've just tried to keep it plain and simple: I just gotta do better than last year. I try to always add value every year and do new stuff."

The weekend before we spoke in October 2013, he won a road-bike race up Glendora Mountain and picked up $1,000.

If the continued stream of victories, big and small, someday isn't enough for Cannondale, and Juarez loses his sponsorship, Plan B kicks in. "Everyone gets to the point where they are too old, and someday I will have to accept it," he said. "But I guess I haven't gotten to that point yet. When I do, I could get by with owning a bike shop and be happy.

"When I was in BMX as a kid, I thought: 'How cool it would be to wear a helmet the rest of my life!' So for me, right now, this is as good as it can get. But regardless of what happens, I'll always be wearing a helmet, no matter what."

longevity. Regular strength training can help you slow the body's natural rate of decline of muscle mass (normally 1 percent per year after age 35), fast-twitch fibers, oxygen-processing capacity, power, reaction time, human growth hormone production, and, if you are male, testosterone.

Note: To allow for muscle recovery, you should not lift with the same muscles more than once every 48 hours. A successful strength-training strategy also includes a warm-up set with light weights; rapid contractions with heavy weights to build muscle and maintain power; heavy circuit training with no rest between sets to spike HGH; a recovery workout following a hard workout; and periodizing (changing) your routine to keep your muscles fresh.

The Exercises

The strength-exercise routines described below, put together by Chris Drozd, are separated into three categories: (1) those that develop cycling-specific muscles; (2) those that develop the muscles ignored by cycling; (3) those that undo the damage cycling does. The exercises can be done with dumbbells, a weight bench, a Swiss inflatable ball (yoga ball), or weight machines, making it possible to do most of them at home.

"You're a cyclist, not a bodybuilder, so you don't want to be in the gym much," said Drozd. That's why he favors a "less is more" philosophy that trains complex movements—not individual muscles. Squats, deadlifts, and other multijoint exercises give you the best bang for the buck, get you out of the gym (or your garage) quicker, and are thoroughly natural. Humans function with multijoint movements: the hip, knee, and ankle joints all work together as you run and jump.

How Many Reps?

For all exercises below, for general strength do 3 sets of 10 reps to failure (the point at which you can no longer maintain form). For stamina, do 20, 25, or even more reps; for power do 1 to 6 reps, all out. Be careful with *all* of these, especially if you're new to weight lifting. Hire a trainer—a good one—to get you started. To warm up, use lighter weight for the first set. Always warm up well, for about 10 minutes, at least. (Warm up when riding, too.)

A Word About Timing

There is debate as to the best time of year to lift weights. Throughout the early 1990s, the common belief was that weight lifting was strictly an off-season endeavor for cyclists. Late-season weakness, however, led innovative triathletes, such as Mark Allen, to maintain strength training throughout the season, and their performances improved as a result. *Bike for Life* recommends that all cyclists—except possibly top-level racers concerned with having too much muscle mass—follow Allen's lead. One caveat: Don't do any heavy lifting, especially with your legs, within a week of an event you've been training for. Six-time Ironman winner Dave Scott blames his fifth-place finish and poor bike ride in the 1996 Hawaii Ironman on lack of recovery time from a heavy lifting session three days before the event.

Cycling-Specific Strength Exercises

The following exercises will build more power on the bike by strengthening the cycling-related muscles.

1. Barbell deadlift

Benefit: One of the best cycling-specific movements, the deadlift develops the calves, quads, hams, glutes, lower back, midback, and forearms and adds midsection stability.

Description: Standing with feet at hip width with knees and hips bent and back flat, hold the barbell with hands about shoulder width and stand up, careful to unbend at the hip joint—*not at the waist.* Keep your back flat (neutrally aligned), not rounded, at all times. The deadlift can also be done with dumbbells and a kettlebell.

2. Decline sit-up

Benefit: This sit-up conditions the hip flexors and abdominals, which together are integral to a good pedal stroke.

Description: On a slant board with your hips beneath your bent knees, sit up and lean back with a smooth, controlled motion, keeping the midsection stable. To keep this exercise safe for your back, keep it straight and unarched. Draw your navel in toward your spine the entire time, from top to bottom position. Perform reps to failure.

3. Push-ups

Benefit: Push-ups condition the midsection and strengthen the "pushing" muscles of the upper body, including the triceps and chest. Cyclists use all arm muscles while climbing; holding a line while mountain biking requires good stability on an unstable surface. Staying stable while pushing up from a ball is more challenging than a simple ground push-up or a machine or free-weight bench press. To increase the ground push-up challenge, do them with hand positions altered (one forward, the other back), with different sizes of balls under each hand, and with feet elevated on an exercise ball.

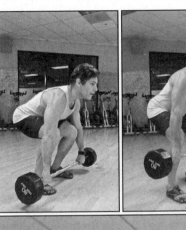

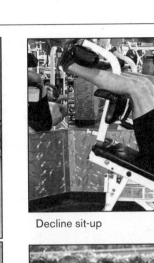

Decline sit-up

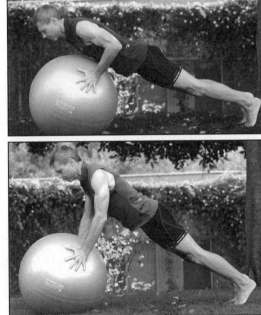

Push-up on ball, positions 1 and 2

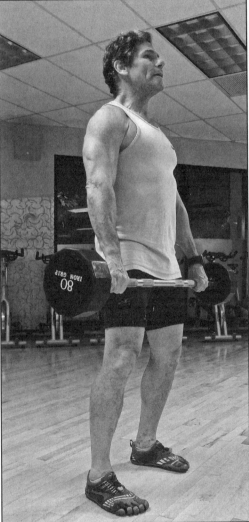

Barbell deadlift

Description: Keep your back and legs flat and aligned, so your whole body moves as a unit. Tilt your pelvis back, draw your navel into your spine, keep your butt low, and switch hand positions to increase the instability factor. Perform reps to failure.

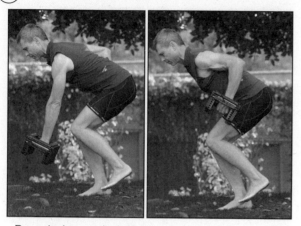

Row: single arm, single leg

4. Single-arm or single-leg dumbbell/cable rows

Benefit: This exercise works the back and mid-section in a cycling-specific position under conditions that require balance and build stability and alignment. Balance is important on a bike, especially as you age.

Description: Warm up with conventional double-arm rows with both feet on the ground. (This works the back well but requires little stability, especially if performed on a row weight machine.) Then release the right dumbbell/cable handle, hold on with the left, stand on the right foot, and pull the left-hand weight toward your body as your left elbow moves straight back.

5. Leg curls

Benefit: Leg curls strengthen the hamstrings and calves. Although not a multijoint exercise, the leg curl resembles the cycling upstroke and develops hamstring and butt strength, which is necessary to balance a cyclist's often overemphasized quads. This exercise will help you avoid pulled or torn muscles.

Description: Lie belly down on a leg-curl, weight-stack machine. With your heels beneath the pads and knees aligned with the hinge, bend your knees, "curling" the weight toward your butt. As you do this, press your hips into the bench if you feel them start to rise from the bench. Lower your feet slowly. Do one-legged curls to gauge and fix discrepancies in the respective strength of each leg.

6. Single-leg leg presses or step-ups

Benefit: Single-leg presses and step-ups allow for a concentrated effort on one leg at a time, providing for strength symmetry. The leg-press position is quite cycling specific; the ability to load weight onto the legs in such a position, without the need for stability, is of great use in building high local strength and stamina. Conversely, step-ups require great balance, and large loads cannot be easily used. This makes for far better three-dimensional conditioning, improving your stability and alignment under load. You can increase the height of the step to target specific strength-range deficiencies, if needed.

Description: Sit in a leg-press machine and only push with one leg. Concentrate on staying aligned. Keep your knee, hip, and toe all on the same plane. Avoid twisting to the side and avoid allowing your knee to collapse to the inside.

Step-ups (standing on a step and pushing up, as if walking up the stairs) accomplish the same thing but ramp up the difficulty by adding imbalance. Drozd says they condition stability from "ankles to ears." Do them with or without weights in hand. Do not let your right foot swing behind the left.

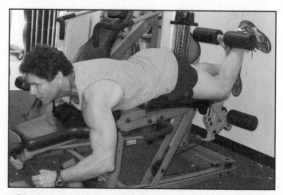

Single-leg leg/hamstring curls

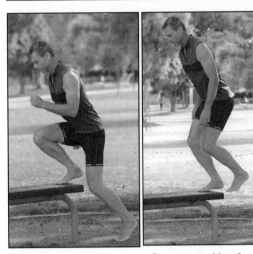

Step-up, position 1   Step-up, position 2

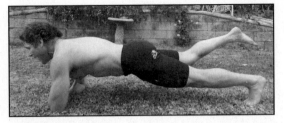

Plank: leg raised

7. Calf raises

Benefit: This exercise helps to prevent injuries by extending the range of motion in your feet, ankles, and lower leg. The stronger the connection between the foot and the leg, the better your power transfer will be.

Description: Standing on the edge of a step on the ball of your foot, with the heel down as far as it can go, push up on your toes and raise your heels as high as you can. This move conditions the full range of motion of the involved muscles and gives you strength at the end of the range. Avoid bouncing. Make sure your knees are bent about 25 to 35 degrees, and keep that bend throughout the movement. You can use any steps

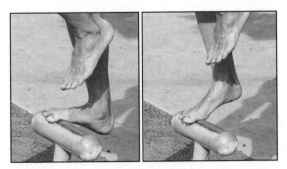

Calf raise: heel down   Calf raise: heel up

or even a jungle-gym bar (as shown in the photo). Hold onto any structure to stay balanced during both double-leg and single-leg calf raises.

8. Modified plank with leg raise

Benefit: This type of plank will help you maintain the aerobar position in cycling. More importantly, it develops midsection stability and stamina, especially when you raise one leg, supporting yourself and remaining aligned with only a single leg.

Description: Get in a flat-back push-up position, but rest your upper body on your elbows instead of your hands. Then raise one leg at a time as high as it can go. Hold it as long as possible, up to a couple of minutes.

9. Squats

Benefit: Done with or without weights, squats increase the strength of your hip, knee, and ankle muscles in a fairly cycling-specific manner. They rely on your body's natural ability to stabilize and align itself, rather than neglecting that three-dimensional aspect, as leg machines and Smith squats do. Because of its difficulty and the whole-body involvement it requires, this exercise encourages overall strength and stamina and works the core and lower back.

Description: Standing erect with a barbell over your shoulders, bend the knees, lean forward slightly, and lower yourself, then return to a standing position. This exercise has front and back versions depending on how the barbell is

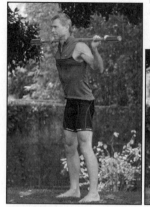

Back squat:
up position

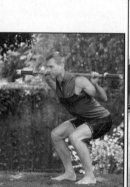

Back squat:
down position

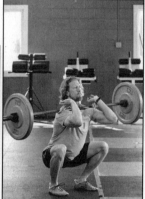

Front squat:
down position

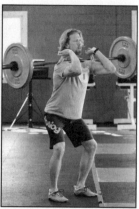

Front squat:
up position

positioned (see photos). Don't go beyond the point where your butt is lower than your knees until you are an advanced weight lifter. This exercise can also be done on a squat machine.

Muscles That Don't Get Worked in Cycling . . .

. . . but that you need in order to be a balanced person.

1. Glutes

Benefit: While not completely neglected in cycling, the glutes, in a phenomenon known as "reciprocal inhibition," release in response to hip-flexor tightening. As the hip flexors reflexively shorten, their opposing muscles, the glutes, have to stretch to accommodate, and they can become saggy, flaccid, soft, and weak as a result. This exercise tightens the glutes and restores their power. Ideally, it is done in conjunction with the hip-flexor stretch (described below).

Description: Using a leg-press machine, press through your heels (not your forefoot, which uses more of your quads than your glutes).

2. Upright rows

Benefit: The shoulders are largely ignored in cycling. Pulling up a barbell, dumbbell, or bar from a low pulley also replicates the pulling you do on a handlebar, especially while climbing.

Description: Bracing yourself on a low bench with one hand, lean over so that your back is relatively horizontal. With the other arm straight, grab a heavy dumbbell and hoist it up as high as possible toward your chest. Try to bring that elbow to shoulder level. Avoid shrugging.

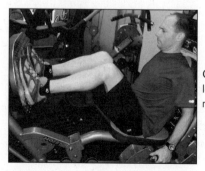

Glutes:
leg-press
machine

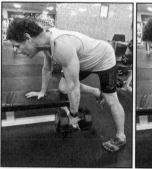

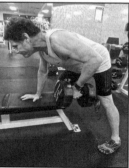

Dumbbell rows, position 1   Dumbbell rows, position 2

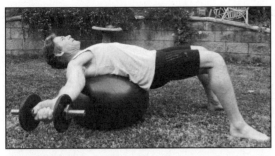

Pec flys on ball, down position

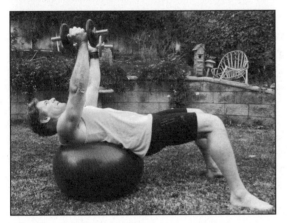

Pec flys on ball, up position

3. Pectoral flys

Benefit: Flys build the pecs (pectoral muscles), which are ignored in cycling.

Description: Lay face up on a Swiss ball, with the dumbbells directly over your chest at about the nipple line. With your palms facing each other, slowly lower the weights out to the side, still keeping them directly in line with the chest. Pause briefly at the bottom, elbows just below the ribcage, and, without shifting or twisting, raise the weights back to the starting position. There should be a slight to moderate bend in your elbows throughout the motion. In a gym with no balls, use the pec-fly machine.

4. Triceps

Benefit: These rear upper-arm muscles are actively worked during climbing and stressed from balancing your torso as you lean on the handlebars. They can become sore during long rides.

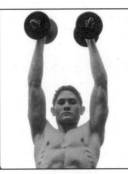
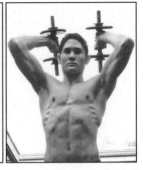

Triceps, up position   Triceps, down position

Description: In a standing position, with the dumbbells straight overhead, palms facing each other, lower your hands to ear level, then arc the dumbbells back to their original position.

5. Pull-ups (or lat pulls)

Benefit: The "king of the back exercises" strengthens the connection between rider and bike and upgrades form, posture, and power transfer. It works the arms and protects and strengthens your back by hitting the massive lat muscles.

Description: Jump up and grab a pull-up bar with hands in any manner—forward, backward, or handshake position—and hang. Pull up until

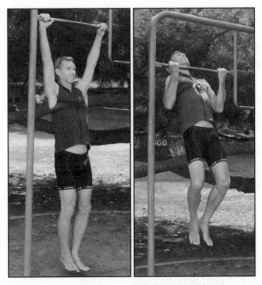

Pull-up: position 1   Pull-up: position 2

your chin clears the bar. Return slowly, under control, to a complete hang. If pull-ups are too hard for you at first, use a seated lat pull-down machine at the gym. Pull the bar down to the bottom of your ribcage while keeping your chest high and shoulders back.

6. Deltoids

Benefit: Delts mainly are used during standing climbs in cycling, and otherwise for body symmetry and balance.

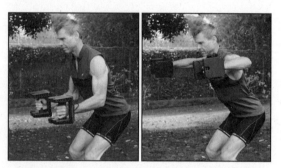

Deltoid raises: position 1   Deltoid raises: position 2

Description: In a crouched "action position"—with knees and hips bent, back straight, and head forward—hold the dumbbells out in front of you and lift them 90 degrees out to the side. The motion is similar to flapping bird wings. Keep your shoulders from elevating or shrugging. Your hands and elbows should stay aligned with each other and on the same plane throughout the movement and end up level with the shoulders.

Exercises That Undo the Damage Caused by Cycling

1. Back raise

Benefit: Cyclists tend to have weak backs, as the typical riding position stretches out and fatigues the small muscles that line the spinal column. The fix includes bridges, back strengtheners like pull-ups and lat pull-down that build the massive latissimus dorsi muscles, and the simple back raise, which gently works the spinal erectors.

Description: From a prone position on the floor,

raise your head and chest off the ground a few inches and hold for two or three seconds. Don't hyperextend your neck. Perform reps to failure.

Note: Overdoing back exercises or doing risky ones can injure you by putting excessive compression and shearing force on the disks, which become more vulnerable as we age. For this reason, many PTs will warn you to avoid the back-hyperextension bench at the gym (in which you hook your feet onto pads), the bicycle sit-up, which involves touching opposite knees to elbows in a fast, torqueing motion, and all sit-ups done without a flat back and rigid core.

2. Hip flexor lunge stretch

Benefit: This stretch lengthens the hip flexors, which are shortened by cycling and by sitting at a desk, in a car, et cetera.

Description: Kneel on one knee and place the other foot directly out in front of you with the knee bent at a 90-degree angle. Align the knee of the front leg vertically with the same-side ankle. Place both hands on top of the forward knee, and keeping the upper body upright and vertical, slide the rear knee backward until a stretch is felt on the top front of that leg, near the hip and lower ab region. The stretch will feel "deep." Sink further into the stretch with each deep exhale. Back off a bit if the stretch is "burning."

3. Swimming (crawl and backstroke)

Benefit: Swimming, which elongates your posture through repeated overhead reaching, is

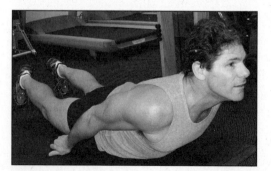

Back raise

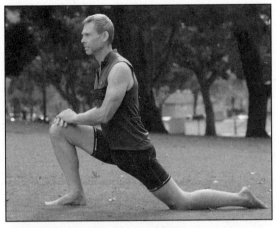

Hip flexor lunge stretch, position 1

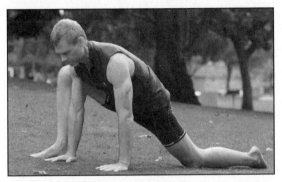

Hip flexor lunge stretch, position 2

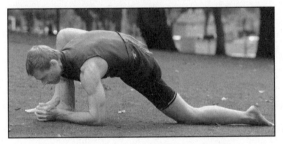

Hip flexor lunge stretch, position 3

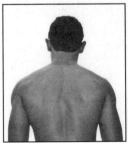

Chest stretch, position 1   Chest stretch, position 2

the antithesis of the protracted, hunched cycling position. Also, this stroke's pronounced hip twist works the midsection, which is largely ignored in cycling. Swimming also is a terrific means of resting cycling muscles while still conditioning your heart and lungs, and it is great for adding condition to the upper body, which is typically ignored by cyclists. Also, swimming develops a proprioceptive and kinesthetic sense that, though not specific to cycling, can have some neural carryover, improving positional and spatial awareness. Swimming a couple of times a week for 15 to 30 minutes each time is ideal for cyclists.

4. Chest stretch

Benefit: The chest stretch restores lung capacity and expands and lengthens the chest muscles, which shorten over time because of cycling's hunched position.

Description: Standing erect, straighten your arms and hold them at your sides; then pull them behind you by pinching the shoulder blades together. Focus on holding an imaginary pencil between the shoulder blades. Perform this stretch frequently—at the gym, in the elevator, and when you get out of bed or your car.

5. Scorpion tail raises

Benefit: This exercise restores strength to the spinal erectors, gives the proper curvature to the lumbar spine, and de-humps the upper back.

Description: Lying face down on a Swiss ball, raise both legs while arching your back, lifting

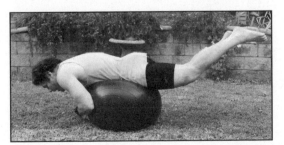

Scorpion tail raise on ball

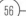
your legs as well as your upper body as far as possible up into the air. You balance on your hands and abdomen. Perform reps to failure.

QUICK PRE-RIDE WARM-UP ROUTINE

Don't hop on your bike cold. While everyone else is sipping coffee and bragging about the good deal they got on bar tape at Mickey's Cyclemania, do these three body-weight exercises from Dr. Michael Yessis, a former consultant to several Olympic and Los Angeles pro sports teams. Yessis is a proponent of active-isolated stretching, which moves the muscle through a range of motion that includes contraction (strength) and elongation (stretching). They'll help you start the day feeling loose and flexible, not tight, with all the right neuromuscular pathways firing. (Note: If it's really cold, add push-ups.)

1. Calf raises

Benefit: Warming up the calf and Achilles tendon provides ankle flexibility.

Description: Stand on the edge of a step or curb on the ball of your foot, then raise the heel as high as possible and lower it back down below the plane of the step. Initially perform it with both legs, then switch to single-leg reps.

2. Good mornings

Benefit: This movement strengthens a cyclist's weak back muscles while stretching and strengthening the glutes and hamstrings.

Description: While standing, feet about hip-distance apart, arch your back and bend forward at the hips until your upper body is parallel to the ground, keeping your back flat and your legs straight. Then straighten up slowly, keeping your back arched as you lift your torso up by focusing on pulling through your glutes.

3. Air squats

Benefit: The king of body-weight exercises, the squat strengthens quads, hamstrings, and glutes.

Description: Standing with feet wider than shoulders and at an angle, keep back arched, head forward, and butt back as you lower your body. Bring your butt to within a foot of the ground, keeping heels down, knees aligned over your feet, and arms in front of you. If your knees hurt, double-check the angle. If it still hurts, stop this exercise.

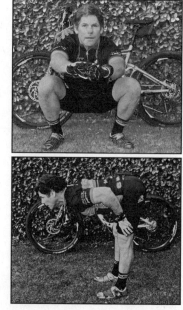

Air squat, from front

Good morning

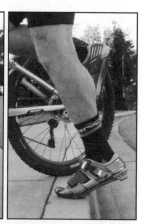

Calf raise, down position

Calf raise, up position

A CYCLIST'S SECRET WEAPON: MAXIMUM OVERLOAD

It's radical. It's new. It's a hard, heavy, time-saving strength regimen that delivers sustainable power that'll keep you fast throughout the race—and the decades.

Cameron Wurf squats—and jumps. He squats again—and jumps. Eighteen more times, the 30-year-old Australian, in his fourth year on the Cannondale Pro Cycling team and the only pro rider in history to have been an Olympic rower (Athens 2004), squats down so low he can touch his hands to the asphalt, then blasts off as high as he can, 18 inches or more off the ground. It's January 2014, and he and his teammates, including two-time Giro d'Italia winner Ivan Basso and super-sprinter Peter Sagan, two-time green jersey winner at the Tour de France and runner-up at the Tour of Flanders and Milan–San Remo, have just gotten back from a three-hour training ride in the Santa Monica Mountains in this early-season training camp in California.

But Wurf, a domestique who was given the green light to "go for it" when he started getting results, doesn't just limit his jump-squats to winter; he does them all season long. And he doesn't do them alone. Half of his teammates, noticing his steady progress into the top 20 and 10 in races, now do them too—with the approval of the team's German trainer, Sebastian Weber.

"I brought the engine and discipline of a rower into this sport—and also the cross-training," said Wurf, a native of Hobart, Tasmania. "Rowers run, lift weights, and do jump-squats. We know pain. When I was on the national [rowing] team at 19, I used to do 120 jump-squats in a row. I could squat a 330-pound barbell 10 times. In 2011 and early 2012, when I was now only doing cycling, I found myself getting a little soft, a bit stagnant. So I went back and adapted some of my rowing cross-training, and it made a big difference. You've blasted your legs so hard with the weights and jump squats

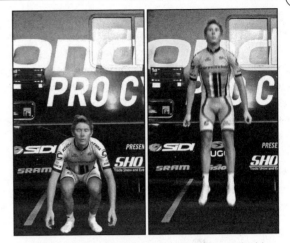

Cam Wurf says his jump squats develop sustainable cycling power.

that they don't hurt on the climbs any more, from the first climb to the last."

Technically, that's what's known as "sustainable power." And whether Wurf ascends to the elite of the sport in the next few years or not, the in-season weight training he does is a very efficient way to get sustainable power—and, I think, might well be the wave of the future for all cyclists. That's because 30 minutes of strength training, especially used with movements like squats and leg presses that functionally mirror the movements of leg-centric sports such as running, cycling, and even rowing (which is 70 percent legs), can concentrate more stress on sport-specific muscles than hours of the sport itself.

This "overload"—repeatedly taking muscles to the point of "failure" (the point where you can't lift the weight any more without breaking form, and thus where microtears occur in the muscles)—is the key to fully mobilizing the body's natural self-improvement mechanisms. The process, known as "super-compensation," rebuilds the microtorn muscles and makes them even stronger.

All aerobic activities, including running and cycling, elicit some muscle-strengthening and hormonal response, but overloading your muscles way beyond normal with strength training—even just with body weight, as with Wurf's jump-squats—causes the extreme stress that will cause them to adapt (grow and strengthen) more rapidly and thoroughly. Done right, these overloads add little weight and bulk.

Is there a best way to achieve overload? For instance, if you did Wurf's jump-squats with your body weighted or holding dumbbells, wouldn't the super-compensation effect be even greater?

A few weeks before I interviewed him, Wurf spent an afternoon talking with a high-profile pro cyclist who actually did something like that: David Zabriskie, five-time US national time-trial champion, three-time Tour of California runner-up, and the first American to win stages in the three biggest international grand tours (France, Italy, and Spain). Zabriskie had retired at age 34 after a crash in May the previous year. But until then, having nothing to lose after a six-month suspension for admitting to drug use back on Lance Armstrong's 2003–2005 US Postal Service team, Zabriskie tried out a radical training regimen developed by West L.A. and Santa Barbara trainer Jacques Devore. It included a low-carb diet and a unique weight program that took the concepts of overload and super-compensation to a new level.

Devore calls it Maximum Overload.

Maximum Overload (M.O.) is heavy, controlled, high-volume lifting with built-in rest, making it very different from conventional three-sets-of-10 circuit training and high-intensity programs like CrossFit. M.O. takes multijoint exercises that target cycling prime movers, such as deadlifts and squats, and performs them in small, heavy batches in an increasing progression in both weight and quantity.

"It's simple: If you want better performance, you have to train at maximum output—not at sub-maximum output," said Devore. "That means you must push very heavy weight—repeatedly. By definition, you improve your performance when you raise your *maximum overload*—i.e., push that same weight more often in a session or do the same reps with a higher weight."

So that's what he had Zabriskie do. In the gym twice a week through the fall and winter of 2012–2013, and once a week from January forward, Zabriskie maximally overloaded his deadlifts, one-legged leg presses, and jump-squats, which were performed on a special air-resistance upright squat machine with padded shoulder posts which you blast upward against.

I drove to Santa Barbara and did the workout myself. It was different, intense—and exhausting. And it was working, according to Devore, who was giddy over Zabriskie's uncharacteristic early-season hill-climbing prowess at the seven-day Tour of Catalonia in Spain that February. Zabriskie didn't win the race or ride near the front; he actually dropped out on the last day. But Zabriskie did do something unusual for him in the early season: Although not a great hill climber, he did not fall off in hill climbs in the latter part of each day. Late in the day, his leg muscles still had gas in the tank.

"At DZ's level, it isn't necessarily how fast you can go," said Devore. "It's how little you can deteriorate throughout the day. For that you need *sustainable strength*."

Sustainable strength is not raw, top-end speed—that, you get from intervals. Sustainable strength, said Devore, gives endurance athletes two things that they need to improve to win: the ability to *hold form*, and the ability to *hold power*.

You see, when muscles fatigue and form fails late in a race, you don't get as much out of each pedal stroke. When power fails on the fourth of seven hills, your momentum falls off the table.

Given his history of being a slow starter, Zabriskie went into the Tour of Catalonia expecting to DNF much earlier. When he didn't, it proved to him and Devore that M.O. worked. As Wurf might say, DZ had blasted his legs so hard in the gym that they didn't hurt when he blasted them later on the climbs.

Zabriskie came home with high hopes for the rest of the year. That ended with a broken collarbone in May 2013 at the Tour of California. He retired after missing the Tour de France and competed on the winning four-man team at the 2014 Race Across America—still following his M.O. strength program.

So Maximum Overload has never been officially tested. But by the principles of supercompensation, it looks promising. And since it is a given that all aging athletes must strength-train to retain muscle strength, flexibility, and power, M.O. should be considered a super-effective, time-saving option that can provide structure and purpose to workouts. If weights are an anti-aging weapon, M.O. is an atomic bomb.

The math for M.O. is easy: Find your point of failure for six reps in any exercise, like the squat. Let's say it's 100 pounds. You just squatted 6 x 100 = 600 pounds, and could not do a seventh squat. Rest a few minutes, do two more sets, then add up the total: 600 x 3 = 1,800 pounds. This is your baseline.

Now, in M.O., you will exceed that total by breaking up each set into mini-sets of only three reps (instead of six), but do each mini-set five times. Resting in between each mini-set, you will squat that 100-pound bar 5 x 3 = 15 times per set, instead of only the six times you would do in a regular set. So, in one set, you'll have lifted 1,500 total pounds instead of 600. For the second set, you again try to do five mini-sets, but fatigued, you may do only four sets (1,200 lbs.). By the third set, you may be so wasted that you can only do two mini-sets (600 lbs.). The total: 3,300 pounds.

How will you know when you are stronger? When you exceed 3,300 pounds by doing five mini-sets on both your second and third sets. At that point, you have officially raised your sustainable strength and power level, so you need to add more weight. Add 5 or 10 pounds and find your new six-reps-to-failure weight. Remember that each exercise is computed individually. You may progress rapidly in the deadlift, but not so fast in thrusters.

How do you get rest between mini-sets? You pair the squats with an exercise that works non-conflicting body parts, like a bent-over barbell row. That way, you rest your legs but don't waste time.

With Devore's advice, *Bike for Life* simulates and simplifies Zabriskie's M.O. workout with four cycling-specific exercises that hit the legs, core, and upper-body pulling muscles: the deadlift thrusters, cable torso twist, bent-over rows, one-legged leg presses (see photos this page and next). Popularized by CrossFit's "Fran" workout, thrusters are a combo squat/push press done at explosive speed that can mimic the effect of the pneumatic air-resistance jump-squat machine Zabriskie used in Devore's gym.

Of course, if you find yourself in a hotel room without access to a gym or weights, you can

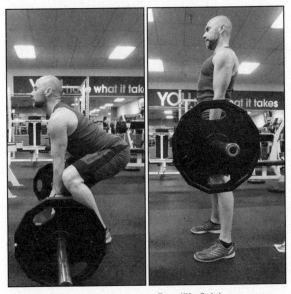

Deadlift, start   Deadlift, finish

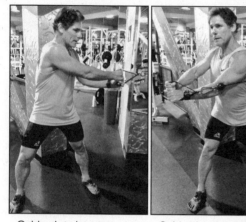

Cable ab twist, start   Cable ab twist, finish

Thruster, start   One-legged leg press

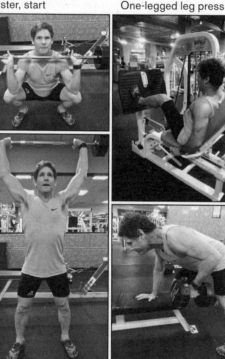

Thruster, finish   Dumbbell rows

always spend a couple of minutes a day doing Wurf's jump-squats. Just 20 will leave you heaving. They'll quickly build explosive and sustainable power and strength as you do increasing numbers of sets before reaching fatigue.

As of late 2014, apart from Zabriskie, cyclists hadn't yet heard of Maximum Overload, but I suspect that will change soon. In the meantime, if you see any cyclists jumping up and down in training or even before races, don't be surprised. Jump-squats are here to stay. And they are the tip of the iceberg.

HIGH-PERFORMANCE YOGA FOR CYCLISTS

Ten yoga poses from fitness guru Steve Ilg will strengthen your cycling—and help you repair the damage it does.

Steve Ilg knows a cyclist when he sees one. "Three out of four who first come into my classes are not flexible—and that hurts them big-time," said the USA Cycling coach and inventor of high-performance yoga. A high-level road cyclist, cross-country skier, snowshoer, and rock climber, Ilg was once dubbed "the world's fittest human" by *UltraCycling* magazine and was pictured on a 1992 cover of *Outside* magazine next to the headline: "This man can break you—and build you up again." Two decades later, at age 53, Ilg remains as chiseled as a bodybuilder, as flexible as a yogi, and, as I saw while teaming with him at the Furnace Creek 508 relay races in 1996 and 2004, in possession of an aerobic engine worthy of a champion half his age.

"Flexibility is huge for cyclists for two reasons: proper bike fit and quality of life," said Ilg. "Yoga can open up your power and get your flexibility back fast."

The problem with cycling, he said, is that it is "strange on the body; it can suffocate it. "The sport mandates long hours of intense exercise in an imbalanced position with a constricted range of motion, a closed kinesthetic loop that does not fully extend legs or arms and shortens connective tissues," he said. "So when cyclists come into my yoga classes, I immediately see a number of muscular weaknesses and biomechanical inefficiencies: weak midsections and undeveloped *internal flotation*, humped backs and slumped shoulders, and stiff and weak hip flexors, top of the feet, ankles, and knees."

Internal Flotation

If you were stopped by the yogic term "internal flotation," as I was, don't be surprised. I don't understand half of what Ilg says, anyway, but it eventually made sense. (When I went to his classes, I just copied the girl in front of me.) Ilg describes internal flotation as "a natural, fluid state of inner mobility and support based upon appropriate breathing." It's a key concept for cyclists to understand and use, given that the sport unwittingly has a tendency to work against it.

"When we are internally supported," said Ilg, "we breathe and move from a mobile core—our abdominals, hips, and lower back. When we are internally supported, our breath becomes a turbine; it creates a fusion of powerful breath and physiology that creates and radiates action from the inner toward the outer. All animals move this way; think of a starfish and you've got the idea."

The trouble is that cyclists often don't move this way. "Most cyclists are overly concerned with their leg strength and speed, and remain untrained in yogic breathing," said Ilg. "As a result, we are grossly unbalanced throughout our core. We have super-strong hip extensors and virtually nonexistent hip flexors. Just have cyclists perform a standing backbend with their arms extended overhead and see how far they get. This imbalance weakens our riding—and our postures. We tend to skeletally brace ourselves on our bike with locked-out arms, shoulders pinned close to our ears, our spines unable to maintain a flat, low, aerodynamic position." So without internal flotation, "cyclists collapse inward and restrict their most powerful forces from within. When we internally float our postures with turbine-like breath, we are in 'attack' mode more often instead of 'survival' mode."

The yoga poses that Ilg prescribes below, taken from his recent book *Total Body Transformation*, are designed to erase those cycling-specific restrictions on a cyclist's body. He says they'll maximize power transfer, elongate the vertebral chain, and stabilize pelvic alignment for enhanced biomechanics and riding technique.

The Mental Spotlight

The poses are also designed to take you beyond purely "physical" fitness. "These positions will enhance '*ekagrata*'—the ability of 'one-pointed' mental concentration," said Ilg, referring to another yogic concept that has important applications to cyclists.

"In the mental-training sciences," he said, "mental energy can be directed in two primary ways: one-pointed concentration [OPC] and high-perspective mental energy [HPME]." The latter can be likened to a traffic helicopter; the vision is all-encompassing as it looks down onto the ground to see which freeways are congested and which are clear. To cyclists, HPME is required while riding in a large peloton. Bike racers must process a lot of incoming data while sensing surges and attacks from all around them. OPC, in contrast, is like a narrow-beamed spotlight at night from that same helicopter; the spotlight deletes everything save for whatever is in that narrowed beam of vision. A cyclist needs OPC while descending at high speed in the rain, or when opening up a final sprint to come around opponents. If HPME is a floodlight, then OPC (*ekagrata* in yoga) is like a surgeon's laser scalpel. HPME is peripheral awareness, and OPC is focused awareness.

Now that you know more about yoga than you probably wanted to know (go to wholisticfitness .com for Ilg's Wholistic Fitness online training), it's time to, as Ilg said, "feel the *chi*"—the life force. Here's his yoga workout designed specifically for cyclists.

The 30-Minute Yoga-for-Cycling Workout

The following 30-minute *asana* workout (defined as "conscious breathing while sustaining postures") consists of moving deliberately, with little rest, through 10 challenging traditional yoga poses. Ilg says the workout can be used on in-season recovery days and more regularly throughout the off-season. It starts with a general warm-up routine, adds important core poses, and moves on to cycling-specific poses.

Important rules:

1. Perform all yoga poses barefoot in a draft-free, clean, warm space where you will not be interrupted.

2. Hydrate before and after, but not during, a session.

3. Allow at least three days of recovery time between sessions.

4. Hold each pose for a minimum of 45 seconds and up to a maximum of 90 seconds, unless otherwise prescribed.

5. Consciously engage in deep nasal breathing (technically known as Ujjayi Pranayam in the yoga world) throughout the entire program. "Do not move without the presence of conscious breathing," said Ilg. "Breath dictates movement. When your mind wanders, draw it gently back with deep breathing."

Step I: Warm-Up Exercises

This dynamic sequence, which flows unbroken from one pose to another, generates internal heat to promote elasticity of connective tissue, helps remove cellular toxins, and focuses the mind within the body, according to Ilg. Cycling-wise, it builds postural strength on the bike.

1. Downward-facing dog

In this classic yoga position, the body looks like an upside-down V. Standing with your feet flat on the ground, bend down, place your fully extended hands flat on the floor, and walk back 3 feet. Put your butt high in the air. Let the spine lengthen by keeping the thighs firm, as if you were trying to lift the kneecaps up to the thighs. Lift your toes to lower your heels.

This pose loosens restricted shoulders, lengthens the spine, and stretches the Achilles tendon, hamstrings, and arm muscles. It also bathes the brainstem with oxygen and nutrients.

Hold for three breaths, inhale, and move on to . . .

2. Plank pose

This simply is the "up" position of a push-up, with arms vertical, hands flat, feet resting on the toes, and the back and legs in a straight line. From the downward-facing dog, simply lower your butt, rock your head and shoulder forward, and walk your feet back a little further.

The plank builds your midsection and shoulder strength. Hold it, exhale, and lower halfway down to . . .

3. Chaturanga

This is the "down" position of a push-up. It works your midsection and arms. Keep your elbows pinned to the sides of the ribs. Hold it, inhale, and move to . . .

4. Upward-facing dog

Rock forward, lower your legs and the tops of your feet to the ground, and push your head and torso straight up by fully extending your arms.

Hold it, exhale, and push back to . . .

5. Chaturanga

Hold it, inhale, and press back to the plank; hold it, exhale, and move back to the downward-facing dog.

Repeat the entire five-exercise sequence five times, recover for 30 seconds, and then move on to the core sequence.

Step II: Core Sequence

6. Navasana/Ardha Navasana superset (repeat two or three times)

The following two poses condition a cyclist's upper and lower abdominal muscles and gastrointestinal tract, adds to core strength and balance, increases mental focus, and builds strength and power by developing internal flotation.

"These are killer ab exercises—they make ab machines at the gym seem easy," warns Ilg. "Just

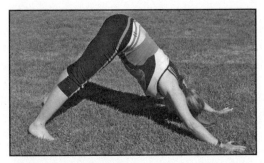

1. Downward-facing dog

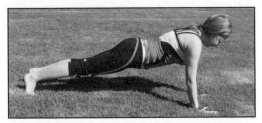

2. Plank pose

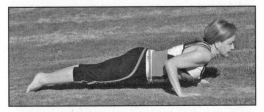

3. Chaturanga

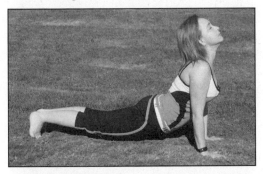

4. Upward-facing dog

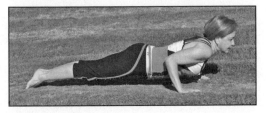

5. Chaturanga

do your best until the strength comes online, which happens remarkably quickly."

6a. Ardha Navasana (half-boat pose)

From a sitting position with your legs stretched out in from of you, raise both hands so that your arms are parallel to the ground with your palms forward and your fingers outstretched. Imagine that your spine is growing longer. Then exhale as you lean the upper torso away from your feet; at the same time, raise both legs off the floor, knees slightly bent, until your feet are at eye level. Spread the toes and draw them and the inner arches of the feet toward you, and press the balls of the feet into the air. Balance on your sacrum (tailbone) and experience the burn of the abdominals. Breathe for a few moments before moving into...

6b. Paripurna Navasana (full-boat pose)

Inhale and draw both legs higher while simultaneously raising your heart-center toward the knees, straightening your legs to take the shape of a V while still balancing on the sacrum. Keep raising the feet until they are above or even with

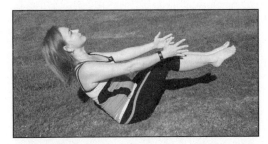

6a. Half-boat pose

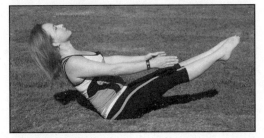

6b. Full-boat pose

the top of your head. Do not round the back; it should slightly arch as you seem to move the navel toward the upper thighs.

Exhale into Ardha Navasana and *repeat* slowly back and forth between the two for 30 to 90 seconds. This equals one superset.

Step III: Cycling-Specific Sequence

Sustain each of the following postures for 60 to 90 seconds of deep, nasal breathing before moving on to the next one. This sequence targets cycling's power-chain musculature, releasing the tightness and strengthening the weaknesses created by its imbalances.

7. Utkatasana (chair pose or fierce warrior pose)

"The worst biomechanics that I see in cyclists of all categories—rounded spine, weak torso stability, scrunched-up shoulders, knees and feet out of alignment—can all be solved by this one yoga pose!" said Ilg.

Stand with your feet pedal-width apart. Bend both knees deeply until the tops of your thighs are parallel to the ground. (Don't sweat it if you can't go parallel; you will eventually.) Do *not* allow your heels to come off the ground. Point your toes forward, in alignment with your knees.

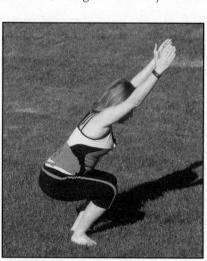

Fierce warrior pose

Raise both arms overhead; you should feel a backbend in the back of your heart area. Do *not* allow your elbows to bend. "Your arms are your warrior swords!" said Ilg. "Make sure your swords are strong and long!" Press back your head and keep soft eyes, looking forward. Nasal breathing only. Hold for 60 to 90 seconds.

Note: If your heels can't touch the ground in this pose, it is because cycling has shortened the connective tissues in your calves and hamstrings. If so, widen your stance until the heels do touch. Over time, you will close the gap.

8. Virasana (hero pose)

"When cyclists come into my yoga classes, they are notoriously stiff (which means 'weak') in their hip flexors, tops of the feet, ankles, and knees," said Ilg. "Weakness is not something I want my athletes to carry into their cycling. This one pose, hero pose, excels at removing stiff, brittle, and weak trigger areas of a cyclist and replaces them with strength, suppleness, and life energy. I call it a 'gateway pose' because it opens the gate to making other postures more available to you."

Sit on the ground in a kneeling position. Press your knees together and splay your feet apart so they rest beside your hips and you are sitting between your heels. Turn the soles of your feet directly behind you, and point your toes backward

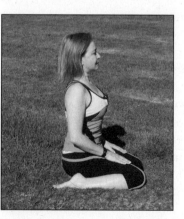

Hero Pose

as well. (If this is too much for you, options include sitting on the heels, sitting on the inside edges of the feet, or crisscrossing the feet under your buttocks.) Make your spine beautiful—tall and erect.

Rest your palms on top of your knees, puff out your heart-center slightly, and gaze softly in front of you. Breathe and dance your edge here for the prescribed time (that is, "strike a balance between effort and ease," Ilg says). After doing one, you may repeat the pose or move on to the next pose.

9. Eka Pada Sarvangasana (one-legged all-parts pose)

This difficult pose counteracts the limited range of motion in cycling that causes waste-product buildup and shortening of connective tissue. "It trains the body to become more 'lymphatically fit'—to better process exercise-induced cell toxins while providing a beautiful full range of motion for the entire spine and lower body," Ilg explained. "It also benefits heart rate, reduces tension, and improves thyroid and parathyroid functioning—meaning more strength endurance for cyclists."

Lying on your back with your arms at your sides, bend your knees and draw both heels into your buttocks, press your fingertips against the ground, and raise your torso and legs simultaneously as you roll back into a shoulder stand (head and shoulders do not move). With knees still bent, quickly bring your palms into your lower back and use your elbows as small support pillars. Walk your hands down closer to your armpits. With thumbs placed on the side ribs, press the back ribs toward the spine with your fingers. Now you should be looking straight up into your mid-thighs.

Exhale and push your legs and torso straight up to the sky. Press your hands deeper into your back as you move your sternum toward the chin. Relax your face and work on steadying your

entire body. ("As your 'internal flotation' strength develops, you can try removing your hands from your lower back to an overhead position," said Ilg. "By doing this, you will quickly discover why it is called "all-parts pose." It requires great strength to do this movement purely!")

After 60 to 90 seconds in this pose, exhale and arc your right leg down behind you until all five toes touch the ground. Keep both legs fully extended. Exhale, raise the right leg back, and repeat with the left.

After working both legs, slowly bend your knees toward your forehead and then straighten both legs until your toes touch the ground. Exhale. Then remove your hands from the lower back and clasp the fingers from each hand around your two big toes. Slowly, keeping your legs straight, roll your upper spine, then the middle spine, then the lower spine, down on to the ground, all while keeping your legs close to your torso. Exhale and squeeze both knees into your chest with your hands. Breathe, then relax and extend your legs to your original supine position.

Note: You may find this pose to be quite a bit more challenging than the others, especially if you have neck and shoulder problems. An easier approach I tried was a reverse sequence in

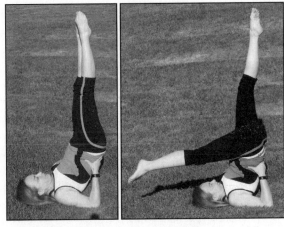

Modified headstand   One-legged all parts

which, starting on my back, I rolled my legs overhead, then supported my back with my hands and raised one foot high in the air. In the end, the position looks the same and has a similar effect.

Step IV: The Grande Finale

10. Savasana (corpse pose)

"Learning how to relax into the body is, without a doubt, the pivotal quality of champion athletes," said Ilg. "Learning how to mentally 'let go' is precisely what is needed when high-end suffering is trying to convince your ego to quit. This pose, your final relaxation posture, is crucial for relaxing your mind and body, the only way we gain better health, healing, and self-knowledge."

Lie supine, facing upward, with both legs stretched out in front of you to complete extension, hip-width apart. The heels are facing in, and your feet fall out to the sides like an open book. Stretch both arms, with your fingers outstretched and your palms facing upward at a 45-degree angle from your torso.

Inhale and raise your chin to your chest. "Take one loving last look at the body that has served you so well in the last few minutes," said Ilg. "Thank it, close your eyes, gently lay your skull down, and calm the inner war. Namasté."

(In case you were wondering about that last word, it's what they say in India instead of hello or good-bye. "Namasté means that the sacred space that lies within me recognizes and honors that same sacred space that lies within you," said Ilg. "When you and I communicate from that space, we are one.")

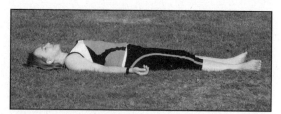

Savasana (corpse pose)

THE GLORY OF GOALS

THERE IS NO INCENTIVE TO TRAIN WITHOUT A DREAM. HERE ARE THE STORIES OF TWO MIDDLE-AGED DREAMERS WHO SET LOFTY CYCLING GOALS AND ACHIEVED THEM IN IMPRESSIVE FASHION.

PERIODIZATION POWER: TRANSFORMING AN OVERWEIGHT MIDDLE-AGED NON-RACER INTO A STAR

In 2004, Rich MacInnes, then 44, experienced what he calls his "rebirth." The traveling operations efficiency expert and father of three from Louisville, Kentucky, lost more than 30 pounds, went from a non-bike racer to Cat. 3, and from watching Masters races to winning them.

MacInnes was a high-school and college runner who got heavy after he wrecked his knee in a church softball game. A cyclist friend dragged him into the sport and he fell in love; after three and a half years, he owned a $5,000 road bike, did tandem trips with his wife, and could ride a century in five and a half hours. Then, when he saw a buddy race at the 2003 Masters nationals, he said to himself, "I can do that. I just need a coach."

MacInnes was 206 pounds when he first visited the offices of Carmichael Training Systems (CTS). His program started out as all should: finding where you are now and setting future goals. His were moderately ambitious: Drop 20 pounds, ride a century in less than 5 hours, climb L'Alpe d'Huez (he often flew to Europe for work), and do a bike tour from Louisville to Upper Peninsula Michigan.

To do that, CTS gave MacInnes a five-word plan: periodization with a fast cadence.

"CTS works on the cardiovascular system first—strengthens your heart and gets you processing oxygen well," said MacInnes. "The fast cadence is difficult at first, but it takes the stress off the legs. Then it slowly builds your power and

(continues)

THE GLORY OF GOALS *(continued)*

has you practice active recovery. It plays real well for an aging athlete."

Before MacInnes got down to work, he did a field test to measure his wattage output. The test involved 2- to 3-mile intervals with a 10-minute rest in between—an ordeal, he said, that "left me with my tongue on the ground." Also measured: lactate threshold, maximum heart rate (174), and body-fat percentage. A bike fit revealed that MacInnes was sitting too far back; as advised, he got a longer stem to put his weight more over the front wheel.

After that, he was given a diet plan from a nutritionist and a training plan from a coach, Colorado Springs–based Kate Gracheck. He signed up for Expert level—four hours per month, $150 per month. For that "dirt-cheap amount," said MacInnes, Gracheck gave him a monthly schedule in advance and modified it based on his travel plans, such as a business trip to Abu Dhabi. Likewise, when he wanted to run and swim, train with weights, or do yoga or Pilates, she would build that in.

"Initially, my bike handling was much improved from the bike fit; I could instantly corner better," said MacInnes. "But the training plan they set me up with was very frustrating—too easy. Kate had set me up at 90-minute rides—half of what I'd normally do on my own—at no higher than 135 to 142 heart rate. I rode at a cadence of 95; normally, I ride at 85.

"I'd download my files and send them to her— and she'd verbally (or by e-mail) spank me. 'You're not racing now—you're training,' she'd say.

"I started to get it after a couple months when I noticed I dropped 10 pounds and felt stronger. It was amazing! But then, instead of letting me go faster, Kate told me to rest, shorten my rides even more, slow down, and pedal faster. . . . A while later, I did a field test; it was crappy. I was mad, but Kate just laughed. 'What'd you expect? We haven't done anything to strengthen you yet.'"

Over the winter, strengthening commenced. Two months later, MacInnes's tests showed a quantum leap. In February 2005, he tried his first Cat. 5 race. In March, he won two of them. Entering Masters races, he began learning that the strongest riders often do not win—team tactics are key. By July, a year after he began the CTS program, MacInnes was doing his sprints in the hills instead of the flats and training 9 to 12 hours per week. He then rode a hilly, 25-mile time trial at over 26 mph with a maximum wattage of 1,200— double what he could do a year before.

By then he was down to 172 pounds, the lightest he'd been since college. "Watching my body literally morph has motivated my then-wife [they since divorced], who started doing aerobics three to four times a week and did her first triathlon," he said. "The training kept me out of bars at night and out of trouble. When I was at an account, they all know that I wouldn't eat late. I get up early now. I shaved my legs—went through the whole thing—Nair, razor blades.

"I was once a top-level athlete, and I'd always wondered if I could get back to that level. Well, overnight it seemed, I was a Cat. 3, placing high in multi-day races in the 1 and 2 levels. I'd rediscovered the old Rich."

MacInnes got fitter and fitter over the next few years. By age 50, he was the second-strongest member of a four-man time-trial team that won the 50-plus age group at the US road nationals in 2010. The next year, with the nationals to be held in Louisville, he wanted to podium as an individual—and so he was training hard. Then a month before the big event, he crashed. Bad.

MacInnes was unconscious for three or four minutes. His lacerated lung filled with 3 liters of fluid. Brain shear, where the skull doesn't move but the brain does, left him with secondary auditory memory loss. He had two herniated disks impinging on 40 percent of his spinal column. And he was leukemic, meaning that his red blood cell count had dropped by half.

After only three weeks off the bike, MacInnes limped out of the house and began walking. Then he began jogging. Then he hopped on his bike.

(continues)

"I'm gonna do that 25K TT at the nationals, just like I planned," he said. "Just to finish." His doctors thought he was nuts.

The time trial started on a steep uphill climb. MacInnes was so weak and winded that he thought he'd pass out. "It seemed hopeless," he said. "Halfway through, my muscles and lungs had nothing left. All I had was the will—and that's what pulled me." Only when the route circled back to the final descent to the finish did he breathe a sigh of relief.

"I'm in the tuck, doing 30 or 40 miles per hour, all I could think was, 'This is it. This is what I came here for.' It was one of the greatest days in my life."

The accident, a divorce, and his years of non-stop work forced MacInnes to take stock. He decided to take a year off from work, to mentally and physically recover. Then, in 2012, he moved, taking four bikes—including a Trek Madone 7.9, a TT bike, and a Superfly mountain bike—to Boulder, Colorado, to be closer to his daughter and grandchildren.

Instantly, MacInnes was enthralled with the active biking-hiking-running lifestyle in the foothills of the Rockies—and socked by the altitude. "Here, you're straining to keep up with old ladies and guys with hairy legs and backpacks," he said. "I used to be an aging athlete with an attitude. Now I'm an aging athlete with an altitude."

For a normal person, the accident might have been an excuse to slow down, to reduce the goal to "fitness" rather than "competition." But MacInnes, who turned 55 in 2013, said that wasn't enough for him.

"I'm happy I'm alive. But if you're gonna play this game, you have to go for it. To compete at that level, you have to take risks. I respond better to intensity, so training and competing work for me," he said. He's back with Kate Gracheck, his old CTS coach. And his sights are set on the time trial again.

He knows what to expect. "Jack LaLanne used

to say, you can be 50 and in shape or 50 and out of shape. Either way, you're going to be in pain.

"We're all going to die. But not all of us are going to live."

YOUNGER EVERY YEAR:
DAN CRAIN WAS A NON-RIDER AT 50, AND ENDURANCE LEGEND AT 60

In March 2004, Dan Crain got up at 4 a.m. every day and rode a century before work. "I was fatigued all the time, all month long. But it paid off," said the corporate insurance manager from Irvine, California, whose 3,100 miles won him the March Madness competition of the Davis Bike Club, of which he was a remote member. "After a few weeks' rest, I was surprised to feel like I was supercharged. I came back stronger than I'd ever been—at age 59!"

Crain, a long-distance legend in Southern California, was thoroughly amused by the unlikelihood of a near-60-year-old being at his peak, especially with his history. For the first half-century of his life, he did no aerobic activity at all. He surfed in college and skied regularly in his 30s, period. At 50, worried his legs were getting weak, the father of two began cycling and joined the Bicycle Club of Irvine, one of the largest clubs in the area. Crain gradually moved up to double centuries, and he participated on a four-man team and two two-man teams at the famed Furnace Creek 508. A double-century aficionado, he has competed in 106 of them in his riding career, including all 18 doubles in the series in 2000.

Over time, to maintain leg strength, Crain added kickboxing and twice-a-week lower-body strength training—low reps and heavy weights one day and high reps with light weights the other. He did tons of squats and deadlifts—but no upper-body exercises. That oversight would hurt him when he put his neck on the line—literally—at his first solo 508 in October 2004.

Three-quarters of the way through the race, after 380 miles—the longest ride of his life—Crain was in fourth place in a field of 61 solo riders and

(continues)

feeling invincible. Not only had he traversed an immense, forbidding swath of Southern California against 40-mph winds, but he'd also traveled light-years from 1995, when he was a non-athlete. Now he was an entirely different person—and about to join the endurance gods: the 500-mile club.

He didn't plan, however, on "Shermer neck."

"With less than 100 miles to go in the 508, I could no longer hold my neck up," he said. "It was falling forward like a rag doll. I literally couldn't see." It was a classic case of the condition that was first suffered by Race Across America pioneer Mike Shermer, in which riding in an aerobar tuck causes the muscles of the hyperextended neck to collapse.

Crain's crew tried in vain to keep him riding. First they cut a 4-inch strip of sleeping pad and fashioned it into a neck brace, but it didn't work: "I couldn't breathe and it compressed my aorta—it was stopping blood from getting to my head," Crain said. Next, they hooked bungee cords from the back of his helmet down to a strap under his arms and around his chest and back again. "But it didn't feel safe to me," said Crain. "I could feel the vertebrae in my neck being pinched—felt like I was going to damage myself." After 420 miles, with his legs still feeling great, Crain had to drop out of the 508.

But there was a silver lining. "I DNF'ed but had the ride of my life!" he shouted. "So I was very optimistic for the next year. I added neck exercises to my training, did wrestler's bridges, raised my handlebars an inch or two, and planned to be back even stronger."

He carried out that plan. Crain put his neck on the line twice in June 2005 with teammate Fred Boethling, with whom he set a new record in the two-man 60-plus age group at the 3,052-mile Race Across America, riding from San Diego to Atlantic City in 8 days, 13 hours, 34 minutes. In 2006, he set a 24-hour course record of 399 miles in the 60–69 age group at Big Canyon, and in 2007 he set another 24-hour course record (of

387 miles) at Cobb Mountain. Ultimately, he was a seven-time finisher of the Furnace Creek 508, once as a soloist, four times on a two-man team, once on a four-man team, and once on a mixed team. He finished the brutal California Triple Crown (CTC) stage race seven times from 1997 through 2007 and amassed 106 double-centuries and 13 California Triple Crowns (for doing three double-centuries in a year). He and teammate Anny Beck won the tandem division of the California Triple Crown in 2001, and took second in 2004.

For his efforts, Crain was inducted into the CTC Hall of Fame in 2001 after riding 50 doubles dating from 1996, into the 100 Double-Century Club in 2007, and into the Furnace Creek 508 Hall of Fame the same year.

When he was inducted into the Hall of Fame, Crain gave these tips to new double-century riders:

1. Don't accept pain from riding long distances—work on the problems.

2. Don't try to make up time on descents. The risks aren't worth the rewards.

3. Enjoy the ride and share the experience with others. Life is better experienced as a shared journey rather than as a race to beat others.

Relentlessly upbeat, Crain's philosophy, he said, was to "celebrate life and share the celebration with others." His long years in the non-athletic wilderness gave him a perspective to which many late-blooming cyclists can relate: "Is it possible to continue improving as you get older? Yes—I'm proof of that," he told *Bike for Life*. "My body is far younger than it was two decades ago."

Note: Tragically, Crain did not have a chance to ride to age 100. On a Tuesday evening, August 3, 2010, he was cut off and rear-ended by a Toyota Land Cruiser while climbing from Irvine over Newport Coast Drive to the beach. Two weeks later, following two spine surgeries, he had a sudden cardiac arrest in the hospital and passed away, provoking a massive outpouring of grief from the Southern California endurance cycling community.

Rebecca Rusch

THE OLDEST ROOKIE

"There's this girl out there who is so stiff, so uncoordinated, that it's actually painful to watch!" a photographer told me halfway through the 2006 24 Hours of Adrenalin Solo Mountain Bike World Championships in Conyers, Georgia. "I can tell she's not a cyclist. She muscles the bike like she's lifting weights—riding solely on strength. The rest of the girls are smooth and flowing, but she's a barbarian! Who is she? What is she even doing here?"

She was nearly winning. At an age when most pro mountain bikers are long retired, Rebecca Rusch, then 38, was a rookie rider who barely knew single-track from a singles bar. She was a paddler, a climber, a runner, and, most famously, a world champion adventure racer who'd specialized in weeklong races like the Eco-Challenge and the Raid Gauloises. Like many who competed against the then-unknown cyclist at her first adventure race in Malibu in 1997—a 24-Hour Eco-Challenge qualifier she helped her team win—I was not surprised that a stellar professional career followed. Rusch went on to captain Team Montrail in adventure races in Borneo, Vietnam, Nepal, and all around the globe for nearly a decade. The Gregory company even named a special lightweight backpack the Arreba, a play on her nickname, Reba.

In 2006, when her adventure racing sponsorship suddenly dried up, Rusch decided to try pro mountain biking—and as onlookers pointed out, it wasn't

pretty. Instead of riding quickly over an obstacle, Rusch was so scared that she'd hop off her bike and carry it. But the lack of basic bike-handling skills—not required on the nontechnical fire roads of adventure racing—was balanced by a monster endurance. She'd stunned the bike world earlier that year with wins at a local 24-hour race in Spokane, Washington (including beating all the men), and the 2006 NORBA 24-hour nationals. And now, against the best in the world at the 24 Hours Solo in Conyers, she shocked herself by taking second place.

"She's got the engine. Wait till she learns how to ride," said her mountain-biker boyfriend Greg Martin, licking his chops.

It was a prescient warning. Rusch learned fast, quickly becoming nearly unbeatable, and was soon a role model for all latecomers—especially 40-plus women—trying a new sport. Starting with learning how to hop a curb ("a skill little boys learn when they are six," she noted), she quickly raised her technical game and dominated: In 2008, she won her first of three straight World Solo 24-Hour Championships. Then she won three straight Leadville 100s (2010, '11, and '12)—and nearly everything else in sight over 50 miles long. Barreling into her late 40s, she wasn't slowing down.

A common theme in Rusch's story is "the right place at the right time"—she was a rock climber when the indoor-climbing boom hit, a paddler recruited for adventure racing when it got hot, an endurance machine hungry for work when 24-hour solo mountain biking was at its peak, and a siren for women when their interest in the sport was skyrocketing. With long-distance events more popular than ever, Rusch, 45 at the time of her Bike for Life *interview in September 2013, is arguably the No. 1 female mountain biker in the world. Here the "Queen of Pain," as she's known, talks about her journey from rock climber to mountain biker, the trauma and head games that won't let her quit, her late-bloomer skill acquisition, and her plans for staying on top and motivated past 50.*

I GREW UP in the Chicago suburbs, ran track and cross-country in high school, graduated from the University of Illinois with good grades and a marketing degree, then learned how to rock climb—and that changed everything. I hopped in the car and drove across country to hit all the best climbing spots—basically, a six-month party. My mom, a high-powered executive in a man's field, probably wasn't very happy about it.

I ended up in California, teaching climbing and eventually becoming a part-owner and manager of my own rock gym, Rockreaction, in West L.A. I was one of the first investors in the chain.

In what seems to be the theme of my life, I was in the right place at the right time. First, through a boyfriend I was dating who had been an Olympic rower, I found this great group of girls who were outrigger canoe racing; I ended up joining the outrigger team and the US women's whitewater rafting team. Then, I met all the adventure racing people in L.A. who were coming into the gym to learn to rappel. It was hilarious; they were all wearing tight Lycra. Soon, finding out I could paddle as well as climb, they'd say, "We need one female on our team. And you can do two out of the four sports, so—you're in."

I could actually do three out of the four: I could climb, paddle, and run. But I'd never mountain biked. No matter. My team won a 24-Hour Eco-Challenge qualifier in Malibu in 1997, which got us an all-expenses-paid invitation to go to Eco-Challenge Australia. All I thought was, "All right, it's a free trip, I'll go." And lo and behold, that launched an entire career as an adventure racer that lasted 10 years. I left the rock gym and ended up becoming something I never would have dreamed of: a pro athlete. One, I never considered myself that good an athlete; two, I have asthma; and three, adventure racing just seemed outrageously insane and expensive—How could you really make this work? I ended up making it work by living out of my car for five years; that was the only way to be able to afford to go on these great trips, and not have to worry about paying rent.

I ended up managing the team, soliciting sponsorship, and making it all happen. It was definitely not lucrative. I would laugh my head off when I'd fill out forms where you'd have to list your job. I was a professional athlete, just not making much money. Just think of the expense of getting four people plus climbing, paddling, biking equipment to a place like Morocco. If you have a $100,000 sponsorship package, there it goes out the window in two or three races.

Like my father [more on him later], I just wanted to travel, and thought this was a really good way to go all over the world: Yeah, I'll ride this wave, try to make it happen. We ended up putting together the best team in the world for a number of years.

I got lucky. I was a jack-of-all-trades in a sport that required that, and I never got hurt. I have no idea how many adventure races I did. I raced for 10 years pretty much full-time. There were always three big expedition races a year and a bunch of little 24-hour ones to fill in.

Then it suddenly was over—and I had to think of something else to do . . . like mountain biking.

I remember it distinctly the day it all came to an end. It was October 13, 2006, and I got a phone call from the CEO of Montrail, who'd been our title sponsor for three or four years. "I'm just giving you the heads-up: Montrail's been bought by Columbia, and the sponsorship's done," he said. I was already sitting there planning our budget for the next year, thinking Montrail had no reason to drop us. So I called up the team and just said, "The party's over. I can't land another title sponsor like this." I remember feeling really lost. Like, "Okay, what am I going to do with my life?" I was in my late 30s. What am I going to do? I'd been on the fire department in Ketchum, Idaho, for several years. I did a lot of soul searching.

Then, I called up Red Bull. I had one more year left on my contract with them. They said, "We're not going to take the money back. You've got a year, so find something to do with it." They were really cool about it. I told 'em, "Look, I don't have a team or a sport anymore." I made some calls to other teams, but I didn't really want that; we had such a great relationship with our team that I didn't just want to jump in with another one. Red Bull said, "Do whatever you want."

This was October, so I went with a bunch of girlfriends to the 24 Hours of Moab, just for fun. They said, let's just go do this event, we've never done anything like it. We all went knowing that cycling was my worst event—had always been my worst event in adventure racing. And I never really liked it. We went just for fun—you know, a party weekend. We ended up winning the women's expert division, and I ended up having the fastest lap time of any female in the race.

The funniest part was that I had to get off the bike and run a bunch of the technical sections. I couldn't ride very well, but I sure could get on and off my bike. From adventure racing, I learned how to do that while trying to keep up with the guys. That sparked something. Red Bull had told me, "Do whatever you want for another year," and my first thought was ultra-running, because I knew I needed endurance. But the longest thing I could find, I realized after the 24 Hours of Moab, was 24-hour solo mountain-biking.

A month later, I did a 24-hour solo in Oregon. And I ended up beating the entire field, including the men. "All right, I guess that this is it for the year," I said to myself. My second race was the US national championships—and I won it!

My third race is where you saw me in Conyers, Georgia, at the 24 Hours of Adrenalin Solo World Championships—and you wrote that article for *Mountain Bike* magazine about me finishing second without basically knowing how to ride a bicycle. That day launched a whole new career.

So I called up all my old sponsors, telling them I wanted to do more biking. "Well, okay, we'll stick with you," said Red Bull. Specialized renewed at a higher level. Seven years later, I'm still at it, with three solo world championships and four Leadvilles.

Mountain Biking 101 at Age 38

AGAIN, I'M COMPLETELY surprised. Me, a professional cyclist? Anyone who adventure-raced with me knows how badly I sucked on a bike. They all told me how much I sucked on the bike. You know how bad I sucked on a bike. I'm going to be a bike racer? It was a friggin' joke!

I wasn't a good rider and I'm still not. I'm okay, that's it. But I've done all right because I worked hard to bring my skill level up, and I can keep going for a long, long time.

Regarding the skill issue, I already mentioned how I'd run my bike around obstacles during adventure racers. That was okay if I wanted to take second, as I did in the '06 worlds. But I had to raise my skill level to win, and that meant learning the basics. To give you an idea, I couldn't even hop a curb at that time, meaning I couldn't clear large rocks and drop-offs. Now, after years of practice, I can hop a curb. But it's still not natural; I really have to stop and think about it, gear up for it, and say, "Okay..."

Little boys on their Stingrays learn how to hop a curb. I had to learn in my late 30s what they have wired by the time they are eight and nine. It takes an incredible amount of forgiveness in yourself to do this, because learning as an adult is hard—especially something that is scary.

This is why I understand how to motivate and teach other women in clinics nowadays. I get it. Because I'm terrified a lot of times when I'm riding my bike, because it's not a natural thing that I learned when I was five years old. As older learners, and especially as women, we think it all through, and have to process and know exactly what it is we are supposed to do. With the speed of mountain biking, there's not enough time to actually think, "Okay, lift up on my feet and lift up on the fork and lean back and do this." By the time you thought all that, it's too late. So trying to go from an intellectual learning to something that you just feel and is intuitive is a very slow learning process. Then you throw fear in the mixture, and it's really hard to get any better, because you have to fail. And you have to keep getting up off the dirt and trying again. That's scary. Then you have to fail again—and try again.

The progression needs to be really slow. When you are thrown in a bike race, unfortunately, the way I did it, I didn't get a really good learning process. I think it was beautiful luck that I rode 24-hour races, which are half at night. Because a lot of times I rode better technically in the dark, where I couldn't see all the scary stuff and think about it. I also think I rode better the more tired I got, because I really just couldn't fight it anymore.

It's hard to learn something as an adult. But I also say that it's never too late. If someone like me, who really did not have an aptitude for mountain bikes or other high-speed sports like downhill skiing can do it, anyone can. The biking anyways feels really fast to me. Having my brain catch up is what's been the biggest challenge.

The Queen of Pain

LUCKILY, I'VE BEEN able to make up for my poor riding technique with, for lack of a better term, "pain management." The magazine *Adventure*

Sports, during my last years as an adventure racer, called me the "Queen of Pain," and I liked it. It was my first and only magazine cover, and the nickname just sorta stuck. I'd never heard of it before, but I took it as a compliment. I was the captain of a team in an ultra-endurance sport that went 24 hours a day for a week or more at a time. Yes, there's lots of pain involved.

Pain is a huge part of adventure racing and endurance mountain-biking, which is what makes them so mental. Oftentimes the fittest, fastest person out there does not finish first, because they can't handle the pain. It takes a lot of brainpower to ignore the pain, put it aside, and forge forward when you don't feel like it. You have to ignore the demons and the voices in your head that are saying, "It hurts," or "I have blisters on my feet," or "This is too hard."

The very first Eco-Challenge qualifier that I did in Malibu in 1997, I was terrified. I was a rock climber, a runner, and had done a bunch of outrigger canoeing. But the thought of doing something for 24 hours straight was really daunting to me. I ran cross-country and track in high school, and was always better at the 2-mile than the 50-yard-dash—always better at longer stuff. That's like 12 to 14 minutes in high school. But 24 hours?

I remember telling my boyfriend at the time, "You know, I can't do anything for 24 hours. I can't even sit on the couch for 24 hours. I don't know how I'm going to do this." Of course, I was a terrible bike rider. So I remember thinking that I was going to be the weakest link, the worst one, that everybody was going to come down on me. But that didn't happen, due to my ability to manage the pain.

We were riding in the middle of the night, way up one of the huge canyons in Malibu, and one of the strong guys on our team was having so much trouble that the other two guys were having to push and pull him. So although I was in pain, all I had to do was keep up. I did it by counting pedal strokes. I'm not going to get off the bike for 100 pedal strokes. Then, okay, I'm going to count to 100 again.

That was my first experience with how to mentally ignore the pain in my legs, ignore that it's hours to go until we see the top. I still play number games. In 24-hour bike racing I would calculate, "If there are four more hours to go and I'm going this many miles per hour, how many more will I finish in 12 hours?" I'd do math. Then, if I'm in, say, New Zealand, I'd have to convert it to kilometers. I'm not real good at math. So I'd make mistakes. And it took a lot of time. And in that time, you've just gone another 20 miles.

The overall theme of all this is distraction. Instead of focusing on the pain and how long you have to go, you play games to get your mind off it. Adventure racing was cool that way, because you're with people, so you could talk and tell stories. Louise Cooper, one of my teammates, would sing. The Australian guys would tell really off-color jokes. So the trick to being "mentally tough" is actually not even thinking about it—distraction.

At the same time, you can distract yourself by being in the moment and not looking ahead. In a 24-hour race, I'll break it down by one lap. Can I keep the same speed that I did the last lap? So instead of thinking, "I have 47 more laps to go," I'll think, "How can I make this one lap really good?" So break it down in chunks. I use the same approach in a race like the Leadville 100. I think, "Can I climb Columbine as efficiently as possible?" Or, "Can I maintain 10 miles per hour going up?" Don't intimidate yourself by thinking, "Oh god, this is only mile 35 out of 103."

The High School Anti-Quitting Epiphany

I NEVER QUIT. The counting, the math distractions help ensure that. But at the root of it, quitting repulses me. That's because I quit one race in my life of my own free will, and it was so traumatic that I vowed never to do it again.

It was in high school; I was a junior, and it was the conference championship. Normally, I was the number one or two runner on our team, but on that day, I was behind girls I shouldn't have been behind. I was just having a bad day. It was an important meet to qualify us for the Illinois state championship. I was just having a bad day. I was pretty bummed that I was in the middle of the pack, and I just stepped off the course—and quit. And I remember it so vividly: My teammates, and my mom, and people all coming up to me, and saying, "Are you okay?" And my coach. And I had nothing to say—I had no good reason, other than my ego, that I was bummed that I wasn't up farther in the pack [where] I should have been. And this one girl on our team really stepped up that day and had the race of her life, so we still qualified for state championships. But had she not done that, it would have been my fault that we wouldn't have gone.

I remember the shame I felt of just quitting and having no good reason. I've thought of that many times over the years. I would rather be carried down the finish line in last place than have to explain to my friends and my family why I quit. Unless you have a broken leg or something, it's not acceptable. And that has really stuck with me—out of shame or pride or ego, I don't want to tell people that I quit.

I don't want to let my friends and sponsors down. So I keep going. A lot of times in endurance sports, that's enough. You're the last one standing.

Every single Leadville I've won I have not been in the lead at the start of the race. I've been as low as fifth place. But I won those four races because I didn't give up and I kept going, plodding along.

I'm kind of glad I quit that day in high school, so early on in my sporting career. Because it scarred me for life, and helped me become a stronger person.

When teammates of mine have quit, it hurts me down to my soul. When you feel good, and you put in all this preparation into your race, and then . . . somebody got a blister, or just gives up, it's hard to be understanding. It's the good and bad of adventure racing: You have people to share your successes with, but you also have to share their failures. You have to take it all, like marriage.

A teammate dropped out of Eco-Challenge Morocco in '99, the first race that I captained. Mark Burnett (Eco-Challenge race founder and a TV producer, now known as the godfather of reality shows such as *Survivor*, *The Apprentice*, and *Shark Tank*) had encouraged me to put together a three-woman, one-man team. We ended up with someone for whom it was too much mentally and physically, and she quit during the race. She wasn't hurt, she could have kept going. And that was pretty hard for me, and I tried all my skills of persuasion and coercion, and trying to get her to step up to the plate. And then I just got mad. I tried everything, but she quit, and the three of us finished the event unranked.

I miss the team aspect when doing the solo mountain-biking I've done, but in some ways it's also really cool to do the 24-hour solo stuff, where it really is just you, with nobody there to hold your pack or hold your hand, to celebrate your successes and tough out the failures. You have to pat yourself on the back at the end, and no one can really understand what you've been through—like the Kokopelli Trail, which I did this year [2013] by myself. It was a huge achievement. But no one will understand what I went through on the trail, other than me.

Finding New Challenges

BESIDES DOING ESTABLISHED events, like Leadville, a big part of my motivation nowadays is coming up with my own challenges. Also, Red Bull, my longtime sponsor, always pushes their athletes to come up with projects. So I proposed trying to set a new self-supported women's record on the Kokopelli (a 142-mile trail from Fruita, Colorado, to Moab, Utah), which I did by over half an hour: 13 hours, 34 minutes. This was a culmination of my adventure-racing experience and my cycling career, putting the two together. I had to carry my own stuff, filter water, find my way. I was in my own head the whole time, with no people cheering me; [there's] nobody saying your name, no personal friends to give you food, to let you chase a rabbit. Just me, alone, with my Garmin, and the time splits I wanted to hit. I knew by maintaining a certain mph, I'd break the record. I was just focused on the splits, saying, "Can I go a little faster? Should I be eating, should I be drinking? Where's the next water stop when I can filter?"

In my mind, that's the best situation: Where your mind is occupied the whole time, so that you don't necessarily have to play those games of counting and that kind of stuff. If the route is really exciting, you're really engaged and happy to be there.

Kokopelli was one of my greatest achievements. It was the first time I combined everything I know. I think I'll have more adventures like that.

The next one might be to ride the whole Ho Chi Minh Trail in Vietnam, 800 miles, to visit my dad's crash site. It was August 25, 1968. Dad was a colonel in the air force. He never came home. I was two, so I have no memories of him. It would be a pretty cool journey in many ways.

From what I hear from my grandparents and mom, my dad was a wanderer who loved to travel. He played the banjo, lived out of a converted mail truck, and played at coffee shops. I think my wanderlust—traveling to places and living out of my car for five years off and on— might come from him. My organization and independence comes from my mom, who raised my older sister and me alone and has traipsed around the world supporting us.

Promoting Women and Idaho

ONE OF THE most rewarding things I've been able to do is promoting causes and events I think are important, like Gold Rusch—women's clinics, women's events—and a new gravel race called Rebecca's Private Idaho.

In 2011, I launched the SRAM Gold Rusch tour, because I saw an opening. I saw women like me, who get intimidated by riding or when their boyfriends take them riding and leave them in the dust. Because I remember what it's like to be a beginner. In a lot of ways, I still feel like a beginner. So I can relate to them and the fear. Sometimes, you just need somebody to show you, and give you confidence. Then they can go back to their boyfriends and show 'em up!

With the Gold Rusch tour, I go to about six different places and events a year and try to encourage women. The idea came about a couple years ago at Sea Otter [the Sea Otter Classic] when I was trying to get into the booth of SRAM, a sponsor, to get a bike part. And basically, I was intimidated, even though they were a sponsor. I didn't feel welcome. There were a bunch of guys hanging around, all talking shop. And I wasn't really confident to go in and ask for this bike part. I thought, "If I feel this way, probably a lot of other women would feel this way too—and what can we do about it?"

I talked to SRAM about it, and at the next Sea Otter they set up a Ladies Lounge right next to the main mechanics bay—a place where women can come in, talk to the pros, talk shop, have a mechanical clinic. We added wine and cheese to make it a welcoming atmosphere. Now, every year, I pick and choose certain events and we create women's rides, mechanical clinics. I invite media, I give female athlete pros some media exposure. The whole idea is to make connections, inspire women to go home and stage their own clinics, start their own women's mountain bike clubs, become a cycling journalist. It's a snowball effect. In Pennsylvania, a high-school girl who came to my event started hosting her own girls' rides. It's just great the way this happens: You give somebody a little confidence and a boost, and then they run with it.

This support can be very beneficial for a lot of women in my age bracket and even older, who, when they were in school, only were offered sports like cheerleading and maybe track and field. Today, sports are wide-open for women, and they have the time and freedom to do them—and are loving it. That is the demographic that is really fun to ride with. It's like riding with a 12-year-old kid, feeling that freedom and joy. But there is a difference. As kids, everything is new, and you're always learning new stuff, so it's not such a big deal to be a beginner. But as we get to be a doctor, or a Fortune 500 company CEO, you don't want to look like a fool. You're a high-powered executive in your regular life, so it's hard to try something new and look like an idiot at it. In mountain biking, you have to fail to be able to learn, but you don't want to fail as you get older. You're supposed to be good at everything. You're in your 40s—you're not supposed to be a "beginner." You have to be humble enough to say, "Oh man, I'm a total beginner, and I really suck at this." It's easier to do that in the company of other women, because we're supportive of each other.

Rebecca's Private Idaho, which I staged for the first time in September 2013—and it was awesome—is a gravel road event. They're really catching on now. It came about because I love Idaho. Over a decade ago, after living in my car and traveling all around for so many years, this place really grabbed my heart, and I haven't left. People always say, "Idaho? What's there? It's just potatoes?" So I wanted to do a bike event here to show it off, share it. I always thought I'd put on a mountain bike event. But last year [2012], I went to two events that really clued me in as to how I could get more people here: the Dirty Kansas 200-mile gravel road event. I didn't want to go—Specialized made me. As a mountain biker, I thought, "What could be more hellish than 200 miles of gravel road?"—but the gravel, I realized, is the great equalizer, putting together the skills of mountain biking and road biking in one place.

The gravel keeps your attention, believe it or not, for 200 miles. Plus, no need for a Forest Service application. Then I went to Levi's Gran Fondo event in Northern California and saw what it does for his community. I talked to Levi [Leipheimer] and sponsors, and they all said do it, do it, do it.

The timing is really good. Gravel is trendy now and people want to ride for a cause—all fundraising for charities I care about. We had 250 riders. And they showed up in the aftermath of the fire.

My plan for the next 10 years: Keep using my name and my influence to help inspire people and do good things. Get people riding, into the backcountry. I do think the bicycle and being outdoors make the world a better place.

Staying Fit and Looking Ahead

I TRAIN LESS now as I get older, but I train better, so I get faster every year at Leadville. I try to eat healthy, but not obsessive. I Nordic ski and back-country ski in the winter. It's a healthy break for me and gets my upper body and core strength. I think it's boring to only ride or do one thing year round, and that the multisport thing is really healthy. It's the reason that in 20-plus years of being an athlete I really haven't had a major injury. I do no weight lifting per se—no squats in the gym—but I do lots of body-weight stuff. I'm remodeling my house, so I move big pieces of wood around, and I'm on the fire department. So there's lots of real-life strength training built in to what I do. It's kind of the same thing as a gym—just more fun. I'm on call at the fire department. For the big fire here (in September 2013), I worked three 17-hour shifts in a row, then it ended. We also do backcountry rescue, all the medical, so a lot of opportunities here for me to use my athletic skills.

I sometimes go to a gym—more in the winter. People look at my arms and think I work out at the gym, but it's just life. I don't rock-climb much anymore. I'm very focused on my bike training—because I have to compete against women who are 25 years old.

I'll always do events, but I'll also be looking for the next inspiring thing, such as the Koko-pelli self-supported bike/adventure-racing mix. Variety is the spice of life, and doing different things motivates you. If you dread going to the gym, then you are not doing the right thing. If it becomes a chore, then the passion is gone. All my career decisions and trajectory changes happened because I followed something that sparked the passion. All the coolest stuff has been kind of scary and risky, but worth it.

At this point, I can't foresee switching away from riding the bike, due to two things: I love how far you can go and how much you can see. It's a great way to travel, do adventures, get outside your one-block radius. If you're a runner, you can only go so far. And cycling is something you conceivably could do until you're 100. You can take it at any level, and it doesn't hurt, doesn't have to be painful. So those two things make me think that I always will be riding. I don't think that this sport is going to be one of those that fade away. I will always find new places to go and new challenges to take on two wheels.

When people say to me, "Oh, you're so lucky to be doing what you do," I say, "No, I chose this, I created this. It's not luck necessarily." The bike is a machine of unlimited possibilities, but it doesn't pedal itself. Whether it's riding in the Alps, or coming to Sun Valley, or being with a group of friends who you really love to ride with, it's up to you to find that inspiration to do something with it. You always have to find joy and passion as if you were a little kid the first time you got on a bicycle and went "wheee!" when you went down the street. Once you lose that, it's all over.

3

TECHNIQUE

Skills to get you there faster, safer, and in style

"Jam the outside foot down. Don't just let it hang there. Jam it down!" Those words reverberated in my brain as I tore down twisty, treacherous Northern California mountain roads one day in June 1994 at speeds that would have scared me out of my gourd two months earlier—before I took a weekend course at John Howard's Cycling School of Champions in San Diego. I had no choice but to use what I'd learned from the US Bicycling Hall of Famer. Due to misreading the map, I'd arrived 90 minutes late in Santa Rosa for the start of the Terrible Two, one of the world's hardest, most beautiful double-centuries, featuring 16,500 feet of climbing through Napa and Sonoma counties. I spent another hour taking wrong turns. My only hope of catching up to the pack and winning my fourth consecutive "California Triple Crown" T-shirt (representing the completion of three double-centuries in a year) was to throw caution to the wind.

Yet as I let loose and heeded Howard's instructions—"Lift the inside foot, lean into the turn, and drive the outside foot straight down with most of your body weight"—I surprisingly felt safer, not riskier. Just as John promised, "sticking" the outside foot gave me remarkable control at high speeds, virtually gluing my wheel to the road like a slot car in a track. For the first time in my life, I wasn't nervous on the steeps and was making up huge amounts of time on them. After four hours of being told

repeatedly by organizers that I should quit, I began catching some of the laggards.

By 10 p.m., after 14 hours of one of the best rides of my life, maybe the first time I actually felt like a competent cyclist, I had conquered all four major climbs, some with up to 11 percent grades, and was homing in on the finish when I was spotted in the darkness and pulled from the course for safety reasons. Damn—I had done the work: 201 miles. But that year was the last time the Terrible Two measured out at 211 miles; it was shortened to exactly 200 thereafter.

So I drove 600 miles up from L.A., did all this work, and didn't get my Triple Crown T-shirt. But at least I learned a couple of valuable lessons about efficient cycling that day: No. 1, I better figure out how to read a map, and No. 2, technique works.

The previous chapter gave you a blueprint for building a high-performance machine. This chapter gives you the technical skills to drive that machine. The brief clinics outlined below will help transform you from dilettante to connoisseur—from mere "bike rider" to a true "cyclist." At any level, whether you do charity rides or centuries, ride a $200 Costco cruiser or a $7,000 custom carbon fiber–titanium dream machine, it comes in handy to know the basics of riding a bike—how to stop, climb, corner, descend, and draft. Ultimately, it's not just about the extra mph they confer; it's about the safety of being in control of your newfound power, the pride of mastering real skills, and flat-out fun, pure and simple.

1. HOW TO STOP

"Sooner or later," said John Howard, "you are going to come face-to-door-handle with a distracted soccer mom who is talking on her cell phone and screaming at her kids. What you need is a Hot Stop."

A Hot Stop is an emergency technique that can save skin, bones, and, possibly, funeral-home paperwork. It is the nearest thing to stop-on-a-dime braking. Done right, you won't skid out and will live to ride another day. Here's what you do:

1. Shift your weight rearward. At the first sign of trouble, slide your glutes very far back and low, behind the seat. This lowers your center of gravity, improving rear-wheel traction and preventing an end-over.

2. Level your pedals. This keeps you from pulling to one side or clipping a pedal if you do lean.

3. Grab the front brake hard, the rear easier. Apply far more pressure to the front brake than you otherwise think would be safe. The correct percentage of braking bias is two-thirds front and one-third rear; in the rain, use equal braking pressure. It will probably take several tire-sliding sessions before you can get the hang of it. If you don't lock up the wheel and catapult into a truck, you'll stop amazingly fast and under control.

4. Get ready to bail. Find an escape route or stopping point and focus on that, rather than on what you want to miss. The bike will naturally follow your eyes.

2. HOW TO TURN

Good cornering skills not only make you faster—allowing you to make up time without working any harder—but also make you safer, less likely to crash. Here are the basics, according to Howard.

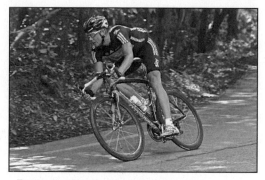
Fast cornering: jam the foot down

1. Push your butt back. Your hips should be slightly to the rear of the saddle, and your back as flat and parallel to the top tube as possible.

2. Raise the inside foot. If you are making a right turn, put the right pedal/foot up, in the 12 o'clock position on the crank, and shove the left leg straight down on the pedal in the 6 o'clock position. The right knee should fall out toward the turn as you lean, providing a lower center of gravity and more stability. To handle higher speeds, drop your shoulder, or even your head, slightly.

3. Have one finger over the brakes at all times. Be ready to use a light, feathery brake. Don't grab the brakes hard, which would risk a skid.

4. Enter the turn wide and cut in. Be at your preferred speed 10 feet before the turn. Drift to the outside of the straightaway before entering the turn, then cut an arc toward the apex. (Enter the curve on the inside, and you may have a date with the hay bales on the outside curb.) The flow is: outside, inside, outside. The idea is not to steer the turn, but to set up for it, then adjust your body weight so that your knee comes out in the direction of the turn.

5. Weight the outside pedal. The more weight you shift to the outside pedal, the more traction you have. Drive your body weight into that pedal. "Jam it!" Howard said. You'll stick like glue to pavement.

3. HOW TO CLIMB

Don't dread the hills—relish them. With proper hill-climbing technique and strategy, climbing can actually be relaxing (see John Sinibaldi interview on page 123). In fact, climbing can be a time-efficient staple of training, providing superb conditioning in an hour or less. It can even help you make a name for yourself, as it did for Tom Resh, one of the best-ever American climbers. At one time, Resh, now retired, held records at three of the toughest hill-climb competitions in North America: Mt. Baldy in Southern California (4,700 feet of elevation gain in 12.7 miles; Resh's time: 56:15); Mt. Charleston, Nevada (5,700 feet in 17 miles; time: 1:16:05); and the world's longest-known-climb event with the greatest elevation gain, Maui's Mt. Haleakala (10,000 feet in 38 miles; time: 2:45:32). Here's how Resh rushed 'em.

1. Big gear, fast spin. Generally, be in the biggest possible gear that will allow you to keep the pedals spinning above 85 percent of your flatland rate. That would be above 76 rpm in the hills if you pedaled 90 rpm on the flats. Any slower than 60 to 70 rpm and your heart rate, energy use, and perceived exertion jack up.

2. Beware Armstrong-style spinning. A super-fast spin rate isn't the answer if you're not trained for it. Spinning may save your legs, but it leads to a high heart rate and heavy breathing. "The key to climbing is to achieve a cadence which balances the pain in your chest with the pain in your legs," said Resh. Let experience— and the 85 percent rule—be your guide.

3. Bigger isn't necessarily better. For short climbs under a half-mile long, it's okay to use an extra-large gear. But for longer distances, smaller gears will be faster, more efficient, and less tiring. If you struggle in a big gear for too long, your legs will wear out before the hill ends.

4. Match your body position to the steepness of the hill.

a. *Shallow grade: Sit.* Stay in a normal or aero position. After all, you don't want to fight the wind as well as the hill.

b. *Moderate grade: Push your butt back.* The back-of-the-saddle position provides extra power by increasing the extension of your leg, utilizing the glutes, and boosting the effectiveness of the calf muscles. A good blueprint to follow: Drop your heel at the top of the pedal stroke, then push through the ball of the foot. Scoot your butt back and forth to alternate the focus on the glutes and the quads, respectively. Flex your elbows. Don't hunch your shoulders or round your back; try to fold forward at the hips.

c. *Steep grade: Stand up.* As the hill becomes steeper and your cadence slows, the sitting position may not deliver enough power. You'll need to stand. Standing also can provide relief during long climbs or that extra burst of power you need to drop an opponent.

5. Standing technique. Grip the hoods of your brake levers while still seated, and stand up by putting your weight on the pedal that is traveling downward. At this point, rock the bike side to side for leverage, using your body weight and arms to push the pedals down.

If standing gives you more power, many wonder, why not stand for the entire climb? Simply because you use more energy standing. You have to support your weight as well as push the pedals. Again, it's a trade-off between speed and efficiency.

6. Don't weave. Studies show that a 3-degree change in your steering angle makes you work up to 30 percent harder. It also increases the distance traveled.

7. Hill-training intervals. Heading for the hills is a fast way to develop power. Find a hill 2 to 3 miles long. It doesn't have to be really steep, because you can always make it steeper by using bigger gears. "Two or three times up the hill are enough as long as you make a hard effort the entire way," said Resh. "Just pretend your archrival is up the road." Use the ride downhill as your recovery. Constantly monitor your body while climbing. Go as hard as you can without blowing up.

8. Join an expert climber. Try this virtual ascent with Tom Resh:

To show you how it's done, *Bike for Life* asked Resh to create a simulated climb. Clip into your virtual pedals, imagine a tall, thin rider next to you, and heed his words:

"Get ready, rookie. Up ahead of us looms a 1-mile-long hill. But notice as we approach that I don't shift gears. I wait until the hill slows me before I shift.

"Now we are starting to go up. I move my hands to the top of the handlebars and slide back on my saddle to give me a little more leverage.

"Now my pedal cadence is beginning to slow, so I stand up to get a little more power and keep my speed up.

"Even with the extra power, however, my pedal cadence is still slowing down. So I sit back and finally shift to an easier gear. My goal is to keep my rpms within 15 percent of what they are on the flats.

"Now, just as I am starting to adjust to the increase in effort, I look ahead to see a short, steep section. Rather than shift down to an easier gear, I stand up and power over this section.

"After the steep part, I sit back down. Immediately, I monitor myself: How do my legs feel? How is my breathing? Can I go faster and drop you, or should I be nice since this is our first ride together?

"Whew! This is getting to be a long one. So I'll stand up once in a while to stretch the legs.

"Thank god, the last 100 meters. I stand again. Standing up uses more energy, but there is always a rest on the downhill. See you at the bottom!"

Mountain Bike Climbing Technique

Off-road climbs are very different from asphalt ascents. That's because the main concern is traction on the loose ground, or rather the lack of it. These conditions all but eliminate standing while climbing, as the seat must be weighted to keep pressure on the rear wheel. Do this:

Steep Climbs

1. Scoot your butt rearward for back-wheel traction, but bend at the hips and elbows; drop your chest toward the handlebar to maintain front-wheel control.

2. Raise your chest away from the bar for more rear wheel traction. to keep the front wheel grounded, lower your chest. Don't move your butt.

Super-Steep Grades

1. Perch your butt on the tip of the saddle.

2. Lean waaaaay over the bar to keep the front wheel from popping up.

3. Forcefully pull down and back on both ends of the handlebar along with each downward pedal stroke. Perfect timing adheres the back wheel to the trail, while your weight keeps the front wheel down.

4. Do upper-body training at the gym. Otherwise, you won't last long. Your shoulders and arms will fatigue—it's tiring.

4. HOW TO DESCEND

Tearing down twisty mountain roads involves the same skills described above in the "cornering" section. But mountain biking is a whole different animal.

1. Get back. Push your butt back and drop your chest to lower your center of gravity. The steeper the descent, the farther back and lower you should be, to the point where your rear is floating behind the seat altogether. Make the mistake of straightening up, and you'll eventually be launched over the bars.

2. Momentum is your friend. Inertia will carry you over most minor obstacles without a problem, but those same rocks and roots can knock your front wheel sideways if you slow to a crawl and ride over them timidly. So learn to lay off the brakes, build some speed, pick a line, and go for it.

3. One-digit braking. Put just one finger on each lever. The best mix of steering and braking control comes when your index fingers loop over the levers and your other fingers hold the bar.

4. Front-brake-centric. Use the front brake for 70 percent of your braking power; use the rear on more technical sections to avoid skidding the front wheel.

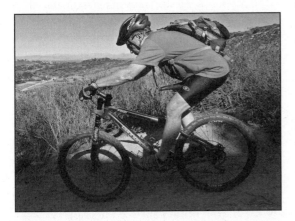

5. HOW TO RIDE IN A PACELINE

Riding behind others, front wheel to rear wheel in a formation known as a paceline, helps you cheat the wind. This "drafting" is part of the sport, even in casual riding and touring. Some say it can save up to 40 percent of your energy, especially if you are riding into a headwind. Here's how to do it:

1. Hook up with a group. Hey, break out of your shell. You can't draft by yourself, unless you've got a thing for 18-wheelers.

2. Pick a wheel. Stealthily latch on to a rider who's steady and smooth. See how long you can go without him or her noticing you.

3. Stay close. Start about 3 feet away; work up to within an inch of the wheel. Modulate your speed with brakes; or instead, use soft pedaling or sit up to slow yourself with wind resistance.

4. Keep a steady pace. Aim for 20 mph, a good speed for first-time drafters. Don't go any faster at first; you'll get tired and lose concentration.

5. Factor in the wind. In a headwind, stay directly behind your mule. In a crosswind, position yourself on a line between your mule and the rider behind you (who is using you as a mule).

Downhill and hot stop: shift your weight back

STILL A SLOW CLIMBER?

THE HECK WITH TECHNIQUE; JUST LOSE WEIGHT.

HERE'S HOW:

Spanish cyclist Miguel Induráin was an awesome time trialist who fell off in the hills; then he dieted off 12 pounds before the 1991 season and won five straight Tours de France. Lance Armstrong was a one-day world champ who lagged in mountainous stage races; then he lost 20 pounds to chemotherapy in 1997 and one seven straight Tours de France (until he was caught doping). See the pattern here? If you want to ride faster—especially climb better—just lose weight.

For several decades, coaches have known that there is a proven demarcation line that separates champions and also-rans: a power-to-weight ratio of 6 watts per kilo of body weight for a sustained 45 minutes. Below that point, said BMC Racing team doctor Max Testa, a pro can't keep up in both the flats and the hills; but above it, he's a potential multi-time Tour winner. Thanks to James C. Martin, PhD, assistant professor of exercise and sports science at the University of Utah and a 1988 national Masters track champion, we even know how much faster you'll climb.

(continues)

STILL A SLOW CLIMBER? *(continued)*

His study, "Validation of a Mathematical Model for Road-Cycling Power," published in the 1998 *Journal of Applied Biomechanics*, estimates that every 5 pounds of weight loss will help you ride 30 seconds faster over a 3.1-mile, 7 percent hill climb.

Of course, a proven way to melt the fat is to increase your mileage and reduce your caloric intake, but this may be difficult for those with limited time, and can also risk weakening muscles, according to David Costill, PhD, retired director of the Human Performance Lab at Ball State University. "Don't start hard training before you have your body weight where you want it," he said. "You lose weight only by burning more calories each day than you eat, and if you do that while training hard, you will not only be burning fat, but causing a sizable breakdown of muscle protein."

Although this issue may be less acute for noncompetitive and heavier athletes, experts like Dr. Arny Ferrando, former director of the performance lab at the University of Texas Medical Branch at Galveston, say the safest weight loss is gradual, not rapid. "You won't jeopardize muscle mass if you drop the pounds gradually—no more than a pound or two a week," Farrando said.

Below are 10 ways to help you lose weight gradually and painlessly—off the bike. These dietary and lifestyle changes are so easy to incorporate into your daily routine that you may forget you're doing them—until the day you realize that you arrived two minutes ahead of your riding buddies on Hell Hill, rather than two minutes behind.

1. Do a light workout the moment you wake up. "It is a fact that you burn more fat before eating breakfast," said Asker E. Jeukendrup, director of the Human Performance Laboratory at the University of Birmingham School of Sport and Exercise Sciences in England. "Although there is no scientific evidence yet, we assume weight loss."

With a minimum of easy-to-access fuels like muscle glycogen or bloodstream sugar in the system (your body utilizes a good deal of glycogen during the night), the body reaches for "intermuscle" fat, the plentiful but hard-to-access fat within the muscle, according to Dr. Gabrielle Rosa, the coach for many of Kenya's top marathoners, who are known for their early-morning runs.

Intensity is not important. "There's no need to work out hard," said Max Testa, the BMC doc. "A 20- to 30-minute light jog, spin, or even brisk dog-walking increases your metabolism and primes you for a better workout later in the day." Jeukendrup recommends no more than 70 to 75 percent of maximum heart rate.

That jibes with studies indicating that you should exercise hard later in the day, not earlier. Building on previous findings of increased afternoon body temperature and metabolism, Dr. Boris Medarov at the Jewish Medical Center in New Hyde Park, New York, found that resistance in air passages decreases as nightfall approaches, increasing air-gathering capacity in the lungs by 15 to 20 percent.

2. Walk after dinner. "A 20-minute 'dine and dash' immediately after dinner burns up to 100 calories and helps you burn more later," said Carl Foster, PhD, of the Department of Exercise and Sports Science at the University of Wisconsin–La Crosse. "That's because, while slow enough not to interfere with digestion, briskly walking one or two miles raises your metabolism." It also cleans your pipes and clears your head, he adds, reducing by 20 percent the glucose and insulin that flooded into the bloodstream with the meal.

3. Eat more dairy. Studies led by Michael Zemel, PhD, author of *The Calcium Key*, show that diets high in calcium appear to set off a chain reaction that prompts the body to metabolize fat more efficiently. Calcium supplements aren't nearly as effective, he adds, as a high-calcium

(continues)

STILL A SLOW CLIMBER? *(continued)*

diet. Dr. Robert P. Heaney, professor of medicine at Creighton University in Omaha, said three or four servings of low-fat yogurt or milk a day could help Americans lose an average of 15 pounds a year. Another factor, many researchers say, is that dairy makes you feel full, so you eat less.

Those who are lactose intolerant can eat dark, leafy greens (such as kale and collards), which have high levels of calcium.

4. Don't starve. Low-calorie diets lead to bingeing and kick the body into survival mode, which encourages fat storage.

5. Graze. Eat more small meals throughout the day. Long stretches without eating—e.g., going from a noon lunch to a 7 p.m. dinner—also kick the body into survival mode, which encourages fat storage. Eating and digesting numerous smaller meals "prevents blood sugar spikes and costs lots more energy," said Dr. Arny Ferrando of the University of Texas. To avoid junk food, keep fresh fruit like apples, grapes, pears, and bananas around. They're low in calories and portable, said Suzanne Havala Hobbs, a registered dietician and faculty member at the School of Public Health at the University of North Carolina at Chapel Hill.

6. Avoid liquid calories. A Coke won't make you feel as full as an orange will. Studies show that your body doesn't register a feeling of fullness from liquid calories, which helps you gain weight by leading to overdrinking and overeating later. So, instead of a soft drink, slurp zero-calorie, noncarbonated water. (Beware carbonation: It leeches calcium from bones. See Chapter 9.)

7. Eat mindfully. "It's hard to overeat if you follow a holistic approach and eat slowly and elegantly," said Los Angeles performance yoga and fitness trainer Steve Ilg, the author of *Total Body Transformation*. That means sit with an elegant posture, back erect, cross-legged in a chair or on the ground. Put the fork down between every bite, consciously breathe between every third bite, and chew the first bite of food 30 times. "Doing this, an astounding insight arises: Digestive secretions give the body a deeper feeling of satisfaction," said Ilg.

8. Don't eat much after 8 p.m. A large meal before you go to bed, especially one high in carbs, stimulates insulin, changing your sleep time to fat storage instead of fat-burning and inhibiting the body's production of muscle-maintaining growth hormone. If you must snack late at night, go for a piece of turkey breast, not an orange. "It seems odd at first, but it's better to eat lean meat than fruit before bed," said nutritionist Betty Kamen, PhD, the author of *Betty Kamen's 1,001 Health Secrets*. "Fat-free meat is all protein."

9. Cut fat, not carbs. "Reducing fat intake is the most important step for weight loss," said Jeukendrup. "For exercisers, it is not a good idea to cut carbs; that simply reduces the fuel for your workouts and increases the risk of overreaching/overtraining." Example: Eat a salad with your burger, instead of fries.

10. Change—don't cut—your carbs. Switch the majority of your daily carbs to low-glycemic-index carbohydrates such as yogurt, fruit, nuts, and bananas, which are broken down slowly by the body. They provide you with an appetite-curbing feeling of fullness that you don't get from high-GI foods like bagels, cereals, and rice cakes that are burned quickly as sugar.

11. Cut down on alcohol. Booze is a double whammy: a dead calorie with no nutritive value that has a negative domino effect. The liver has to pay attention to it first in the metabolic sequence because it's toxic. While being stored as fat, it crowds out good calories and gets them stored as fat, too.

12. Read before you eat. Look at a $0.99 bag of corn chips. One serving is 150 calories. Then read further: There are five servings in a bag. That's 750 calories—one-third of an adult's daily requirement.

BIKE COP SKILLS

I once learned some valuable mountain bike skills at the Dirt Camp mountain bike school, and some priceless road skills at John Howard's School of Champions. But I didn't realize how incomplete my bike-handling was until I hung out with cops. Not just any cops, but . . . bike cops.

On assignment for *Bicycling* magazine, I attended a four-day boot camp staged by the International Police Mountain Bike Association (IPMBA). I emerged with a certificate qualifying me to be a bicycle policeman as well as huge respect for the job that cops do and the skills they have on bikes. They can dismount at high speeds to tackle fleeing perpetrators. They can shift into "stealth mode," threading silently and safely through crowded streets and auditoriums at 1 mph. It turns out that these urban-riding skills, which allow them to catch surprised bad guys right in the act, also can make any cyclist a better, safer rider. I use them almost every time I ride. Here's a sampler:

SKILL NO. 1: ULTRASLOW RIDING

To maintain supreme control and balance at less than 1 mph, bike cops simply apply the brakes as they pedal. By keeping constant pressure on the crank, this technique lowers your center of gravity from the seat to the bottom bracket, greatly aiding balance.

Benefit for Normal Cycling: On the road, the ultraslow technique helps you stay clipped in at red lights and aids in negotiation of clogged city streets; on dirt, it allows for trials-like handling through a technical single track and for more confident turning on tight switchbacks. It also allows you to ride comfortably and get a workout while riding with much slower riders, such as young children.

SKILL NO. 2: LEFT-HAND BOTTLE GRAB

To simultaneously stay hydrated and in control on crowded streets, bike cops are trained to access their water bottles with their left hands. This forces them to use their right hands—and rear

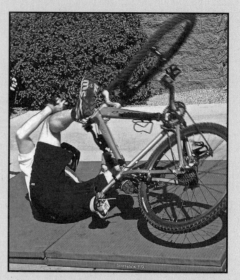

How to fall: roll on shoulder

brakes—when an obstacle (like an open car door) suddenly appears.

Benefit for Normal Cycling: During sudden stops with the rear (right-hand) brake, you won't go over the bars or wipe out as you might by jamming only on the front (left-hand) brake.

SKILL NO. 3: INJURY-FREE FALLING

As you fall sideways, hold onto the handlebar and stay clipped into the pedals. Try to let the bar-end hit the ground first to absorb the shock, and simultaneously tuck your shoulder so that you roll onto your side, spreading the force of the landing over the mass of your body. If you do this right, the bike arcs upside-down above you as you roll over on the ground and click out.

Benefit for Normal Cycling: Doing a "Heisman Trophy"—sticking your arm straight out to brace yourself—puts extreme stress on a small area of your hand that can easily torque, and you can end up breaking your collarbone. By keeping your hands on the bar, you greatly reduce the chance of injury.

SKILL NO. 4: DESCENDING STAIRS

Cops can't afford to slow down and dismount

(continues)

BIKE COP SKILLS *(continued)*

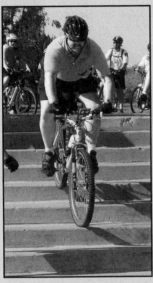

Descending stairs and dropoffs

when chasing perps down stairs. So they push their butts back and off the saddle to lower their center of gravity and de-weight the front wheel, keep their pedals even and their hands feathering both brakes equally, and aim the bike perpendicular to the steps. This combination allows the front wheel to float (not "thunk") while gravity carries them forward and downward, but still gives them control of the bike.

Benefit for Normal Cycling: This is a good practice to adapt for off-road drops and steep declines (not to mention showing up the kids outside the local library).

SKILL NO. 5: HIGH-SPEED DISMOUNT

Chasing a perp at high speed, a cop will cross his right leg over the top tube and plant the right foot to the left of the front tire, so that he can step off the bike in full running position. He then will push the bike to the right and out of the way or fling it forward into the perp's legs, knocking him over.

Benefit for Normal Cycling: Use this move to attack a too-steep-to-ride incline with running momentum, or to quickly put your bike between you and a threatening animal.

SKILL NO. 6: SPLIT A CONE (AVOID OBSTACLES)

Bike cops like to say that nothing wrecks the mood on a crowded sidewalk like a knocked-over bike cop. To survive unavoidable obstacles that you can't see until the last second, IPMBA developed a drill called "split the cone." You set out a cone or similar obstacle (e.g., a rock or shoebox); roll the front wheel just to the right side of it; and then, at very slow speed (using the ultraslow riding technique), turn the handlebar sharply to the left so that the cone passes between the front wheel and the down tube. The key is to keep the outside (right) pedal in the up position as you begin the turn. To "split" a line of several cones, decrease the initial angle of attack and maintain the pedal in the up position, using half-pushes and returns.

Benefit for Normal Cycling: An excellent all-around coordination-builder, this drill can be used to clear small obstacles in tight spaces—and impress your friends. At bike-cop school, I saw instructor Jeff Brown of Dayton, Ohio, split a line of seven cones. When I told that to Hans Rey, the famed trials guru, even he was impressed.

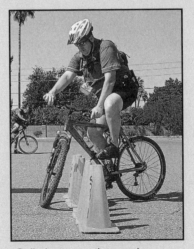

Split the cones: the amazing Officer Brown does seven

Johnny G

HE TOOK CYCLING DEEP INSIDE

Bodybuilders don't ride bikes. And cyclists don't bodybuild. But a South African immigrant named Johnny Goldberg did both with such passion and charisma and vision that he single-handedly changed the health-and-fitness industry and improved the fitness and outlook of millions around the globe. In the early 1980s, Johnny got into the Los Angeles personal-training phenomenon at the ground floor, then took himself to the limits in the 3,000-mile Race Across America. Frustration over the un-bike feel of standard exercycles led to his hand-welded invention, the innovative Spinner stationary bike, which uses a heavy flywheel and standard cycling bottom bracket and pedals. That morphed into Spinning, the cycle-to-the-music group workout sensation now used by millions in America and in bike-crazy Europe, where massive outdoor Spinfests have attracted over 500 Spinners at a time in the Netherlands and 1,000 in Italy. Perhaps millions have used Spinning as a springboard to outdoor cycling. Spinning fundamentally altered our view of group aerobic exercise class from organized dancing and jumping to a quest, a challenge, a journey into heart and soul that could be appreciated by men, not just the largely female crowd who attended standard aerobics classes. But as the man now known simply as Johnny G told Bike for Life in his interviews in March 2004 and December 2013, he

couldn't have come up with it until he'd been on his own amazing journey first.

I WAS FOUR years old when I got my first bike and fell in love with cycling. A bike was more than a workout tool. It was a place to sink my sorrows, to dream. It was a place to break through boundaries, to get myself out of this box or cage. It was a place for me to liberate myself, to find peace and harmony. To take that trip on to the coattails of God. To find the sense of freedom that lots of people find using the bike. It has always been a staple in my life. The martial arts and the swimming and the squash and the music—they were all cool. But none of them made me feel the way the bike did.

We were very primitive in South Africa. My dad was a pharmacist and we had very little money. I used to work on my bikes for hours. When I was 12 years old I put on ape-hanger handlebars. When I was 16, I actually rode across South Africa for an organization called TEACH—Teach Every African Child.

At 12 or 13, I met Arnold [Schwarzenegger] when he came to see Reg Park, who won the Mr. Universe a couple of times in the 1960s. I was best friends with Reg's son. He and I watched *Pumping Iron* together. We went through all the magazines—*Ironman*, *Muscular Development*. I met Frank Zane and some of the all-time greats, and started getting into bodybuilding. I was very much excited about the prospects of health and fitness, as it was just starting to unfold in South Africa.

About 1978, when I got out of the army, I was running a gym for Reg. I was like a sponge to him. Over the years, I'd practically spent more time with Reg than his own kid. He and I used to talk bodybuilding at length. Exercises. Philosophy. Diet. His fears. Reg was extraordinary. He hit the gym every morning from six to eight. He wasn't just a bodybuilder; being in the fitness business, he'd say he was a "physical culturist." That was the beginning of my search for self-development and understanding. The first building block.

I wanted to come over to the States. My big dream was to go over to California to go to Venice Beach, to Muscle Beach, and to train at the Gold's Gym.

In June 1979, at age 23, I came to the US on a 30-day tourist visa. Went right to Gold's, worked out, then got held up. Welcome to America.

I hadn't really found out what I was looking for, but I wasn't going to leave. Soon, I met a guy in Venice Beach who was selling Ginsu knives—possibly stolen merchandise. He would drive the car with product and I'd walk in and visit the shops. He paid me a dollar per sale.

One day I walked into a health club on Motor Avenue in West L.A. called World for Men and World for Women. It had separate wings, which was a big deal—they could work out at the same time. Back then, most clubs had separate hours for the sexes, so the owner had his own niche in the market. I told the head guy that I had experience running a health club and that I could raise their business by 10 percent—and they hired me. I worked for a month, and when it came to pay day, there was no pay.

So I've got no money. I'm eating sugar cubes to stay alive. Sleeping on a couch. I've got my fair share of challenges.

But I stay working there, making my $3.25 an hour, and finally get paid. We run a successful "two memberships for the price of one" ad campaign—my idea: one man, one woman—in 1980 and get a lot of traffic.

At Ground Zero of the Fitness Revolution

My big break came in 1981, when I answered a phone call from a huge Hollywood agent named Sandy Gellen, who handled the biggest names in the industry—Cher, Dolly Parton, Barbra Streisand. He was looking for a private trainer to come to his house. At the time, personal training was almost unheard of. There were no fitness organizations, no exercise-physiology classes. You just had a background in bodybuilding or sports or something. I went up to Sandy's house in Beverly Hills, gave him a workout, and sometimes ended up training him seven days a week.

I was making a hundred bucks for two hours—pretty good money. With my $3.25 per hour at World for Men, plus commission on sales, I was bringing home about nineteen-hundred bucks a month.

Soon, I started picking up all the celebrities and started working the Hollywood scene. It was amazing. Victoria Principal, Andy Gibb, Jack Scalia. Soon, I was making $8,000 a month.

Training exploded. Jake Steinfeld—"Body by Jake"—did the first big show, *Entertainment Tonight*. He was training Spielberg. Dan Issacson was doing Linda Evans and Christopher Reeve. The movie *Perfect*, with John Travolta and Jamie Lee Curtis, came out.

My style was always different, real world. My clients were always ultra-skinny and ultra-fit. I'd run them on trails in the Santa Monica Mountains, up the stairs at UCLA, and combine it with weights.

I started getting a reputation—that I was really tough. If someone really wanted to go to another level, almost a sportsman with philosophy, I was the guy.

All this time, I'd never stopped riding my bike. I got into triathlon and bike racing in 1984. My marriage started to fall apart in about 1985, and I needed out. I needed space. Cycling gave me space.

Everything in cycling was pedigreed—Cat. 3, Cat. 4, certain distances. I hadn't made Category 2 yet, and I was having a lot of conflicts between traveling and my clients and the races and sponsorships. It was tough. And family and kids and responsibility was really difficult. I dealt with it by putting in more miles.

Then I went to Texas and did the Spenco 500. Five hundred miles from Waco to Comfort and back. A thousand cyclists from all over the world. Pro teams. 7-Eleven. Schwinn-Icy Hot. Thomas Prehn. Ultra-distance cyclists—Pete Penseyres. Mike Shermer. Randonneurs. I had no idea about long-distance riding, no support, no proper gear. Specialized gave me a pair of slick tires. I tried a liquid diet. Carried my stuff.

I took a seventeenth in that race. There was prize money to twentieth, and I won $280, maybe $320, which was pretty cool. Took me a week to recover and get back to L.A.

I'd never gone over, I think, 105 miles before. But here I went 500 miles at that pace! With packs and motorcycles and copters! I mean this was the real thing. The real deal—my first ultra. It gave me such a sense of awe. It was incredible. There was something about the distance. It was about facing my weaknesses, about being totally exposed and limited. My brain started to fly.

The Concept: A Stationary Bike Workout

IN 1985, I opened the first "Johnny G Cross-Training and Nutrition Center" at Matrix 1 on Westwood Boulevard. I started [leading] 30 minutes of high-intensity drills on a stationary bike—which was very different. The stationary bike had always been used as a warm-up, not for workouts. I added combinations of squats with pullovers, extreme supersets, giant sets with no

rest, and ended it by doing their body work. It was sort of an all-in-one workout.

I was inspired by my teenage memories of the Donavet stationary bike, a German-made machine with a built-in heart-rate monitor. At Matrix, we used Windracers, a competitor of Lifecycle. The bike gave the clients a real good sweat. It gave them a feeling of conquering terrain—and fears. I could talk to them like an athlete. And, of course, it gave me my own niche. No one had a bike workout.

Combining the bike workout with the South African accent and my appeal and the whole thing, and it was cool. I got in all the magazines. I was in *Variety*, the opening show of *Geraldo*, *Hour Magazine*, Gary Collins. I trained Melissa Gilbert for a movie. And my results were very dramatic.

The next year, I opened my own Johnny G Cross-Training and Nutrition Center in Beverly Hills. Arnold was there at the grand opening. I hired a lot of guys, including Rob Parr [Madonna's longtime coach]. I set up four road bikes on turbo-trainers, not the old Lifecycle-style bikes.

That was an important step. I was getting really aggravated, annoyed, and frustrated with the old bikes. The pedals were wrong. I wanted to get people into real bike shoes. I wanted them to have this experience of what it felt like to get out of the saddle. To sprint, to do intervals. To sit back and close their eyes. To create a really cool environment that could help me get people into a really athletic state. If people weren't going to go outside and actually ride the bicycle, I had to take them there indoors. I had clients I was taking out on bikes on the weekends, triathletes and other guys who already had 10-speeds, but from a commercial point of view, this wasn't where the business was. The business was in being able to take people on this journey where I could get into their heads and talk to them. They would look into the shadows of themselves in the mirror, and I started to give them visualizations. With the music—and I was using Pink Floyd and the coolest music, not just typical aerobic tempo—it was incredible! It was a very exciting time.

It was really the start of Spinning. The name and the specially designed Spinning bike and 40-minute training session weren't there yet, but the concept was.

Aerobics had limited a lot of people. It never gave them an opportunity to be self-expressed. Aerobics was becoming very dance, very choreographed. So guys and people who weren't very coordinated started to find a different sense of power on the bike. And this was a great thing, because I could tap into them using the bike as a tool, as an analogy. I wasn't sophisticated, I never understood what I was doing, I never had the wisdom or the experience or the foresight to know what would happen later. But at the time my instincts were sharp and I was coming from a very intuitive place. This place was spot-on for where people needed to go. I was definitely on the right track.

Spinning worked for super athletes and it worked for average people. In 1985 I had met pro triathlete Brad Kearns while out on a training ride. I asked if he wanted to ride with me, and eight hours later we were near Santa Barbara before we turned around and went back home. Brad was in third place in the Desert Princess duathlon series. Then I brought him into my cross-training center and helped him visualize, and I made him believe in himself. He saw the winning time, which was 8 minutes faster than his best time. And he beat that time I think by 1.6 seconds. And he became the world champion in 1987. When I met [actor] Jack Scalia, he had just gone through recovery. And he could dream about doing a triathlon. Back then, there weren't a lot of guys who were taking just ordinary people and getting them into sports.

The RAAM Revelation

I HAD NO idea what the Race Across America was in 1985, but in 1986 I was trying to qualify for it. I did the John Marino Open [the 500-mile western states' RAAM qualifier] from Tucson to Flagstaff and back. I was still trying to do a few private clients. I was trying to get a divorce. I was dealing with not being the dad on weekends. I started doing these long miles and the riding started taking over more of my life.

Having absolutely no idea what I'd bitten off and what I'd gotten myself into, I entered the 1987 RAAM with very little sponsorship, very little support. Got a couple of buddies together. I was a raw-food vegetarian and I suffered for eight days in the rain. I quit 400 miles from the finish.

The problem was I never knew at the time that I was bipolar manic-depressive. Sleep was very important. If you start losing sleep and you're not medicated, you start getting really delusional. I started having huge spiritual conflicts and psychological conflicts. Five hundred miles was a great distance for me. Everybody has their distance; you just have to know what yours is. You just have to find it. Well, I outreached my space. I outreached my parameters. I broke my boundaries.

I never had any boundaries before. I was invincible. My mind had no sense of boundaries. I never laid any down. It was just possible. Training would make it possible. No doubt. It's okay to have a very positive state of mind, yet, it also can work against you. For me in this event, it worked against me. It was too much, too hard. I had too many conflicts. Too many emotional things going on, too much chaos going on within myself. These also became huge principles which I used later. Chaos and emotional traumas and how the mind would work in ways that could be far more effective, if the right pieces were put in place. What happened was this RAAM was an extremely fruitful and productive learning experience. Yet athletically it was disastrous. I lost about 26 or 27 pounds. It took a long time for me to recover.

When it was over, I decided I was finished with the ego. I was finished with being the best.

I got in my vehicle and drove to a friend's house who said I could recover at his house. And I drove back to California and began a three-month recovery. I lost my clientele base. I couldn't go back into the gym. I didn't want to go back into the gyms.

To survive, I had to sell everything. There were a lot of nutrition companies sending me a lot of high-tech stuff they were working on—carbohydrate diets, meal replacement. I was sort of selling the stuff to a couple of guys that I knew and cashed out all the money I had, maybe a thousand bucks, maybe twelve hundred bucks. And I borrowed some money to buy a bike and I started training again, because I wanted to go back and get my RAAM ring.

Because I didn't finish RAAM, I knew I'd have to requalify in 1988, put a crew together and get back to the Race Across America in 1989. So I was facing a two-year ordeal to finish what I'd started.

Finishing RAAM was gonna take a lot of work. A lot of planning, getting the crews together, and a lot of guts and courage. Because I wanted to finish it. Ego-wise I couldn't let this thing go. It was the first time I'd really been outmatched. Yah, it was the first time I'd felt worthless. Or acknowledged not being capable of matching up to the mind of the great Johnny G. And it was a really interesting time.

I was doing incredibly long miles. But I was training on a 24-hour cycle, not a normal 12-hour day. Because of my bipolar, I wasn't sleeping a lot—three or four hours every other day. That is why I couldn't talk in sentences. I was just like I was on speed all the time. You get into the manic states, you get abundant energy. You start to fly. You get very scattered. You just become delusional. Graeme Obree [the former World Hour Record holder from Scotland] just wrote a book on his bipolar disorder and how it helped him achieve what he did. If you can channel and focus it, you can harness unbelievable energy. Boundaries and limitations start to disappear. And so I would dream. I would have ideas, a thousand ideas a second. I was always creating something new. And this was my four-day training cycle. What I started to find was Tuesday I would start at 6 a.m. and finish at 6 p.m.—go 200 miles. But I would switch it up. Tuesday I would go into the deserts. Thursdays I would go into the mountains. But Friday night, I would start at 6 p.m. and then I could come back at 6 p.m. Saturday night. Brad Kearns would usually meet me at 6 a.m. on Saturday morning and spend a 12-hour day with me. I'd do my 24-hour ride on the weekend.

In four days I would clock anywhere between 760 and 830 miles. . . . The rest of the time, I had just met a wonderful girl and had fallen in love head over heels. For the first time in my life, true love. And we found a little bungalow in one of my clients' backyard. He let us use it. We had a little futon. An old-fashioned bathtub. A little refrigerator. And that was our life. She would sell sweaters and make jewelry and I would go out and train.

I had given up everything—a complete lifestyle change from big-time trainer to cycling monk. But I had a two-year task. See, this is where life is beautiful. And this is one of the most special parts of the journey. Really about this process, about as an adult being able to say, okay, this is what I need to do.

So I went and did the qualifier—the John Marino Open, otherwise known as RAAM Open West. And I won by four and a half hours in 29:36.

I averaged 18.1 miles an hour, climbing 36,000 feet and with temperature changes from 106 degrees F. in the day to 11 and 12 degrees at night. It was such a severe event, so challenging. And my time was so fast that it was the only time in history, I believe, that there was only one qualifier for RAAM besides the winner. Second place came in just within the 15 percent cutoff—the rule that qualifiers for the RAAMs have to qualify within 15 percent of the winner's time. No one else made the cutoff. This is a pretty cool thing.

So I went into the RAAM knowing I would have a good shot of finishing it. And I rode really fast for the first four days. I was in great shape. I thought I could break eight days—my goal. And halfway through I just realized it wasn't going to happen. I dropped to riding 16 hours a day, not the 22 I'd planned for. I finished in 10 days. But I got my RAAM ring!

And I was happy. In my first RAAM, I thought my athletic god would set me free, get me recognition, love, fame, be the key to a life of accomplishment, to the road to nobility. I didn't know until I finished the second that it was just a race.

I'd first used the term "spinning" in 1985 or 1986 when I had bikes on a trainer in my garage. "Come on over and catch a spin," I'd say. Harvey Diamond, the author of *Fit for Life*, was talking to me about my training once and latched onto the term "spinning."

RAAM was a profound and interesting lesson. The bicycle became a universal metaphor. Talking about headwinds, intensity, the struggle in a way that everybody [in a class] could relate to. In cycling, an individual must be able to participate in the group without being restricted to the group. In 40 minutes of Spinning, people get stuff from the great masters.

The Spinner Is Born

During my RAAM training, I'd put a specialty bike together—the early version of what is now known as the Spinner. Jody was pregnant. I'd ride at night when the air is clean. So that became my race strategy: rock and roll at night, sleep in the day, 2 p.m. to 4 p.m. In the end, I couldn't maintain that plan during the race. But I came away from the training with the basics of Spinning, the rhythm and combinations and movements, the three hand postures, the heart-rate training zones. The principles that would end up in the manual.

After I finished RAAM, Jordan was born.

Now I have to make a living. I took two of my Spinners to the Mezzaplex and told the owner I don't want to go back to private training. I gotta get back to the gym business. I issued a challenge: if anyone can stay with me on a Spinner workout, they get $10. The mirror, the music, it's like Russian roulette. I'm hammering them to death. Nobody can last 10 minutes. It creates a big buzz.

I needed more bikes. I went to Helen's Bike Shop to buy a Schwinn DX 900 stationary bike, but it couldn't handle the standing and the jumping. Or take regular pedals.

At the end of 1989, I built a fleet of my own bikes and opened the first Johnny G Spinning Center, in Santa Monica. I never thought about training people. It was my thing. Training session with my mates. I'd take them on a journey. I built 15 more hand-welded bikes, then moved the class to Karen Voight Fitness in 1992, thinking Hollywood was better exposure. It worked. It was amazing.

When people began trying to rip off the program, I started working on the trademarks and took it back to my garage for a couple of years. I sold bikes and trained people at Crunch. I met John Baudhuin, now my partner. We got a call from Schwinn, made a deal, and launched it at the 1995 IHRSA [International Health, Racquet & Sportsclub Association] trade show. It was profound. In three months, Spinning was in 400 gyms, in 1,000 within a year, and in 1,500 by the end of 1996. We formed Mad Dogg Athletics, traveled to 3 countries every 10 days, and logged a million miles in the first year training instructors.

It was unique—the first time equipment, training, and philosophy were sold together. We've trained 65,000 instructors over the years from Brazil to Moscow. By 1999, I was overworked, dead tired. And Schwinn was trying to rip us off. Luckily, we sued just before they went bankrupt. In 2003, we made a big deal with [equipment manufacturer] StarTrac, and I went traveling again. Went to lots of six-hour and eight-hour events for charity in Italy and Brazil.

I took up surfing and paddleboarding when we moved up to Santa Barbara. Training for a 200-mile ocean paddle right now. Been training for Orlando Kani, a Brazilian martial art, to go along with my black belt in Shodo Kan and study of Chi Gung, a stick-based martial art. Actually haven't been on a real bike in two months.

Update

THE NINE-YEAR PERIOD between the preceding interview and a follow-up in December 2013 was a life-changing journey of both tragedy and creativity for Johnny G. Years of hectic worldwide travel, overnight rides, and 12-hour Spins to promote Spinning led to a compromised immune system, a heart virus, and cardiomyopathy—damaged heart muscles that do not effectively pump blood. He had heart failure in late 2004. "I almost died," he said. "It's taken years of recovery to get back to stretching, walking, exercising. No more high-intensity stuff—ever."

Unable to serve as the spokesman and lead trainer of Spinning, Johnny G sold his interest to his partners and moved to Santa Barbara with his wife and family. Hoping to stay connected to the fitness industry, he revisited an idea about a hand cycle that had struck him in 2002 when he met members of the Challenged Athletes Foundation. In 2006, he built 300 prototypes and pitched the concept to Matrix Fitness, a large industry supplier. Though not a huge hit like Spinning, his KRANKcycles today can be found at the Olympic Training Center and gyms around the country.

Johnny's forced lower-intensity pace and growing interest in yoga and Pilates led to his newest product: In-Trinity, an incline-decline board and related workout program that combines strength, flexibility and balance. "It's the art of universal movement," he said. "It's possibly the best thing I've done in my life."

Johnny G's story may illustrate the irony of all-out intense exercise, which can produce spectacular results (and lead to something as world-changing as Spinning) but leave the body vulnerable. It also illustrates the power of self-motivation. "In early 2006, when I was at the bottom, barely able to move for a year, facing death, losing the will to go on, I read my own interview in *Bike for Life*," he said. "To read what I'd done and what I'd been . . . I was amazed by it. I drew power from it. I drew strength from myself—and it opened up a powerful motivation. I would never be like that again. But in retrospect, this is part of my learning process with life. I still had plenty of life to live, things to learn, to contribute."

4

THE GREAT INDOORS

How to use indoor-cycling classes to be a better outdoor rider

It's a cool and casual 1994 fall night in West Los Angeles, but inside *The Garage* it's a different world. The lights are off. The music is alternately Zen-like, disco, mystical, and throbbing. The air is heavy with perspiration and breathing and incense and a familiar mechanical hum. It's the sound of pedaling—hard pedaling, slow and labored pedaling, standing and sitting pedaling, pedaling so much faster than you've ever gone before that you feel like you're a passenger in flight, sitting atop a spinning, whirling, perpetual-motion machine, your legs a blur, independent of your body. You sweat like you've never sweat, dripping like a prizefighter in the eighth round, grossly, embarrassingly, frantically blotting, hoping to dam the rivers for a few seconds.

Faintly before you, in silhouette, is a circle of people on unadorned, industrial-looking stationary bikes. From one of them, the muscular rider with the mane of wavy hair, comes an accented voice, bold and soothing, pushing, motivating, pulling you with the power of pure conviction. "Turn the resistance up," he commands, and you twist the numberless dial in front of you to the right—too far probably, because you're so swept up in it. "Become one with the mountain, one with the bike, one with your dreams," the faintly British voice implores. "Dare . . . dream . . . hunger . . . to believe . . . to achieve . . . to find . . . to feel . . . the champion within!"

As we file outside into the backyard when it's over, the theatrical setting and relentless intensity

having left me drained but exhilarated, I'm surprised. It's a strange mix toweling off on the driveway: hard-core athlete types and housewives. Everyone is aglow, basking in victory, but for different reasons. The bike racers got an awesome workout, kept up their training. The affluent Westside matrons are more emotional.

They tell of how they never enjoyed exercise before Spinning, how they lost 40 pounds, how they got a deal on clipless pedals and shoes at Helen's, how they just bought their first bike to ride in the mountains, and how they've become something that was never part of their self-image: athletes. They glance over at the charismatic Voice, the leader of the journey, his Superman physique and leading-man cheekbones glistening with the aura of a cult leader. Eyes light up as they clasp his hands. Thank you, Johnny, they say, it was incredible. See you next Tuesday.

A year later, the workout and the bike that Johnny G honed in his garage exploded into the health-club world. Spinning changed fitness as we know it, drawing millions of dyed-in-the-wool cyclists and average Joes and Jills into the same aerobics class for the first time. Serious riders like it because it's a time-saver, packing 2 hours of intensity into 45 minutes. And everyone likes it because it helps them find "The Champion Within."

Cycling begat Spinning. And Spinning begat cycling fitness, confidence, and a sense of achievement. But it doesn't have to stop there. Spinning can help all cyclists develop and reinforce real-world skills that can otherwise take years of outdoor riding to learn—whether they are grizzled veterans who remember steel frames with lyrical Italian names, or newly minted, health-club-honed rookies who are pedaling outdoors for the first time. The skill-building drills outlined in this chapter are designed for just that.

The fitness, of course, is undeniable: Many think Johnny G's claim that a standard 45-minute Spin class is the fitness equivalent of 90 minutes of riding on the road is too modest; one class is worth two or three hours on the road, most say. Coming from a cyclist's perspective—Johnny G did the Race Across America twice in the late 1980s—he designed his Spinner to be the first stationary bike with the fit and feel of a real bike: normal handlebar positions, a performance bike saddle, and a standard bottom bracket (the assembly that houses the pedal spindle) and crankset, allowing for use of clip-in pedal systems. Then he went further, adding a 44-pound flywheel that did not allow coasting. The result, when combined with the music-charged group energy of a Spin class, was revolutionary: 45 concentrated minutes of legs scrambling at a furious, faster-than-normal rate, never coasting downhill or resting at a stoplight. The Johnny G Spinner did more than replicate cycling. It supercharged it.

Word of Spinning's high bang-for-the-buck fitness spread like wildfire to regular folk and hard-core athletes alike. Health clubbers weaned on Lifecycles became addicted to the relentless Spinning pace. Serious cyclists and triathletes, people you couldn't pay to take a step-aerobics class, poured into Spin classes. Superstars could even be found teaching. Six-time Hawaii Ironman champ Dave Scott was a regular Spin instructor in Boulder, Colorado. Former pro mountain biker Tammy Jacques taught once a week in the winter and spun in-season whenever bad weather hit. Emilio De Soto, former pro triathlete and president of De Soto Sports triathlon clothing, packed them in to his classes in La Jolla, California.

Quickly, Spinning and its many knockoffs—Cycle Reebok, SpeedCenter, Road Racers, and others (now virtually every fitness equipment manufacturer makes this style of bike)—mutated to satisfy those seeking bigger challenges. Johnny G led once-a-month two- and three-hour "Super-Spins" that took advanced students on virtual century rides. Once a month in the summer, New York's Reebok Sports Club moved bikes out to the sundeck for a two-hour workout. A small club in New Jersey offered a four-hour "Mt. Everest Spin." In Denver's Rocky Mountain Aerobic Network club, Reebok master trainer Marsha Macro led a "Mountain Bike Spin" that featured "Explosions," which simulated powering over trail-blocking logs and vertical-rise "Lifts" to simulate bunny hops. Several clubs tried to combine indoor cycling with calisthenics, dancing, and aerobics. At the Workout Warehouse in West Hollywood, California, participants lowered their seats, stood for an entire hour, and did one-arm twisting crunches, lat pulls, and handlebar push-ups. Voight by the Sea in Santa Monica added dance-troupe-like choreography.

Individuals used the club setting to make up their own challenges. Part-time indoor-cycling instructor Ruben Barajas, 39, the director of the Scott Newman drug prevention charity in Los Angeles, says riding indoors helped him to qualify for the Hawaii Ironman several years ago. Slipping on cycling shoes right after a swim, he'd teach a couple of cycling classes in a row, then put on running shoes and hit a treadmill. "I called it 'my own private Ironman,'" he said.

While it took hard-core athletes inside, Spinning began to push former non-cyclists outside. "It's a natural progression," explains Johnny G. "Spinning changes you. It gives a non-athlete the mind of an athlete—taking on a challenge, toughing it out to the end. When you get out of a Spinning class, that impossibly steep hill in the distance that used to seem daunting now suddenly begs you to conquer it." That explains Linzi Glass, an L.A. novelist who never rode a bike before she began Spinning in 1997; within a year, she was leading group rides into the Hollywood Hills. After he started Spinning, famed New York hairdresser Louis Licari upped his outdoor mileage from 10 miles a year on an old, beat-up clunker to 200 miles a weekend in charity events on a new $3,000 racer. One of the most extreme Spinning-to-cycling converts may be Phyllis Cohen of Santa Monica, California, who became a twice-a-day Spinning addict under Johnny G's tutelage in the mid-1990s and went on to organize the first team of age 50-plus women to complete the Race Across America. Ironically, there was one downside to her cross-country experience. "When I was training for RAAM," said the granny-gear granny, whose curly gray locks tumble halfway down her back, "I rode so much in a slower cadence that I got out of Spinning shape."

Nathan Micheli, a tile-setter-to-the-stars from Redondo Beach, California, who hadn't exercised in years, became a three-times-a-week Spinning addict in 2004. "I'm a workaholic who couldn't have imagined cutting short a business meeting to catch a normal aerobics class," he said. "But Spinning class leaves me feeling so fit, so fresh, so relaxed and filled with energy, so like I was just born. I plan my day around it. I can't wait to buy a bike—my first since I was 10 years old—and do the Rosarito-Ensenada Ride."

If Micheli ever does the 50-miler down the Mexican coast, usually attended by up to 10,000 Southern Californians, he'll join millions of former non-cyclists who now crowd into organized bike tours and benefit rides. In fact, in the week before the popular Boston–New York and San Francisco–L.A. AIDS rides, instructors report that Spinning rooms often empty out by half as their students practice on the road.

"As people—especially women—get into it," said Reebok instructor Glen Philipson, "they remember how much fun it is to ride a bike." He guessed that 80 percent of women—compared to only half of the men—come into studio cycling with no real cycling experience, and that up to a quarter of those will eventually buy road bikes.

People who Spin three or four days a week have the potential to ride "as good or better" than regular cyclists, said Chris Kostman, who worked closely with Johnny G in the early days, founded the Road Racers indoor-cycling program at the L.A.–based Bodies in Motion fitness chain, and now organizes numerous endurance events in the western United States, including the Death Valley–crossing Furnace Creek 508. "You come out of Spinning with exceptional cycling-specific fitness," he said. "The intensity, the leg speed (pedal turnover), quick heart-rate recovery and lactic-acid flushing after sprints and hill climbs, and the focus on good form is similar to high-level cycling. But once you get out on the road, there's more to learn than switching gears and learning how to reach over and eat an energy bar at 18 miles per hour. It can take some people, especially those who have never ridden before, six months to get truly comfortable on a bike. That's because Spinning is specially designed as an indoor workout—and most of the instructors don't know a thing about cycling."

In fact, most Spin teachers are indeed aerobics teachers in clipless pedals. Many have never even ridden a bike on the road. They know how to select good music and exhort their followers through a killer 45-minute workout. But few can help make you a better cyclist. "Cycling skills are not what people get out of my classes," said Emilio De Soto. "Fitness is."

"That's why you're going to have to develop those skills yourself—in class," said Kostman, a two-time Race Across America racer. "Spinning classes are an ideal place to work on classic, old-time technique—a traffic-free laboratory environment that can go a long way toward replacing the on-the-road instruction once handed down by veteran riders. By the same token, it's a great place

for the vets to refresh their technique—as long as they remember not to ride an indoor bike the same way they do their 'outdoor' bikes."

Here's what he means.

GOING FULL CIRCLE

AUDREY ADLER NEVER SPUN IN JOHNNY G'S GARAGE.
BUT SHE MAKES A DIFFERENCE IN HERS.

"Although I'd always been fit and athletic, I never considered myself a real athlete until Spinning. Aerobics keeps you fit, but doesn't give you skills you can use, like this does. The minute I started Spinning, I felt like I was preparing for something, as if I was training to be an astronaut." Or a cyclist. Or a changer of lives.

Audrey Adler, a Los Angeles mother of 4 and grandmother of 13, bought her first bike at age 36 after six months of Spinning in 1995. She went on her first serious road ride six months later, her first mountain bike ride in the Santa Monica Mountains after another month, and her first all-day ride a few weeks after that. She'd never swum before, either, but in 1997 did a half-Ironman triathlon. She began changing lives later that year.

The new "Road Racers" program at the Century City Bodies in Motion, a Spinning knockoff, needed instructors, and Adler, who kickboxed at the club, was first in line. "It was the first time I'd ever spoken into a microphone," she said, "but I took immediate command." Soon, she was teaching six classes a week, all of them jammed. Her energy was infectious.

"A guy came up to me once after class and said, 'You kicked my butt.' I said, 'No, you kicked your own butt.'" That fellow was a board member at the Santa Monica public school system. And Adler was soon hired to organize the district's first indoor-cycling program for school kids.

"You see, in Spinning, you control the [resistance] dial, so you work as hard as you make yourself work," she said. "The feeling of accomplishment is immediate. Even people who aren't athletic feel athletic. And there's a camaraderie involved. Whether you're an adult or kid, you get swept up in it. You feel like you can do anything."

In 2000, when Adler's brother was struck down in a motorcycle accident, she used indoor cycling to work through it. "In my grief, I decided to set up a three-hour charity Spin to raise money to buy Adaptive Sit Skis for disabled skiers," she said. Her brother was a family physician and an expert skier. She drew in 30 riders, raised $5,000, and presented it and a memorial plaque in the name of Dr. Aaron Pretsky to the National Center for the Disabled in Winter Park, Colorado. The following year, she did it again, raised another $5,000, and bought two adaptive mountain bikes.

A new challenge presented itself in 2001. "People were approaching me more and more about personal Spin training—busy people who didn't have time for a gym. I thought about opening my own storefront, but the costs were out of sight—and would have taken me away from my family too much. As I pulled the car into the garage one day, it dawned on me: This is a perfect studio!"

She discussed it with her husband. "What are you—nuts?" he said.

Thirty thousand dollars and twelve Spin bikes later, "Homebodies Workout" opened for business. Opening day was January 1, 2001. It was oversold.

"I had to throw people out," said Adler. "I had unwittingly uncovered an untapped market just dying for something like this: Orthodox Jewish women. There's a huge population of them in this area. They don't know a thing about fitness and won't work out in a co-ed environment [their religion prohibits it]. Spinning is a very liberating thing for them.

"I lecture them a lot. 'You'd never blow off taking your kid to a play-date. Well, why blow off a play-date for yourself? You're not getting any 'me' time. Just read the papers. You gotta stay healthy."

(continues)

Adler, who has shelved her decade-old, part-time interior-design consultancy and still teaches a few classes at Equinox in Beverly Hills and West L.A., has 30 steady clients ranging in age from mid-20s to mid-50s; dozens more show up at Homebodies on an occasional basis. The fee is $15 per class or $120 for ten classes; the latter "encourages them to make a commitment," she said. All advertising is word-of-mouth. Spinners reserve a spot in class via email.

"I'm not getting rich off this," she said. "But to hear someone tell me, 'You've changed my life,' is priceless."

One of Adler's proudest success stories was a young, overweight mother of two named Darline, who worked a production job at HBO. "She was cute, in her 30s, but getting fatter and more depressed," she said.

"She came over three days a week. It took her a couple of months to get through a whole class without slowing down. And by the time she did, she'd lost three dress sizes. 'You look so hot!' I told her, and she was so flattered. I felt so worthwhile later, when she told me I'd changed her life.

"There is absolutely no reason why a woman in her 30s shouldn't feel fabulous."

Once her clients are fit enough, Adler repeats a deeply imprinted pattern: She takes them out on mountain bike rides.

"It's a thrill for them, as it was for me, to see the fitness and skills learned indoors translate to a real sport," she said. "And very quickly, they learn what I learned: Cycling is a life-changing experience.

"I always get my best ideas when I'm riding, and meet pivotal people. Just the other day, I was riding on PCH [Pacific Coast Highway] in Malibu, cookin' along at 17 to 20 miles per hour, when I slowed down to ask an old struggling 70-year-old guy on a Colnago if he was okay. Turns out he was a retiring psychiatrist who worked in the same building as my [surviving] brother. I ended up getting my brother a bunch of new clients."

In 2003, Adler retired from triathlons and mountain bike racing. "It's not about me proving myself as an athlete anymore," she said. "It's about everyone else."

"The combination of Spinning and my brother dying had a huge effect on me. I realize that people have a lot of living to do, and being able to help them do it is a gift. Making a difference anywhere on this planet is a very good thing.

"You know that old cliché, 'Random Acts of Kindness'? That's nice, but it's not good enough. Why not plan them?"

Feeling her old competitive itch return, Adler turned to randonneuring in 2007 and has compiled an impressive long-distance resume, completing Paris-Brest-Paris (1,200 km), Washington State's Cascade 1200, the 1,200-kilometer Gold Rush Randonnée in California and Oregon, and Australia's 1,200-kilometer Great Ocean Road. She also did the 2007 La Ruta de los Conquistadores mountain bike stage race and a 24-hour fixed-gear race in New Jersey and Pennsylvania, teaches regularly at the Equinox clubs in Los Angeles and Beverly Hills, and runs classes three months a year for the Israeli Defense Force at the Tzrifin army base in Rishon Lezion, Israel.

1. GENERAL CLIMBING
Spreading the Load

If you've ever seen a pro rider climb a hill, you've seen a thing of beauty. Forget words like "plodding" or "inching" or "agonizing." The pros, using all the muscles of their body in a synchronized dance, look like they are gliding. Spinning can help you achieve some of this efficiency.

"There is no greater confidence builder—and time-saver—than good climbing," said Kostman. "And good climbers stay fresh by using as many muscles as possible throughout their entire body to get up the mountain—not just pushing and pulling from the quads, hamstrings, and glutes. Spreading the load saves your legs over the long haul, and the emphasis on other muscle groups can provide a welcome psychological diversion, especially on lengthy climbs. There's no better place to focus on this than indoors."

When Kostman teaches, he stresses two techniques that can aid climbing. In the first, the Spinner hinges forward at the waist, keeping the spine flat and parallel to the ground, then slides a few inches off the back of the saddle and uses arm and shoulder muscles to pull on the bars and exert more leverage on the pedal. In the second, the Spinner slides forward a bit and cultivates the lower abdominals to push the butt into and back on the saddle to increase leverage on the pedals.

"When you add that all up," Kostman said, "you are using the majority of the body to push and pull yourself uphill."

Another indoor method that Kostman advocates for developing outdoor climbing skills is a low-rpm cadence. "It's popular these days for everyone to emulate Lance Armstrong's climbing prowess, which involves keeping a cadence of 90 or 100 [rpm] even on the climbs, which saves his legs. But the fact is that the average person can't do this well without daily training—the high rpm on the hill will wear him out. On a shorter climb, the average guy is actually better off standing up and pushing a low cadence—something a Spin bike is perfectly set up to do."

Spin bikes, after all, only have one gear. In fact, to climb, you don't downshift, as you would do on a road bike, but instead turn the tension up and slow your leg speed down. Kostman recommends that Spinners fight the urge to ease off on the tension. "In fact, the longer you can hold a high tension at a slow speed, the better," he said. "It'll pay off when you go outside."

Seated Climbs: Butt Back, Heel Down

On long climbs, seated climbing is generally more economical than climbing out of the saddle, because it takes the weight off your legs and keeps your heart rate lower. Technically, the bike seat—not your legs—supports your body weight when you're seated, and your legs have the luxury of focusing on pushing the pedals. To further lighten the load on the quads, cyclists should pull up on the pedals on the upstroke. "But they rarely do it for long outdoors," said Kostman. "Either they shift to an easier gear, and therefore stop pulling up, or just lose focus on their pedaling technique altogether."

He said that one relatively simple Spin-class technique can help you keep that focus: lower your heels.

"Suck in your lower abs to help push your butt to the back of the seat, then drive the pedals down with your heels lower than the toes," he said. "Keep the heels low when you pull up, too; as soon as you lift the heel above the ball of the foot, you turn off the calf muscle." Kostman believes that most cyclists sit too high and too far forward on their bikes, often because they don't hinge their torsos forward enough or push their butts far enough back. By keeping their heels up, they are only pulling up with their shins and quads, rather than their shins, quads, calves, hams, glutes, and lower back. The dropped-heel technique that Kostman advocates jibes with what many top bike fitters say. Paul Levine of the Serotta International Cycling Institute said the dropped heel helps you utilize the glutes for more power (see Chapter 7).

Standing Climbs

Because a stationary bike does not angle upward while "climbing," as does an outdoor bike, Kostman said that the indoor cyclist must make a posture adjustment to cultivate the hamstrings, glutes, and back muscles in the same way that they'd normally be used outdoors.

His advice for replicating the outdoor position is to hinge at the hips, keep your back straight and parallel to the ground, push your nose down to within a few inches of your handlebar, and shove your butt so far back that it barely brushes against the saddle. Look down, not forward, to keep your spine in a neutral, comfortable position; in fact, literally lengthen the spine by inching your tailbone back and the crown of your head forward.

"Many indoor cyclists are misinformed about movement of the upper body in outdoor cycling," said Kostman. "Many indoor cycling instructors tell their students not to move their upper body, period. But this is wrong and counterproductive.

"Outdoors, the bike moves side to side beneath the rider," he said. "Since a stationary bike cannot be rocked beneath you, simulate the effect by moving your upper torso side to side." On a slow-cadence "all-body climb," rock your chest from one side of the handlebars to the other with each pedal stroke. The movement is strictly side-to-side, not up-and-down, and the hips and lower torso remain fixed in proper alignment with the feet and knees.

2. SPEED WORK
Standing Position: Running for Your Life
Standing tall on the pedals and doing what Johnny G called "running" looks strange to outdoor cyclists. "But forget about that," said Kostman. "Cyclists used to think lifting weights and yoga was weird, too. Running on a Spin bike can make you a better cyclist, forcing you to go anaerobic, building explosive power, raising your lactate threshold and turnover, and increasing your ability to make hard efforts. Most people working in a gym have had their HR [heart rate] in the anaerobic zone for a couple of minutes at a time or more, far longer than the brief efforts most people do during intervals."

Here's how to "run" while you Spin: Stand tall on the pedals by putting the entire weight of the body on the quads, with ears, hips, and bottom bracket in a straight line. With the upper body stabilized by tensed abs, and virtually no hand pressure on the bars (using only fingertips for balance), use the momentum of the weighted flywheel to blast your cadence up to 200 rpm—far above the 150 rpm most top cyclists can manage outdoors.

"This particular technique skyrockets the heart rate like nothing else," said Kostman, who claims to have recorded a max of 212 rpm with this technique. In fact, he warns, newbies in the Spin room should beware of getting in over their head. "Just do this for 10 to 15 seconds, max. Don't push it." Either sit back down—or read on to the next technique.

Standing in "Hinged" Position: Still Standing
Whereas standing tall and running (the aforementioned technique) can be tolerated only for a short burst of time, hinging forward and standing can be held for an entire song (three to six minutes) at a cadence of 110–150 rpm. To do this, said Kostman, assume a climbing posture, but don't push as far back over the saddle as you would while climbing with a slow cadence. In this position, you're still lengthening your spine when hinged forward, but resistance is light, and leg speed is high.

"As compared to standing tall, this off-the-saddle position won't 'burn' as much," he said. "Therefore you can hold a high leg speed for a longer period of time—raising your endurance, leg speed, and lactate threshold."

Sitting Position
Kostman likes sprinting during each chorus in a song, rather than sprinting for arbitrary periods of, say, 30 seconds. Ideal for building rapid turnover, the sitting technique is easy: Use very little resistance, sit forward on the saddle, suck in your abs to stabilize your hips and upper body, and go like hell. Again, shoot for 200 rpm.

3. GRADUAL WARM-UPS
The one "problem" that irritates Kostman about many non-cyclist Spin instructors is a tendency to force their classes to "redline" from start to finish. "That shoots your heart rate up—and once it's up, it'll never come down the rest of the session," he said. "Consequently, you never train

for recovery—allowing your heart rate to drop—a key to cycling endurance."

Recovery means that a truly fit person will see his or her heart rate drop by as much as 50 beats on a 30-second downhill. That is important because it allows the body to rest. "The problem with charging out of the gate and freezing your heart rate at a high level is that you never train your heart to rest," said Kostman. "You'll burn out."

His advice: Regardless of what your class is doing (unless you've done your own Spin warm-up before class began), ride the first two songs seated with light resistance, followed by a seated and standing climb for one song each. Be sure to warm your muscles in conjunction with a gradually rising heart rate. Never do speed work until 12 to 15 minutes into the class. Then, go for it.

AND WHEN YOU GET OUTDOORS . . .

1. Know your pedals. Before you go out for a ride, repeatedly practice clicking in and out of your clipless pedals comfortably. Otherwise, your first stop at a red light will be terrifying—especially if you land on your hip.

2. Look up. Never look down, as you might when concentrating in a studio. Always keep your head up, keeping hyper-aware of traffic and road conditions.

3. Butt back. Keep the same form taught in class—butt slid to the back of the saddle, straight back, sucked-in abs, relaxed shoulders, with as much weight as possible off the hands.

INTERVIEW
Ned Overend
THE GRAND MASTER OF BALANCE

In September, he's working the Specialized Bicycles booth at the Interbike trade show in Las Vegas, kneeling down and putting shoes on the feet of retailers as if he were a high-school part-timer working at Foot Locker. In March, he's in Washington, DC, in a three-piece suit, lobbying Colorado congressmen for the passage of bicycle-friendly legislation. One moment, he's on the podium at an XTERRA race, the next he's promoting a local mountain bike event, or flying to California to participate in product planning meetings at one of the world's largest bike manufacturers. Originally interviewed in April 2004 when he was 49 and again in December 2013 at 58, mountain bike icon Ned Overend, a member of the Mountain Bike Hall of Fame (1990) and the US Bicycling Hall of Fame (2001), told Bike for Life that he's superfit and busier than ever.

Today, heading into his seventh decade, this son of a diplomat, born in Taiwan and raised in Ethiopia and Iran, seems to barely have time to think about the six national mountain bike championships, the three UCI world titles, and the two XTERRA off-road triathlon titles he's acquired over the years. Aging glacially has always been the modus operandi of the down-to-earth superstar still known as "The Lung" for his prodigious climbing ability. Back in 1988, battling Ned for the national title, a young competitor remarked with relish, "He's 34 and won't be riding much longer." Overend didn't bow out of mountain biking for another eight years,

then was a full-bore off-road triathlete until 2002—several years after his young rival retired.

I GOT MY first road bike in 1973 when I was in high school. While running on the cross-country team, a Dutch teammate of mine got me a Crescent, a double-butted European road-racing bike that had Campy components on it and sew-up tires. I ended up doing the Ironman Triathlon on it in 1980.

It was Bob Babbitt's idea to do that. [Note: Babbitt is a journalist/broadcaster with Competitor Group, Inc.] We met at a rock-climbing class when I was going to San Diego State and he was a teacher. We started doing some runs and 10Ks together and ended up getting a house down at the beach. He read an article in *Sports Illustrated* about the 1979 Ironman and said, "Let's do this." I did it because it was in Hawaii and I'd never been.

Yet even after doing the Ironman Triathlon, I still wasn't a cyclist. I didn't really become one until I moved to Durango and started riding in the mountains here. By 1982, I'd done more triathlons, but what really got me into road racing was the Iron Horse Bicycle Classic, a huge event here in town. It really gave me an appreciation for how important events are for getting people involved in the sport. The Iron Horse is an epic. It's only 50 miles, from Durango to Silverton, but it's over an 11,000-foot pass. Everybody in town knows it, because it's a huge race every

Memorial Day weekend. Everybody wants to do it—even, to this day, my 13-year-old son and his buddies do it on their downhill bikes, because they don't know any better. Iron Horse piqued my interest in road racing.

For me, road racing was more exciting than triathlon—more neck-and-neck. Whether it's a criterium or road racing, the excitement of racing in a pack is incredible. I did quite well quickly. In '82, I was a Cat. 4 [Category 4, beginner-level racing]. In '83, I was a Cat. 1 doing the Coors Classic, riding for 7-Eleven—on the same Crescent bike I got back in high school. In '84, I started racing mountain bikes, and I was good right away—took second at my first national championship that year at Lake Eldora to Joe Murray. It may seem like a rapid rise, but I had the background: before cycling I raced motorcycles and was an accomplished mountain runner. In high school, we had one of the best teams in Northern California. I won several mountain runs around here. Indian Pass. Kendall Mountain. I did the Pikes Peak Marathon—finished second place twice. So the fitness and skills were there.

I didn't plan on being a pro mountain-biker. Actually, I had switched from being a car mechanic and a carpenter to a bike-shop mechanic so that I could be a pro triathlete or road racer. But while I was in the bike shop, I saw these Specialized Stumpjumpers come through. I thought, "Man, this is a great idea! We've got great trails out here." When I found out about the mountain bike racing series, I called Schwinn, because we were a Schwinn dealer. And they said, "Yeah, we want to do a mountain bike team. Let's do it." At first, they just picked up my expenses and I'd get a performance bonus plus prize money. So I worked a variety of jobs. I worked at Pizza Hut, Subway, things like that in the off-season. Eventually came the salaries—started $10,000, plus bonus. I kinda rode the wave from there.

My first national championship was in 1984. I remember being in the parking lot with almost no other cars there. We're wearing jeans and T-shirts; I really didn't have a logo. We are shaking the hands of the promoter and it is snowing. There is nobody but us left there. Those are the early days of mountain biking.

Contrast that with 1990, when I won the world championships—and helicopters are flying around. I've been to races in Spain where there were literally 40,000 spectators. Where you could not walk out of a protective compound to go into the crowd to sign autographs, because there'd be almost a riot.

I had switched to Specialized after I won the national championships in '85, '86, and '87. The meteoric rise in the sale of mountain bikes was on. Mountain biking became a UCI-recognized event. Europe really came on board when car sponsors came in and the big salaries started. No more working at Pizza Hut.

Banishing Burnout with Variety

I THINK IN 1987 someone was interviewing [John] Tomac [two-time world champion] when he said, "Ned is 32 already. So I doubt he'll be riding much longer." Like I was going to be out of there and he was going to be racking up some championships. Well, I retired from mountain biking as my main job in 1996. I wasn't out of there quite as quick as he thought I would be [laughs].

If someone had told me in 1985 that in 1996 at the age of 40 I was going to miss making the Olympic team by one spot, I would have thought that was absurd.

I get asked a lot how I stay so fit at my age. What I manage to do even now is maintain an enthusiasm for racing and riding hard. I think my approach is really important: cross-training and not being obsessive.

Back in the early days when I was battling Tomac, he'd put in 30 percent more miles than I would. He'd come out of the winter months strong. At the Cactus Cup, the first big race of the season in March, I would get my ass kicked. It would almost be embarrassing. I couldn't finish in the top five in the Cactus Cup, even when I'd come off a year when I won the world and national championships.

That's because I would back off in the off-season. I'd get in the weight room. I'd do some cross-country skiing. I'd do some running. I'd do some swimming. And I'd really back off on the cycling.

I'd start up later in the spring and I'd kinda build through the summer. So that by August and September, the most important races—the NORBA (National Off-Road Bicycle Association) nationals and the world championships—I would be fresher than these guys. There's nothing that gets your enthusiasm going like winning, like improving. There are a lot of guys whose best performance was in the Cactus Cup in March. What would be more depressing than having the races get more and more important as your fitness plateaus or actually goes down?

It happens to a lot of athletes. They overtrain. They are too excited. They are super-serious and they get obsessive about it.

What saved me is that I don't have the appetite for putting in huge miles. I didn't have the attention span. Another thing was that I was actually building a family from the late '80s on. I had two kids at home, and the idea of riding five hours and lying on the couch for the rest of the afternoon didn't really work at home. My wife wasn't going to accept that.

The formula I'd use for getting off the bike in the winter was going Nordic skiing and trail running. I think a variety of sports keeps you healthier from an injury standpoint. Overall it makes you a better athlete and gives you more longevity.

I have tremendous respect for guys like Tinker [Juarez] who do 24-hour races. I know they are going long and hard the whole time. That's why it does not appeal to me at all. I know for a fact that 24-hour races will accelerate the aging process. And I'm getting old fast enough as it is.

Post-40: Taking on New Challenges

I RETIRED AT 40, but didn't stop mountain bike racing. There were always a bunch of races that I wanted to do. But because racing was my job, I was locked into the NORBA national series and the World Cup series, with a lot of traveling in Europe and going to Japan every year. So now I was able to focus on some of these events that I missed, like the Wamagans, a classic race in the Midwest. And I wanted to get into some of these off-road triathlons which were just starting up.

In 1996, the year I retired from the World Cup circuit, they had the first XTERRA Triathlon Championship in Maui. I can guarantee you, because it was in Maui, I was going. My wife was okay with that. "We're all going," she said.

Off-road tris [triathlons] fit in really perfectly with my whole training philosophy. Turns out in that first one I ended up getting third to Mike Pigg and Jimmy Riccitello, a couple of accomplished triathletes. I knew I could improve a bunch in the swim and the run.

Specialized covered the expenses for me, which was a risk because there was no press that year. But it was on ESPN, and I ended up getting considerable press over the years. Huge press. *USA Today* wrote articles on it, so Specialized was happy. If I can examine an event to see if it's got any value, I can do it.

It's great to have new challenges. That is one of the great things about triathlon. Trying to be efficient in the swim. Trying to develop leg speed in the run. You have to do it all. As you get older, you do it with an eye toward not getting injured. Because I constantly go from one little overuse injury to the next. That's one thing I think runners and triathletes do more than cyclists.

As you get older, you can't ignore a tight hamstring. You can't ignore a pain in your shoulder. You have to start getting massage, physical therapy, stretching. As you get older you have to pay close attention to nutrition and hydration. If you're going to be successful as an athlete, you have to pay attention to all those things.

I still eat a lot—I'm a skinny guy, 135 to 140 pounds, and never had a problem with weight—but my diet has changed as I've gotten older. In the old days I would maybe restrict the amount of fat I would take, which I think was probably a mistake. I think it's probably more important to restrict the simple sugars and still get quality sources of protein and fat. For recovery, you need protein. In the old days, I didn't care about protein that much. Just a pound of pasta. But now I also make sure I'm getting some lean sources of either dairy or meat. I take pretty complete vitamin and mineral supplements. I'm more careful to replenish after a hard workout with a four-to-one mix—four carbohydrates to one protein.

I'm a stickler on it. But it's got to taste good. I don't like to spend a lot of time using up calories for food I don't enjoy eating. So sometimes I'll do things like Ensure, the old-people drink. It has a four-to-one carbohydrate to protein mixture. It also has a bunch of vitamins. And it tastes good.

The Atkins diet is too strict on the carbohydrates. You need more fuel. I'm looking at a can of Slim-Fast here. Thirty-five grams of sugar and 10 grams of protein. Huge variety of vitamins. It's a premium milk chocolate shake. That's the important thing, I think. And I've always done that. You know. A diet I enjoy. If you put all the work in to burn those calories, you should enjoy the replacement of them.

I work out every day, if possible. In 2002, I did a ton of XTERRAs [off-road triathlons]. Last year, I was involved in this Muddy Buddy duathlon series, helping promote it. Specialized was a sponsor of that. I think it's a great entry-level way to get people who aren't involved in mountain biking in the sport. Because of my recent travel schedule—a week in DC, a week of product meetings in Morgan Hill—I find that it's hard to carve out time and train for the different sports of triathlon. You don't have the time or the energy to swim, bike, and run. Hopefully I can hit an XTERRA at the end of the year. But I'll always still train.

I'll do two workouts a day, maybe two or three days a week. I have a lunch-hour ride at Specialized. That's a 45-minute hammer session. So I'll do that and I might run for 45 minutes after the meeting.

The Ultimate Tip: Don't Fall

YOU RECOVER FROM injuries a helluva lot slower when you're older. So a good rule is: Don't get injured. In my career, I've had no broken bones. I did break a couple fingers. But I've never broken a big bone. No collarbones. I'm really knocking on wood now.

I've been a good faller. I'm looking at my elbows and hips; I've got scars all over me. I've gone down at 45 mph on a road bike. I had one of my worst crashes ever last spring at one of the club rides. We were going like 30 mph on a slight downhill and there was a chunk of wood in the road. I was about five guys back. And nobody pointed it out, because they were all attacking and going so hard. And I pegged the thing and knocked my hand off the bar. That was ugly. I went face first into the pavement and rolled over on my back and slid down the road on my back. Crushed the helmet. But I was all right. My neck hurt for a while. I've been lucky.

On a mountain bike, a lot of injuries happen at slow speed. You don't get time to get your foot out of the pedal. You come to a technical section, your speed slows to zero, you don't make it over this little log or through these slippery rocks, and you start to fall over. Now, if you can balance, if you've practiced doing a track stand—which everyone should do—you can avoid falling to start with. You have this little extra second or fraction of a second where you can clip your foot out and put your foot down. Most people can't balance when they're falling over. Other people break collarbones....

A key: knowing how to set up your pedals. Set them up correctly, so they aren't sticky, so you can get out easily. Clean out the grit—it gets in your pedals and really changes the amount of release tension it takes. People can't get out of the pedals in a crash. That's a dangerous situation.

And when you do fall, minimize impact. Instead of sticking my arm out, I'll just fall and let the handlebar with the bar end on it hit the ground and let the pedal hit the ground first and then I'll let my body hit the ground with a little less impact. We used to actually do drills in the late 1980s—the teacher was a Polish guy named Andre Modgeleski, a truck driver in Colorado

Springs who was a buddy of Eddie B's in the old country. We had a camp and we'd do some tumbling. We'd have mats on the floor and you'd jump, tuck, and roll, and figure it out. You'd never stick a straight arm down. You'd put your hand down and immediately pull it in and tuck.

Look how much an injury like that would set someone back. Just look at [Australian pro rider] Cadel Evans—three broken collarbones last year. Here's someone who has a tremendous amount of talent. Two years ago [2002], he was in the pink jersey, leading the Giro—made him a huge amount of money when he signed his next contract. Since then he's been unable to finish any important tour. He hasn't made it very far into the season without getting injured. He's going down in crashes and busting his collarbone. Note: Evans went injury-free in 2011 when he won the Tour de France—ed.

Beyond Riding

A LOT OF times riders' main passions are just racing. But I gotta say, I love the R&D [research and development] side of it. And the equipment. I'm an equipment geek, ya know? I've got five road bikes in my garage and I'm a mountain bike racer. I've got like seven of my old mountain bikes at the Mountain Bike Specialist bike shop—from early hard-tail suspensions to one of the first Epics in prototype form. They actually have a museum for it. They've got Greg Herbold's old bikes, and Juli Furtado's.... A lot of people thought I was in business with [owner] Ed Zink just because I had so much stuff hanging down there. Not really. Better hanging down there than in my garage.

I have a unique relationship with Specialized, really my only employer. I am staying in Durango, where it's important for me to be able to stay for training and racing, while Specialized is in California. I don't really have a title; I'm involved with R&D and product development, especially cross-country suspensions and shoes and tires. I'm involved with promotions, and with advocacy, and sales as far as dealer relations. When we do a product launch to the media, I'm there

for that. I ride with the dealers and explain the product to them and things like that.

My current job started evolving when I was still riding. It's been 15 or so years now I've been an employee. As I was racing, I gradually got involved in dealer PR [public relations]. I'd go to the bike show and meet a lot of dealers. And as I would travel around the country racing, I'd dicker with them, get to know them on a personal level. At the same time, I'd get to know the magazine people, because they'd be covering the races, so it was kind of a natural transition when I got more involved with product development. Which was also happening while I was racing, because the Specialized racing teams have always had an influential role in product development.

The Bigger Picture

IN MARCH 2004, I was a delegate at the Bicycle Summit, an annual summit meeting in Washington, DC, for 350 bicycle advocacy groups. We do workshops, learn about the specific issues before the senators and congressmen, how to lobby them as a constituent, a business owner, a taxpayer.

Greg LeMond was there [the previous] year. It's always nice to have a recognized name, a world champion. Also, since I'm a citizen of Colorado, I went with the Colorado delegation. We talked to four representatives and both senators.

I think I had an impact. While visiting Senator Wayne Allard's office, I found out that one of his top aides went to school at Durango High— and my poster was hanging up in her history classroom. So she was excited to see me, and we took a picture together, which I signed and sent to her. Yes, stuff like this—"Here's Ned, the world mountain bike champion, the XTERRA champion"—helps, but it really only has limited value. What pulls more weight is the fact that I am involved in fundraising, in the local trails plans, and advocacy issues for mountain and road biking; that I'm a local business owner in Durango [Bouré Ridge Sportswear]; that I'm involved with a local bike dealer [through Specialized]; and also on the board of the Iron Horse

Bicycle Classic. We put on the race on Memorial Day and we put on the NORBA Nationals—the national finals last year, and a World Cup before that. These are the kinds of things that really speak to the politicians.

It gets attention when I say, "Hey, these events take in a million dollars in May with Iron Horse, then another million dollars in August with the NORBA Nationals, and get international media that brings Europeans here all summer long as a destination bicycle trip." They buy bikes, they're in the hotels and restaurants, taking raft trips. Millions and millions of dollars are generated by these events beyond the events themselves, giving notoriety to the whole Four Corners area. And these senators and congressmen understand that. They know how important cycling is as far as a tourist attraction to Colorado.

If you're just there as a do-gooder, talking about cycling only for its health benefits, you're not gonna get too much attention. Yes, there is Senator [James] Oberstar from Minnesota, and senators in Wisconsin and California and Vermont who are avid cyclists themselves. So they are going to support it because they realize how valuable it is. But for most of them, we go in with a several-pronged attack: the money cycling brings to the state, this whole obesity issue, and health.

I'll tell ya what feels good is when they build a county road in this town and they put a three-foot shoulder on it. In Durango, it's better than most towns, because we have so many people involved in cycling living here. Here, the public-works guy for the city calls the cyclists in and says: "How can we help you guys out?" They'll paint stripes to create narrow lanes in town to make a wider bike path.

Oh, I mean, we got money to improve a dedicated bike path along the river. But when you get out into the county, it's a whole different situation. It takes more to get shoulders on the roads, and we don't have a captive audience like we do with the city government. That's where we need to work next. But as I learned in racing, it's early in the season. We'll get stronger as time moves on.

Update

BIKE FOR LIFE caught up with Overend for an update in December 2013—and discovered that it's still pretty hard to catch up with him; at 58, he was as fit and fast as ever. While serving on the boards of the International Mountain Biking Association (IMBA), Bicycle Colorado, and the National Interscholastic Cycling Association (NICA, the high school league) and performing a number of duties for Specialized, ranging from giving product design advice, to recommending sponsorships for high-potential prospects, to scheduling events and training for the company's pro-mountain-bike team, he continues to compete and win. He won the 2010 single-speed nationals outright at age 55, the 2009 and 2010 national cyclocross championships, the 2012 World Masters cyclocross championship, and the Mt. Washington Hillclimb, and took second at the Mt. Tamalpais Hill Climb. He also competes in wintertime fat-bike events in Wisconsin and Minnesota, including the Fat Bike Birkie (a race on the groomed, snow-covered American Birkebeiner Ski Trail) during the first week of March.

"Frankly, for a guy my age to win, the right guys have to show up—or not show up," Overend said. "But now I have to be in shape all year round—not like the old days (when he was a pro mountain biker). Back then, I'd drink beer when the season was over, wouldn't touch a bike, do some cross-country skiing, and come back very slowly throughout the next spring and summer. But today, I'm frightened of that. You get too far out of shape and you can start losing your VO$_2$ max."

"The key for an old cyclist is to stay very active," he said. "That's easier today with the rising popularity of cyclocross (with its fall schedule) and the fat-bike craze, which has blown up. Now, there are races in the snow in Wisconsin and Michigan that draw three- to four-hundred people." Besides cross-country skiing, Overend lifts weights twice a week all year, stretches, and does some running on soft surfaces.

MEALS ON WHEELS

To increase performance and life span, dump refined carbs
and sugar, eat whole foods, and stay hydrated.

In 1999, I rode nine laps and 117 miles in the Canadian Rockies at the inaugural 24 Hours of Adrenalin Solo Mountain Bike World Championship in Canmore, Alberta, half the mileage of the event's winner, pro racer Rishi Grewal. Since I was the only participant over the age of 40, I declared myself the "Veteran Class Champion"—a joke Adrenalin founder Stuart Dorland ran with every year for a decade while introducing me to people as I covered the event.

In 2008, seeking a true title in the 50-plus age group—which now had seven people in it—I was back in Canmore to ride and write about the Worlds, which had become a giant event with 300 riders from 16 countries. The course was longer and harder than in 1999, but I was way, way fitter. I'd gotten dialed into periodization training and a good diet plan, and over the past few years had turned myself into a "fat-burning machine"—meaning that I'd trained my energy system to fuel up largely on my body fat, of which even the skinniest body has a monthlong supply of. I could ride forever on a can of olive-oil-soaked sardines, an apple, salted cashews, and a granola bar every two hours—a whole-food balance of protein, good fat, and low-glycemic carbs. By midnight I'd done six laps and was moving up on the leader. Unfortunately, all the while I'd been sucking down five or six packets of GU every lap. Back home, I never touched these sugary gels, but

the aid stations were stocked with the mocha and chocolate flavors, my favorites. I just couldn't resist. That pure sugar rush seemed to supercharge me.

Then, at about 12:30 a.m., I went out for my seventh lap—and didn't finish it for almost four hours. Ten minutes into it, I was hit by a wave of fatigue that made me feel like I was pedaling in quicksand. This was more than tired; I felt drugged, poisoned. I couldn't climb the shallowest grades. Dismounting, I could barely walk the slightest slopes. As time stretched on, I felt panicked, terrified, paranoid. When I finally made it back about 4:15 a.m., the timing tent workers told me that they had people on the course looking for me, thinking I must have fallen off a ledge and been knocked unconscious.

Well, I was knocked out—by a GU sugar crash. Those 25 packs of mocha-chocolate gel spiked my insulin through the roof and blocked my finely tuned low-glycemic fat-burning machinery. I was so wrecked that I never went out for another lap. I found out later that the 50-plus winner only did nine laps. Maybe I could have caught him, I thought—if only I hadn't violated the basic rule of racing: Don't change your equipment, or your diet, on race day.

Food is fuel—and not any old fuel will do. If your training has built you into a long-distance economy car designed to go a couple hundred miles in a day, you don't want to fuel up like a top-fuel dragster that does a quarter-mile in four seconds. An engine designed to run on relatively slow-burning gasoline may be stressed out when blasted by instant-igniting nitromethane.

Food and training must work hand-in-hand to build your metabolic efficiency and turn you into a fat-burning machine. The science of training detailed in the heart-rate-based periodization of the previous chapter is well established. But unbeknownst to many, so is the science of food. And the science says that a diet based on fast-burning processed carbohydrates—bread, pasta, breakfast cereals, tortillas, fast foods, energy bars, gels, and sugars, including carbo-loading the day and night before a race and sucking down gels all day during the event—is not only inefficient, but harmful to long-term health.

Yes, cycling lore is filled with stories of guys named Lance consuming up to 7,000 calories a day in the Tour de France, most of that from refined carbohydrates. But as we have all seen, not everything that cycling tradition dictates and the pros do legally or otherwise will necessarily help you ride to 100. Carb addiction—that is, addiction to high-glycemic carbs—is one of them.

Let's be clear: Carbs aren't bad, if they're the right carbs—meaning natural, slower-burning ones from whole foods, such as vegetables, nuts, and fruit. For best long-term health and short-term performance, eat them in meals with animal/fish protein and healthy fats, such as from nuts, avocados, and olive oil. In some instances, targeted use of fast-burning carbs will be appropriate—such as in the last stages of an endurance event, or right after a hard workout, to prop open a nutritional 30-minute recovery window (to be discussed later in this chapter). Otherwise, stay away from sugar (soft drinks) and refined grain- and starch-based carbs (white bread, French fries, white rice) as much as possible.

That's because you don't need as much quantity of carbohydrate for high performance as you think, and you shouldn't be willing to pay for high performance with bad health.

The quantity issue first: Just do the math—and remember that the body packs a maximum of only 2,000 calories of glycogen in the muscles for use as fuel and when you use that up, you bonk. That's why you need to become a "better butter burner," as Phase IV's Robert Forster calls it—a fat-burning machine that taps your 80,000 calories' worth of body fat, a near unlimited amount found even on a skinny body.

An average untrained person burns a fuel mix of roughly 65 percent carbs and 35 percent fat at rest; your goal, with training and diet, is to flip that ratio to 65 percent fat and 35 percent carbs—or even more on the fat-burning side. In fact, a landmark 2013 study by a University of Connecticut team found that Zach Bitter, a highly trained "paleo"-eating ultrarunner who that year set the world record for running 100 miles on a treadmill, was actually burning a fuel mix of *98 percent fats and 2 percent carbs* while running at a 7-minute-per-mile pace, his average speed in races. Because of that, he could get away with eating hardly anything during races and not bonk.

The higher the percentage of fat you train your body to burn, the less you will need to burn glycogen, saving it for vital body functions and organs that require it, like the brain. You already know from Chapter 2 that you can build a fat-burning metabolism through long, slow, distance (LSD) base training. But training shouldn't be limited to *physical* training. *Food* training will greatly accelerate the process. In fact, to improve your fat burning, some believe that what you eat is even far more important than how much you exercise. Mark Sisson, a former Hawaii Ironman triathlon star (fourth in the 1980 race), who has emerged as a leading voice in the low-carb/high-fat movement due to his popular Primal Blueprint series of natural diet books, tells me that you build 80 percent of your fat-burning engine simply by adopting an all-paleo diet (low-carb/high-protein and fat, with no sugar, starches, or refined flour products) for 21 days, with the final 20 percent up to your subsequent training.

So your food choices don't just *fuel* the engine; they help *form* the engine. That's because the body is a smart multifuel machine. Eating a diet high in fat causes the body to preferentially use fat for fuel, whereas eating a high-carb diet results in the body relying more heavily on limited stores of muscle glycogen for fuel.

Having an efficient fat-burning engine is very beneficial in events lasting more than two hours—like typical bike rides. One of the first big names to recognize the value of a higher-fat, lower-carb diet was the six-time Hawaii Ironman Triathlon winner Mark Allen, who I interviewed many time as an editor at *Triathlete* magazine in the 1990s. Allen's mostly vegetarian diet (he'd crave a steak and eat one once a week, he said) took on a ratio of 30 percent fat, 30 percent protein, and 40 percent carbs in his base training period—radically different from the conventional 10/20/70 wisdom of the day. Combined with a low-heart-rate periodized program (designed by his coach, Phil Maffetone, to keep him out of what we now know as the Black Hole), Allen built a monster fat-burning engine and managed to stay in fat-burning mode longer than anyone. His results speak for themselves.

Keep in mind that while *Bike for Life* isn't against a vegetarian diet, essential amino acids are tough to get without animal protein. That's one reason why this plan encourages a balanced, back-to-our-roots paleo/primal diet that includes all-you-can-eat protein (to build muscle) and fat from animals and fish, and plenty of "good" complex carbohydrates like vegetables, as opposed to "bad" simple, refined carbs like sugar, pasta, bread, candy bars, and fruit juices. Complex carbs are good because they are rich sources of vitamins, minerals, and fiber; often low in calories due to their fiber content and water; quite filling (a large bowl of salad greens equals the calories of a single energy bar); generally don't lead to overeating; take a long time to metabolize; don't spike blood sugar and insulin and cause inflammation; and don't interfere with fat-burning as much as simple carbs do.

In short, natural carbs will enhance your overall health and longevity—wheras processed high-glycemic carbs do the opposite. In fact, a good general rule is to avoid the white stuff—Wonder Bread, rice, potatoes, sugar. These processed carbs affect your body in three extremely negative interrelated ways: They raise insulin, cause food addiction and overeating, and cause inflammation.

Negative Effects of Refined Carbs and Sugars

1. They raise insulin, *which keeps your body from burning fat and ends up making you fatter.* Here's why: In response to rapidly elevated blood sugar levels, the pancreas shoves it into overdrive and releases a big spike of insulin, the main hormone that tells the body what to do with the food just eaten. Like a traffic cop, insulin tells the muscles and liver to take sugar from the bloodstream and store it as glucose/glycogen, and simultaneously stops body fat from being burned as fuel. On the flip side, you (ironically) will burn more fat when you eat more fat, as the absence of an insulin response leaves glycogen alone and your muscles fuel up with fat instead. Even if you overeat refined carbs just a little bit, you'll get fatter, because the liver and muscle cells have a limited capacity to store glycogen, and the excess gets sent to the fat cells. The trouble is, as you'll see next, it's hard for people *not* to overeat refined carbs.

2. They are addictive, *which keeps your body from burning fat and ends up making you fatter.* Part of that addiction is due to the widespread use of high-fructose corn syrup (HFCS) since the early 1980s, and part of it is due to the inherent addictive nature of sugar itself. HFCS, a Japanese invention that is one-third cheaper than sugar and 25 percent sweeter (87 versus 70 on the glycemic index), poured into the American bloodstream when Coke and Pepsi first used it as a sugar replacement in 1984. Soon it was in everything: energy bars, ketchup, breakfast cereals, steak sauce. The problem: It encourages overeating and overdrinking because it supresses leptin, a hormone made by fat cells that curtails eating by signaling the brain that the fat cells have had enough. Without the leptin stop sign, per capita soft-drink consumption nearly doubled from 350 cans a year to 600 in a decade. Rats fed HFCS gained 40 percent more weight than rats fed the same amount of sugar. By 1994, the Center for Disease Control noted an alarming increase in obesity.

Natural sugar isn't as bad but still gives you a hedonic rush that is wired to the pleasure centers of your brain, creating an addictive-like desire to keep consuming it beyond satiation. This was confirmed in a study published in the December 2013 issue of *American Journal of Clinical Nutrition*. It found that sugar, more than fat, activates the gustatory region—the part of the brain responsible for the perception of taste. Because starches and grains have higher glycemic indexes than sugar, they are similarly addictive. Since you can't help but eat too much refined carbs, it'll be hard not to get fat—and to become insulin resistant. That means your body no longer responds as well to insulin, so it can't get rid of its blood sugar very well, leading to heart disease, diabetes, and other problems linked to inflammation.

3. They cause systemic **inflammation.** In the short term, inflammation isn't necessarily a bad thing, as it helps to heal your body from external cuts and bruises and internal invaders like viruses and bacteria; the painful redness and swelling you see actually is increased blood flow, which moves more immune cells and nutrients to the damaged areas to speed repair. But long-term inflammation is a different story—it's unseen, inside the body, and insidiously dangerous. Modern irritations, such as smoking, obesity, and a diet loaded with

trans-fats and refined carbs and sugar, make the body think it is injured, so it responds with inflammation and floods itself with a constant flow of immune cells. Inflammation creates a real heat and friction on a physiological level, similar to rubbing fabric together repeatedly; eventually, it begins to degrade. The overwhelming numbers of immune cells and the various hormones in release fouls up healthy cells—over time setting the stage for the development of cancer, arthritis, joint deterioration, atherosclerosis (cholesterol-clogged arteries that lead to heart disease, heart attacks, strokes, and diabetes), and/or even Alzheimer's (due to vascular dementia).

Therefore, depending on the situation, inflammatory response agents can be good and bad. Inflammatory cytokines released into the bloodstream help heal a cut. But when a processed-carb diet makes the inflammation chronic, the same cytokines eventually deteriorate normal cells and tend to irritate and wear down cartilage.

Bottom line: What you eat matters—on the race course and over the course of your life. A balanced, natural, whole-foods diet that includes healthy fats and minimizes refined carbs will help turn you into a fat-burning machine and prevent chronic inflammation and insulin spikes. Yes, there are a few small differences between eating for general health and eating for performance. We will get to those after we first look at the basics of a healthy diet plan.

OVERVIEW: KEEP A BALANCE OF NATURAL PROTEIN, FAT, AND CARBS

If you remember one fundamental rule of a healthy diet, it's *back to nature*. Ask yourself: Could our ancestors have found this food item somewhere on a tree, in a field, on a mountain, or in a river, lake, or coastal sea 10,000 years ago? Processed foods, the ones that cause all the problems, have only been on the scene for 100 years—which may be the reason that as consumption of these foods has increased, so has incidence of chronic disease. The good stuff—whole, natural, "paleo" foods—has been with us since we were human, which may be why our systems work so well with animal protein, green vegetables, fruits, nuts, and legumes, and not with processed carbs and sugars.

In general, whole foods have a low glycemic index (GI), meaning that the body takes longer to break them down into blood glucose. Low-GI foods do a host of good things—reduce inflammation, keep you burning more fat as fuel, balance blood sugar, lower insulin requirements, reduce body fat, decrease blood pressure, improve immune system function, promote longevity, and generally enhance well-being.

To get the most out of low-GI foods, make each meal a balance of good fats, protein, and carbohydrates; eat them together in a meal, not separately during the day. That's because the three work better together than alone, maintaining stable digestion and release of insulin and other chemical reactions.

Here's a breakdown of the three nutrition categories, including how much of each you should eat every day:

Protein

Protein repairs, maintains, and grows muscles, as well as provides about 15 percent of your energy.

Sources: Lean meats, chicken, fish, dairy products, eggs, plain yogurt, cottage cheese, hard cheeses, and nuts and seeds as well as nut butters.

How Much: 4–6 ounces (the size of the palm of your hand). The rule is 0.9 grams of protein for every pound of lean body mass (which excludes fat) per day, which translates to 90 grams (about 4 ounces) for a 5-foot-9 man with 100 pounds of lean muscle on him. Endurance athletes should each get from 70 to 200 grams of protein per day, according to nutritionist Monique Ryan.

Good Fats

Sources: Fatty fish, such as salmon, tuna, mackerel, herring, trout, and sardines, which are loaded with anti-inflammatory omega-3 fatty acids; avocado; certain oils, especially olive oil, coconut oil, sesame oil, peanut oil or peanut butter, and safflower oil; and nuts and seeds, including sunflower seeds, flaxseed, almonds, macadamia nuts, walnuts, cashews, pecans.

How much: Athletes should get 30 percent of their calories from fat. Get 2 tablespoons' worth of oils per day, and a fist-sized chunk of fish.

Good Carbohydrates

Sources: Greens (lettuce, celery, etc.); legumes, such as beans (all kinds); seeds (including quinoa, pumpkin seeds, and sunflower seeds, for example); and fruit (apples, oranges, bananas, berries, and so on). Fruit is loaded with sugar but also with hundreds of substances, including vitamin C, that decrease free radicals and other anti-inflammatory agents.

How much: Enough to fill two hands. (Limit processed carbs to one hand.)

Others

Cocoa and dark chocolate: In laboratory studies, chocolate has slowed the production of the signaling molecules involved in inflammation. The challenge is finding them without too much sugar and fat.

Alcohol: Many studies, including a long-term meta-analysis of thousands of elderly residents of Leisure World, California (now Laguna Hills), have concluded that one drink a day of any alcohol—wine, beer, or hard liquor—seems to lower levels of C-reactive protein (CRP), a powerful signal of inflammation. Too much alcohol has the opposite effect on CRP.

Herbs and spices: Turmeric, ginger, garlic, basil, pepper, and many other herbs and spices have anti-inflammatory properties.

BASIC DIET RULES
1. Beware processed carbs.

Processed, refined carbs, such as white bread, white rice, French fries, and sugar-laden sodas, are dangerous for several reasons:

1. They are counterproductive for fat utilization, in that the body will reach for them as fuel before reaching for fat.

2. They spike your insulin and put you to sleep. Example: If you eat a big bowl of pasta, the large insulin spike opens and transports glycogen (a carb derivative) to the cells, removing it from the bloodstream. That makes you sleepy and/or makes you crave more sugar.

3. They create inflammation in the gut, keeping you chronically inflamed and bloated. Inflammation in the body causes all sorts of havoc, including producing cholesterol.

4. Remember that saturated fat doesn't kill you; it's processed carbohydrates that do that.

5. If you do eat processed food, make it whole-grain bread, brown rice, and other whole grains, which will give you a slower rise in blood sugar, insulin, and the inflammatory messenger cytokine.

6. Dilute and delay the quick absorption of processed carbs and sugars by eating them with protein—such as putting peanut butter on your bagel.

7. Beware of gluten. the overproduction and genetic manipulation of wheat has also raised the general exposure to gluten, a protein not tolerated by 15 percent of the population that is linked to fatigue, inflammation, mood swings, and many diseases, allergies, and digestive problems.

2. Don't fear fat—love it.

For many years, saturated fats have had a bad rap—they're a widow maker, a heart attack waiting to happen, one would think from reading popular news over the past couple of decades. But today, views have changed 180 degrees. A big moment came in October 2013, when esteemed British cardiologist Aseem Malhotra released a study in the *British Medical Journal* that concluded that long years of not eating and drinking fat-laden red meats and whole milk *did not* reduce heart disease, and that the real culprits are sugars and processed carbs.[1] In fact, the believes that a high-fat, low-carb diet featuring unprocessed saturated fat from red meat and whole milk actually has a *protective* effect against heart disease, diabetes, and dementia. Saturated fat was actually the body's preferred fuel. Moreover, a previous study by neurologist David Perlmutter said that a diet featuring saturated fat could prevent and even reverse Alzheimer's.

Bottom line: The world has been turned on its head. It turns out that dietary fat won't make you fat; processed grains and sugar do that. Good fat (oil from almonds and other nuts, olives, and avocados, for example) is now widely acknowledged as an essential nutrient and a valuable fuel for athletes who have trained their bodies to burn it. Olive oil can even reduce inflammation.

3. Beware of trans-fats.

Margarine, processed peanut butter, and other processed foods can contain trans-fats, unnatural fats created during food production, such as by adding hydrogen to liquid vegetable oil to solidify margarine. Trans-fats cause many problems in the body, including increased inflammation and increased risk of coronary heart disease. They also lower good cholesterol (HDL) levels and raise the bad cholesterol (LDL). If the label lists hydrogenated or partially hydrogenated oils as an ingredient, run away—that means it also contains trans-fats. Real butter is a better (and tastier) choice than margarine.

4. Follow the two-hour rule.

By eating every couple of hours—a 100- to 200-

calorie snack of nuts or yogurt will do—you will keep your insulin levels stable and prevent yourself from overeating at lunch and dinner. If you don't get any food in your body from breakfast until lunchtime, your insulin levels drop off, and so does your energy. So at 10 a.m., take an almond break.

5. Don't skip breakfast.

Overnight, your metabolism goes down to idle, burning relatively few calories. Raise it by throwing some food in the tank before you leave the house.

6. Periodize your diet.

To maximize the effect of each training phase, you must change the mix of your regular meals and your post-workout recovery nutrition. This next section discusses this in detail.

SYNCING YOUR DIET WITH A PERIODIZED TRAINING PLAN

An ideal periodized training plan also periodizes diet, syncing it to each workout.

Whether you follow a casual fitness regimen for general health or are in serious training for an event, the basic rule of limiting your intake of processed carbs applies across the board. But there are some tweaks to the rule in order to optimize performance and recovery, which means that daily meals will be different from post-workout meals. Post-workout meals must be eaten promptly after the workout to take advantage of the 30-minute "window" during which the muscles are more receptive to refueling. If you miss this window, you won't be fully recovered for the next hard workout. A description of the window appears at the end of this chapter.

On a daily basis, your goal is to keep your metabolism revving efficiently, because that facilitates great sports performance. Here's how to sync your training phase and food intake.

LSD Base Training Phase

Limit carb intake before, during, and after each workout. This will train your muscles to burn more fat. Also limit your carbs during the recovery meal; if you've stayed aerobic during your workout, it should not have used up a lot of carbs.

Power Speed Phase

Increase carbs the night before high-intensity activities. In this phase, you are performing high-intensity activities like hill repeats and interval training that reach for quick-burning fuel like carbohydrates. So you should raise your daily carb intake to three handfuls a day. Try to eat healthy, vegetable-based carbs as well as quinoa, garbanzo beans, nuts, and legumes. If you must have processed carbs like bread and pasta, limit yourself to one handful a day.

Increase fruit. Bring your fruit consumption to five servings a day. The vitamin C in fruit strengthens the immune system, which is heavily taxed during intervals. Since fruit is mostly sugar, it's best to eat it after the meal, so the previous food limits an insulin spike.

Max Strength Phase

Increase protein intake. There are a total of 12 amino acids in the body, and 9 of them are essential to making healthy tissue. All of the essential amino acids are conveniently found in animal protein (fish, meat, and poultry). It's not as easy being a vegetarian athlete because getting these amino acids from non-animal protein sources requires you to become a serious amino-acid analyzer.

Taper Phase

Reduce overall calories. If you don't match your calorie input to your reduced-calorie usage, you'll gain weight. That's not exactly a prescription for a PR on race day.

THE 30-MINUTE WINDOW OF RECOVERY

There's no debate about eating after a workout: Do it, and quickly. Muscles are stressed and they need rebuilding materials. It's commonly accepted that the muscles are more receptive to using those materials during a 30-minute window after the workout. The question is: What materials? Protein, fat, or carbs?

In the new school of thought, hard-core paleo types say you should focus on protein and fat, with minimal carbs. This will force your body to become better at burning fat the following day (which in any case should be an LSD recovery day, which does not require a quick-burning fuel). The fact that glycogen stores are low after a hard workout is considered a good thing by pure paleoists; it'll force you to learn to become a better fat burner, the goal of all endurance athletes.

The old school of thought puts carbs ahead of protein in a 4-to-1 ratio in a scenario that both refills the stores of glycogen you've used up in the workout and spurs protein muscle repair. The carbs (taken as an orange juice or candy bar immediately post-workout) stimulate insulin release, which pushes the window open for another half an hour, allowing the protein more time to get to the torn muscle sites and commence repair. In about four hours, your glycogen will be fully restored.

Which plan should follow? You must experiment and find out what works for you. Cyclists tend to hang on to traditions, and the 30-minute 4-to-1 carb-to-protein window may be one of them. Common sense seems to dictate that the paleo approach, emphasizing proteins and fats, will work for those who have gone to a low-carb diet, in which a fourth fuel, a fat-derivative called ketones, largely replaces glycogen in the brain and for some muscle fueling. The production of ketones in a low-carb environment have caused some to say that carbs are completely unnecessary, anyway, with whale-blubber-subsisting Inuit populations in the Arctic regions being proof of that.

In any case, the 30-minute window is well-established at this point. The sooner you get food in, the better your recovery the next day.

HYDRATION

Why you must drive yourself to drink

Hydration Calamity No. 1:

It was August 2007, Brest, France. I'd ridden all the way from Paris to the Atlantic Ocean, exactly 600 kilometers, with plenty of time to spare. Then, after getting my time-card stamped at the check-in table in the town of Brest, the halfway point of the 1,200-kilometer Paris-Brest-Paris randonnée, I walked over to the grassy lawn where I'd laid my bike... and fell over, passed out.

I woke up a few minutes later surrounded by men in white coats who were lifting me into an ambulance. They spoke no English, but managed to let me know that the race I'd trained all year for was over. Now, I couldn't ride the 600 kilometers back to

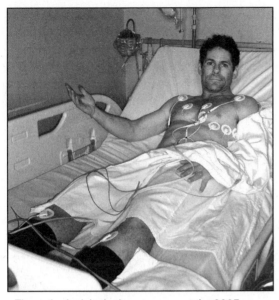

The author's dehydration screw-up at the 2007 PBP led to this.

Paris if I wanted to. They wouldn't let me out of the hospital for 14 hours.

My problem? Severe dehydration. That was a shock, given that I'm normally a hydration maniac and that it had been bone-chilling cold. In western France for 37 hours in the middle of summer, it was freezing cold and rainy, all the way to Brest. Bundled in a rain jacket, sweating inside like a fat man in a sauna, I was unwittingly losing far more fluids than usual, but not replacing them—because it was so cold that I didn't feel the urge to drink much. I had no idea that my radiator was dry until I woke up on the stretcher. (See Hydration Rule 2, below: "Drink before you're thirsty.")

Hydration Calamity No. 2:

It was odd that John Rodham didn't show up on the second day of the 1997 La Ruta de los Conquistadores, the fabled mountain bike race across Costa Rica. The 35-year-old New York schoolteacher was the top-finishing American on Day 1, impressive given the 80-mile ride through jungle, mud, and humidity. By the end of the day, we got the grisly news:

Rodham had gone to bed and never awakened. A hotel maid opened the door at noon and found him in a coma. He fluttered near death for four days until he woke up.

Of course, we all figured it had to be severe dehydration. You easily could under-drink in a race with this heat, this distance, and this intensity. That's why it was a shock to discover, months later when I called him, that Rodham hadn't gotten dehydrated at all. He'd slurped plenty of water from his hydration-pack hose—too much, in fact. He'd developed hyperhydration, medically known as hyponatremia, or "water intoxication," which is caused by drinking too much water without replenishing crucial electrolytes—the salts and minerals, lost in one to three quarts of sweat per hour in the tropics, that function to distribute water to muscles and organs. Hyponatremia's symptoms can include nausea, dizziness, cramps, confusion, and a life-threatening swelling of the brain.

Moral of the story: You can drink like a camel, but you'll need more than water in your Camelbak. (See Hydration Rule 7, below: "Restore sodium levels.")

Too little water, too much water. Hydration seems like the easiest thing in the world, until you mess it up—and it messes you up.

For athletes, water is often the most common nutritional deficiency. You can ride all day without food, especially if you're a well-honed fat-burning machine—but not water. It's too crucial. Humans can live a month without food, but only three to five days without water. In hot conditions, a sedentary person can lose 1.5 quarts of fluid in sweat and respiration within an hour, and dehydration can set in with no water. A cyclist working hard in the heat without replacing fluids can actually die in a period of several hours from the unchecked rise in body temperature, which stresses organs and can lead to heat stroke. Drinking water will cool you down and lower your core temperature.

A young male athlete's body is typically 60 percent water, a female athlete's about 50 percent. About two-thirds of this water is in the intracellular areas—mainly muscles, with most of the rest in the blood. Sweating leads to dehydration; even a deficiency of less than 1 percent can cause poorly functioning muscles, blood, and organs. At 5 percent dehydration—between 6 and 8 pounds of fluid—your body begins to deteriorate. As your blood thickens, the heart works harder as your natural cooling mechanisms of sweating and evaporation become impaired.

Don't wait for your sense of thirst to signal that it's time to drink. Thirst is sensed only after dehydration has started, and once you are dehydrated, it may take up to 48 hours to properly rehydrate. This is why so many athletes are in a constant state of dehydration. Just make sure you top off your electrolytes as well.

So remember to drink—a bottle an hour, at a minimum. To jog your memory, it might be helpful to remember all the things that water does: It burns fat, suppresses hunger, renews your skin, and saves your kidneys and liver from chronic overwork. When your kidneys are taxed from too little water, your liver has to take over, and it can't do its regular job.

With that in mind, drink in these hydration rules from Fred Matheny, longtime fitness editor of Roadbikerider.com.

Hydration Rules

1. Prehydrate. Drink the moment you get up the day of the ride, including a 16-ounce sports drink an hour before the start. Down at least eight big glasses of water the day before the ride. Most of us are chronically dehydrated, so keep a bottle on your desk and sip all day.

2. Drink before you're thirsty. Your body's sensation of thirst lags behind your need for liquid, so grab your bottle every 15 minutes and take a couple of big swallows (about 4 ounces).

3. Bottle an hour. Most riders generally need at least one big bottle (16 to 20 ounces) per hour, depending on conditions—temperature, intensity of the ride, and body size.

4. Hydrate after the ride. No matter how much fluid you drink while riding, in hot weather you'll finish the ride depleted. Your stomach doesn't empty fast enough to keep up with the demand.

5. Weigh yourself before and after the ride. Compare the figures. If you've lost weight, drink 20 ounces of fluid for each pound of body weight lost. Keep drinking until your weight has returned to normal and your urine is pale and plentiful. Rehydrating is especially vital during multiday rides. If you get a little behind each day, by the end of the week you'll be severely dehydrated, feeling lousy, and riding poorly.

6. Practice your hydration. Don't go into a long event without knowing your sweat rate. Some people sweat a lot; others much less. Some lose a lot of electrolytes. Know your body's needs and plan accordingly.

7. Restore sodium levels. Those white stains on your clothing and helmet straps after a long, hot ride come from the salt you've sweated out. It needs to be replaced. Low sodium levels are associated with increased incidence of cramps. Heavy sodium losses lead to hyponatremia (water intoxication), the potentially lethal condition that affected John Rodham at La Ruta. On long rides, get the salt back by nibbling on salty nuts and snacks, adding a half-teaspoon of salt to a water bottle, and regularly gulping a sports drink (it should contain at least 100 milligrams of sodium per 8 ounces—check the label.)

8. Beware the ubiquitous hydration pack. A hose is so easy to drink from it that you can overdrink—and exacerbate the risk of hyponatremia. The solution: Carry a couple of water bottles filled with electrolyte drink on your frame—and use them.

THE TEN COMMANDMENTS OF COOKING

"With proper nutrition and training your endurance could—and should—actually improve well into your 40s," said Phil Maffetone in *Eating for Endurance*. "Eating habits directly affect your fitness."

Maffetone, the famed coach of legendary triathletes Mark Allen and Mike Pigg, said that how you prepare food affects digestion, absorption of nutrients, hormone balance, and energy production. An ideal diet would include lots of raw and uncooked foods (loaded with nutrients), but would not include hydrogenated oils (they create problems for the body) or ground meat (which is laden with bacteria). That and more can be found in what he calls his Ten Commandments of Cooking, listed below. "There's no downside to healthy eating, he said; it's not only better for your body, but tastes better, too."

1. Avoid hydrogenated fats and transfats: Hydrogenated or partially hydrogenated fats such as margarine and highly processed vegetable oils aren't good for your body, as they interfere with normal metabolism and cholesterol balance and promote inflammation. "Stick with high-quality, unsalted butter," said Maffetone.

2. Don't cook with vegetable oil: "Heating the oil causes unhealthy chemical changes in vegetable oil, including converting it to archidonic acid and increasing the amount of free radicals," said Maffetone. Instead of sautéing your food in oil, steam your vegetables, bake or broil meats and fish, or pan-fry using the fat naturally found in the food. Also use butter and olive oil, stable monosaturated fats that don't break down when heated.

3. Steam with a teeny bit of water: "Many vitamins and minerals are lost in the water in which foods are cooked," said Maffetone. "Steam rather than boil, and drink the water—as tea or soup—to reclaim the minerals."

4. Don't overcook: "Many nutrients are unstable in heat," said Maffetone. "Take glutamine, the amino acid; if you cook a steak medium, you lose half the glutamine. If you cook it well-done, almost all the glutamine is destroyed. When fish is cooked, valuable EPA fatty acid is destroyed."

The rule: The rarer, the rawer, the better. No worries about hygiene, either, considering that bacteria, found only on the surface in solid (non-ground) meat, is killed quickly by heat. Part of our diet should be raw. EPA, a fatty acid in fish, gets destroyed when cooked. Raw fish is ideal, as long as you *make sure that it's fresh, that it does not have parasites, and that it is handled and prepared properly to avoid bacterial contamination.*

5. Use whole foods, not processed: Raw foods—uncooked fruits and vegetables—are jammed with disease-fighting bio- and phytonutrients such as bioflavonoids and vitamin E that are often destroyed in cooking and processing.

6. Avoid ground meat: Bacteria, initially only on the surface of solid meat, becomes intermixed throughout when the meat is ground up, said Maffetone. At a restaurant, order ground meat well-done, with no red-colored uncooked section in the middle. To kill harmful bacteria such as *Escherichia coli*, the US Department of Agriculture recommends that you cook all cuts of beef, veal, pork, and lamb to a temperature of 145 F, as measured with a food thermometer before removing the meat from the heat source, with a three-minute rest time before carving or consuming. Outbreaks of *E. coli* are usually traced to ground beef. Ground beef and pork must be cooked to a temperature of 160° F, and poultry to 165°.[2]

7. Use fresh foods first, then frozen, and canned as a last resort: "Same story," said Maffetone. "The more the processing, the more the nutrients lost. Lots of nutrients are lost sitting around. Eat all food quickly. An old, sour orange means the natural chemicals inside are breaking down."

8. Have raw food at each meal: Avocado, soft-cooked egg yolk, tomato, greens, radishes, and carrots come packed with the stuff nature gave them.

9. Use coarse sea salt: "Traditional sodium chloride has other ingredients in it—even sugar sometimes," said Maffetone. "Sea salt has a better balance of minerals—and the best chefs use it

(continues)

because it tastes better. And since we evolved from the sea, you can argue that it is more compatible with the body."

10. The presentation of a meal is important: "Making the environment lovely and dishes healthy, tasty, and attractive to the eye prepares the brain and the rest of the nervous system to digest," said Maffetone. "It's like foreplay in sex—preparing the body for what's to come. Good music, known to add to the enjoyment of a meal, actually helps you digest better and get more nutrients out of it."

THE TIMELESS TRUTH OF THE MEDITERRANEAN DIET

A study published in the *Journal of the American Medical Association* (*JAMA*) on September 22, 2004 (and followed by many similar studies since) detailed evidence that a Mediterranean-style diet, combined with 30 minutes of daily exercise, significantly boosts longevity. For 10 years, the study followed 2,300 active elderly Europeans, aged 70 to 90, whose diets emphasized whole grains, fruits, vegetables, legumes, nuts, and olive oil and were low in saturated animal fats, transfats, and highly processed grains. (Although pasta and bread are common components of the Med diet, they are usually a small proportion of the overall calorie intake.) They died at a rate that was more than 50 percent lower than those who didn't exercise and ate poorly.

The same issue of *JAMA* also cited a study that looked at the Mediterranean diet's cardioprotective benefit, suggesting that it may inhibit inflammation in blood vessels, which is believed to be a major player in heart disease and type 2 diabetes. According to a WebMD (www.webmd.com) news report, "Patients at high risk for these diseases who followed the Mediterranean diet for two years showed more improvements in weight loss, blood pressure, cholesterol, and insulin resistance—conditions that promote heart disease—than a similar group placed on a conventional diet. Adherence to the Mediterranean diet was effective in reducing inflammatory blood markers, which have been linked to a high risk of heart disease."

ATTENTION VEGETARIANS: HOW TO AVOID THAT "DEFICIT"

With rising health fears associated with *E. coli*, salmonella, mad cow disease and listeria contamination of meat and poultry products, coupled with increased revulsion at how cattle—a "food delivery system"—are penned, fed, drugged, and slaughtered, vegetarianism is gaining adherents—and not just in green meccas such as Berkeley, Cambridge, Madison, and Boulder. Twenty million Americans call themselves vegetarians. But vegetarian athletes are especially at risk due to certain deficits in their diets.

Does a vegetarian diet leave some important nutrients out? Do vegetarians need a booster shot of meat once in a while—or at least a booster shot of supplements? Most dieticians agree that protein and minerals such as zinc and iron, all found in important quantities in meat, are necessary for a healthy diet. If you follow a vegetarian diet, here are some ways you can fill these non-meat-linked nutritional deficits with beans, pasta, and rice, or more extreme measures.

DEFICIT: PROTEIN

Besides eliminating fat and cholesterol, a meatless diet reduces protein, which is loaded with nine essential amino acids the body uses to repair its tissues. That is critical for cyclists and endurance athletes, who are constantly stressing their muscles. There are many ways

(continues)

to make up the protein gap, depending on your brand of vegetarianism:

1. Chicken, fish, and dairy (milk and eggs): If you decide to go cold turkey just on red meat, then you do have animal-based alternatives. Non-beef animal products such as poultry, fish, and milk pack as much protein as red meat, supplying all the essential amino acids you need to make new proteins for the body. But strict vegetarians technically won't touch a drumstick, and vegans (who ban any animal derivative) won't do dairy or eggs.

2. Combining legumes and whole grains (for example, the peanut butter sandwich): Vegetable sources of protein lack some of the amino acids the body needs for renewal, unless you eat grains (including whole-grain wheat, barley, rice, quinoa, amaranth, kasha, spelt, oats, rye, corn, millet, and kamut) with legumes (including chickpeas, black beans, lima beans, pinto beans, lentils, black-eyed peas, and split peas) every day. Find them in vegetables and whole grains—including whole-wheat bread and whole-grain rice. Eat both together or at least on the same day.

3. Eat a lot: For a 160-pound sedentary man to get a minimum daily requirement of 8 grams of protein per kilogram (3.66 grams per pound) of body weight, about 60 grams, he must consume 4.5 cups of pasta, three cups of broccoli, and 1.5 cups of tomato sauce. A same-weight athlete, who burns some protein as a form of energy during exercise, needs to nearly double that amount—taking in about 1.2 to 1.6 grams per kilogram of body weight, which will add up to 80 to 110 protein grams. It's easy to get there with meat; a lean, broiled 4-ounce sirloin steak has 31.3 grams of protein. A non-meat diet requires a lot of eating unless you include. . . .

4. Soybeans: This super-legume is the only veggie that can go head-to-head with milk and meat, offering comparable protein quality and amino acids. It doesn't need to be combined with anything. In addition, soybeans contain antioxidant

phytochemicals that help protect against cancer and heart disease—ailments, not surprisingly, that are not nearly as prevalent in Asian countries with soybean-rich diets that include tofu, tempeh, and soymilk.

DEFICIT: IRON

Red meat is a great source of iron, which is essential for preventing anemia, particularly in women, who lose iron through menstruation. The RDA of iron is 10–15 milligrams (mg) a day. A lean, 3.5-ounce steak has 3.5 mg. A similar portion of dark turkey or chicken has 3.1 mg.

While vegetarian fare isn't hurting for iron—firm tofu (10 mg per 3.5 ounce) and fortified breakfast cereal (12–28 mg), plus lentils, kale, collard greens, and dried fruit lead the pack—plant-based iron isn't as well-absorbed as the "heme" iron of animal foods. One sure-fire way to increase iron absorption is to drink orange juice and eat lots of fruit; their vitamin C aids iron absorption. Or you can make a meal that combines dark leafy greens with, say, tomatoes, which are also high in vitamin C.

DEFICIT: ZINC

Zinc, needed for protein synthesis, wound healing, and proper immunity, is also harder for the body to absorb when it comes from plant sources than when it comes from meat. The RDA for zinc is 12 mg a day. Four ounces of beef have 4 mg, fowl 2 mg. Corn and wheat germ, fortified cereals, beans, nuts, tofu, and other soy products have it in decent quantities, too, but to be safe, you may need a boost if you are vegetarian. Dairy foods and a 10 mg zinc supplement will do the trick.

DEFICIT: CALCIUM

Women need at least 1,200 mg a day of calcium, which builds strong bones and prevents osteoporosis. If you consume dairy products, don't worry—a couple cups of milk or yogurt a day will suffice. If dairy is out, try calcium-fortified soymilk (and other milk alternatives, such as almond, rice, or coconut) and dark green leafy vegetables such

(continues)

ATTENTION VEGETARIANS: HOW TO AVOID
THAT "DEFICIT" (continued)

as broccoli, collard greens, and kale. Easiest route: calcium supplements.

DEFICIT: VITAMIN B-12

Long-term deficiencies of vitamin B-12, found only in red meat, poultry, shellfish, and dairy products, can cause anemia and nerve damage. This essential vitamin keeps blood cells healthy and maintains the covering around nerve fibers. You need at least two micrograms of this nutrient every day, an amount available from 8 ounces of skim milk. Athletes may need double this amount, since they consume more calories.

Unlike low calcium levels and other deficiencies, a B-12 deficiency can't always be made up with dairy. Milk and eggs contain B-12, but vegetarians who eat them often still have low levels of the vitamin. If you've cut dairy, it's even harder to get adequate B-12, even though there are many good non-meat sources: fortified cereals, fortified soy, rice and nut milks, and nutritional yeast. Fermented vegetable products, such as miso and tempeh, contain some B-12 because of the fermenting bacteria.

Your best bet if you've cut all dairy products from your diet is to take a daily 2-microgram supplement of vitamin B-12, especially since it can be more easily absorbed than B-12 in food.

INTERVIEW
John Sinibaldi
THE GRAND OLD MAN OF US CYCLING

John Sinibaldi—who died in January 2006 at age 92 after a short battle with lung cancer—was unlike your normal retiree. He had a full head of mostly dark hair. His eyesight was perfect (although his hearing was slipping in his left ear). He hadn't had a cold or flu since the Nixon administration. He worked in his immense garden for hours every day, shoveling dirt, pruning trees, toting jugs of water. He was up at five every morning. He talked fast—and moved fast. He rode a bicycle five days a week, 30 miles per day, 7,000 to 8,000 miles per year, and could still crank it to 30 mph. In short, John Sinibaldi was what we all want to be when we grow up.

And, oh yeah, there's one more thing: nearly 500 cyclists turned out to ride with him on his birthday in 2003—the year he turned 90.

Sinibaldi, Brooklyn-born, New Jersey–bred, and a resident of St. Petersburg, Florida, since 1975, was the grand old man of American cycling. A member of the 1932 and 1936 Olympic teams, he set a US record for the 100K time trial of 2:25:09 in 1935 that stood for 50 years before it was broken. After not riding for nearly 30 years, he un-retired in his 60s and won 14 national Masters time-trial championships, including in 2003, when he rode 12.5 miles in 47 minutes and 8 seconds (16 mph) to win the 85-and-older division at the USA Cycling National Time Trial Championships. He was inducted into the US Bicycling Hall of Fame in 1997. His multigenerational riding buddies at the St. Petersburg Bike Club called him "The Legend." Still spry and limber at 90, he could jump into the air and touch his toes—literally jumping for joy.

What was Sinibaldi's secret to a long, active life? Here's what he told Bike for Life in his interview in March 2004: "Ride your bike like crazy. Hope for good genes [he had two sisters in their 80s]. Grow and eat your own vegetables. Eat red meat only when it's on sale. Listen to classical music. Avoid television. Read the newspaper every day and do the crossword puzzle. Go barefoot most of the time. When you find a gear you like, stick with it. And get your rest on the bike while you climb the hills."

I BOUGHT MY first bicycle in 1928, paid $25 for it. It was a secondhand one, but pretty good. I was 14. I never rode a bicycle before in my life, but a friend of mine who rode said, why don't you try it? And I did—and liked it.

They said I was always a good athlete, but I never considered myself that before the bicycle. I was short, undersized—about 5-foot-4. I didn't really become full-grown (5-foot-11) until I was almost 20. But on the bike, it just came. I never got tired, that was one thing. And the others did.

I started school in 1918, something like that. But in 1921, my father was laid up in bed, somehow he got better, and then we migrated to Italy.

Vice-a-versa. Since I couldn't speak Italian, I lost all my education, and had to repeat grades all over again.

It was right after the war [World War I], and there was no work there. So my father left us to get work. I went to school, but also had to have a job on the side.

Then we came back to the United States, so I started all over again at 12 years old. They put me in 1A school [first grade]. Imagine, me, that age, with all the little kids? Heh! So I never had no education. I went to school two more years, then I quit. At 14, I lived in Jersey and was working in New York in a factory. I was a laborer.

How could I be an athlete? You couldn't be an athlete at that time unless you went to school, and—you wouldn't believe it, but it's the truth—the only people who finished high school were the ones that their parents either had a business or were well-to-do, like they were doctors. But the poor class never finished school. He quit when he was of age. He was allowed to quit at the age of 14. You couldn't afford to go to school.

Spending $25 for a bike was a lot of money, but I was working in New York, making a big salary. Oh, big! I was making $20 a week moving sheet metal. That was just before the Depression hit. After that, when Roosevelt got elected, they passed what they called the NRA [National Recovery Act], and I was making $13 a week.

Immediate Success

ANY TIME I had time off, it was on a bicycle. It was so much fun. At night, when I came home from work, right on a bicycle. I never owned a car, so I never drove. I took a trolley or subways to work. We lived in Union City—where the Lincoln Tunnel comes out on the Jersey side. Soon as I came home from work, we'd eat, get on the bike, and put in 40 miles. Every night.

We'd go up to the New York state line and back. Lotta hills up there. You go all the way up, then go down to the Hudson River and back. It was like a big rollercoaster. It was nice.

We did it for fun, but it was good training. Soon, we joined the North Hudson Wheelmen and we were training with the pros. They treated us nice. They were human beings—not snobs.

I got into racing when the guys told me to. The club had races on a cinder track. They found out I was better than the other ones, so they began to give the other ones a head start.

The first entries in my scrapbook are about 1930—the first time I rode big races. I rode two big ones—one in 1930 and one in 1931. I was still underage. I became 18 in 1932. That's when I won the big ones [laughs]. That's when I started winning 'em all. As a matter of fact, the first four races in '32, I won 'em. A 100-mile race, a 62.5-mile race, they had a 50-mile race, and then there was a 25-mile race on Coney Island. That was a big race, what a mob. It was a flat course. Only 25. The shortest race I ever rode.

At that time, cycling was the biggest sport in the United States. Not football, not baseball—cycling was it.

It was the greatest sport. Those six-day races in New York—oh god, it was mobbed every night. A two-man team race that goes on 24 hours a day for six days. They keep going around, one of the two team members on the track. They cover around 2,500 to 3,000 miles in that week.

I never did those, because they were only for pros. I never turned professional, but I used to beat all the pros. All the kids I grew up with became pros, and I beat 'em all [laughs]. The pros made good money. They were paid higher than baseball players. But I enjoyed the sport so much being an amateur, believe it or not, that I never turned pro. There's no fun in pros. It's a money affair there. The fun disappears.

At the time, I was doing piecework; it was manual labor. They wanted me to ride the six-day races. One of my friends, he was a pro, he said, "No, you're too young for that." At which he was right. To turn 18 as a pro, it would've been bad.

People ask me a lot: Any regrets, not turning pro? No, none, never did, never came to me, no.

And every time I look at what I won, I've won it all by myself. Nobody helped me: no combos, nothing. All clean. That's how I rode, and I enjoyed it.

The pros was a bad vibe. And some of them did drugs. There were different drugs than today—what you call "uppers." But they didn't die young. They lived to be an old age. Today, bicycle racers reach 40 and they're dead. No, I didn't like that kind of a life. There was no fun in it.

Sports at that time was a fun life. You went to the Olympics, and everybody was a friend there. Not like today, where all the sports people seem to hate each other.

1932: Olympics, Jim Thorpe, and Hollywood Parties

I QUALIFIED IN the New Jersey state elimination. It was tough. Then there was a section elimination, and then they had the final in California—in San Francisco. We rode out there by steam train—that was nice.

California was the most beautiful place. I was gonna retire there because it was so beautiful. Never seen a place so beautiful.

Funny thing, three of the four Olympic qualifiers were from our one club in New Jersey—the North Hudson Wheelmen. Otto Ludecke, Frank Cano, and me. Charley Morton was from California—no, that was '36. The fourth rider was—I don't remember—from California. He was a good rider. Rode in the '28 Olympics.

The week after the trials, we went straight to the Olympics camp. A 500-mile train from San Francisco to Los Angeles.

When we got to the Olympics camp, a woman came around and said to Otto, "I'm your matron. I gotta take care of you. You're underage." He wasn't 16 yet. He lied about his age to get in to the Olympics [laughs].

A sad thing: One day when we were at the stadium [Los Angeles Coliseum], there were two people standing outside, and it was Johnny Weissmuller trying to get Jim Thorpe into the stadium to see the games. Thorpe was banned from the games. He could not go in. We had seats for all of 'em. We had 5,000 seats in there. Johnny was trying to get him in, but it didn't work. Thorpe played professional baseball for money. That was the rule. *[Thorpe, a Sac and Fox Indian, played in the minor leagues before winning gold medals by huge margins in the decathlon and pentathlon in the Stockholm Olympics in 1912. He was stripped of his medals the following year for playing semi-professional baseball.]*

We were right there, walking in. They [Thorpe and Weissmuller] were right there, standing outside. If I would have known about it, I would have taken my jacket off and given it to him, and he could've got in that way, with the athletes [laughs].

The Olympics was pretty private. I mean, there was very little media coverage. They never even knew we existed; we never met any media.

But we did meet Joe E. Brown, the famous comedian. He made a movie, too, *The Six-Day Rider*. He was very interested in us. We met him twice. When we went to Germany [in 1936 at the Berlin Olympics], he was there again. He ate with us at the same restaurant in the camp.

We met a lot of people. We were guests all over, which was very nice. To give you an idea, all the movie stars invited us to their parties. Don't remember who they were. All of 'em dead now.

I do remember one guy, James Agony, with the hatchet nose. He was an official at the bike races at the track they built right inside the Rose Bowl in Pasadena.

We had an official representative assigned to manage us, but the guy couldn't tell us anything. We were self-coached. We knew all the rules. We went through all that at home.

No one told us what to eat. In my time, there was no special food for athletes. We ate a lotta pasta, beans, a lotta bread. And no liquor. It was Prohibition times, but we never drank liquor, anyway. Very little soda. We had some ice cream and different things. But as far as food, meat very little, and a lotta fish. Fish was cheap back then. Only the poor people ate fish at that time. Today, only the rich people eat it. Ha-ha.

We didn't do any warm-up, like these people do today. Stretching? Massage? We never did those things. We'd warm up in the race. Don't worry about it.

We were fast then. I'd say we could pedal faster than the guys today, even though we only had one-speed bikes, that's all. There were no problems with that. The derailleur was rare in '32, as far as I know. I rode a single-speed. When we went down big hills, we didn't let them [people with freewheels] coast. We pedaled hard so they had to pedal to stay with us. So they couldn't rest, believe me. *[Note: The freewheel and a rudimentary derailleur were first used at the Tour de France in 1937, but the modern dual-jockey wheel/ parallelogram design didn't arrive until Tullio Campagnolo's Gran Sport in 1951. Riders in Sinibaldi's era either used a simple fixed-gear or a two-sided- hub wheel that had a freewheel for descending/ climbing on one side and a fixed gear on the other for riding the flats. Races were often won by the speed at which a rider could dismount, loosen the wingnuts on the hub, flip the wheel, and reset the chain.]*

I only participated in one event in the '32 Olympics—the 100-kilometer road-race time trial, 62 and a half miles. We didn't compete on the track—there were four events: four-man pursuit race, 1-kilometer time trial, a two-man event, mass sprint, and a two-man tandem—because the guy that represented us wouldn't let us. We did go on the track for training, though. We rode a four-man pursuit race against the US team to train them, and after three or four laps we caught them. So they weren't that good.

I didn't do too good in the time trial. I was riding good. I drank something that didn't agree with me. Something in the bottle. I still did it in 2 hours, 40 minutes. It was pretty fast, but I still could've done much faster that day. According to the reports, I was in second place halfway. But when I drank, that was the end. No medal.

A New Record, Moonshine, and the 1936 Olympics

MY EMPLOYERS HAD agreed to give me a leave of absence to go to California. I went back to work after the Olympics, getting $7 a week. It wasn't enough, but it was all I was used to.

In 1933, I rode a half a year. I won my first two races, and then I fell and hurt my back. Did not ride at all in '34. They repaired my back with a new operation, a spinal fusion. But I came back in '35 with a steel brace—and was faster. Better than I was when I was younger!

I did the metric 100 [100K] in 2 hours, 25 minutes—took 10 minutes off my old best time and set a new record. In fact, in 1975, I was talking to a girl at a supermarket checkout line who was reading *Bicycling* magazine. She turns to me and says, "Hey, your record from 1935 is still alive." *[Note: It was finally broken 10 years later.]*

I won quite a few races at that time. Nobody could beat me, actually. Oh god, everybody wanted my wheel. If there was a pack ride and I came up there, everyone moved aside so they could get on my wheel and at least they'd get second. "That's a good wheel to get on," that's what they'd all say. They all knew it.

I was doing nothing different. I ate the same thing as I always did. Always working the same. I always went to bed early. I never went out, gallivanting like they do today. Or drink. That was bad. One of our pros used to say, "Don't smoke— it's no good." Things like that we didn't do. Anything that was bad we didn't do. Anybody who tells you to "drink beer, it's good for you," is crazy.

I didn't drink alcohol at all. We made it and sold it, yes. My mother used to make liquor during Prohibition. I used to deliver it. Drink it? No.

I really wanted to go to the Olympics again. It was 1936, and I was still young yet. In fact, I wanted to go to three more. There was nuthin to it [making the team]. Like going downhill. I finished in a tie for second to qualify.

The trip was by ocean liner, which was good. You didn't have to go by train. When I went by train to California, I didn't have the money. I sat for four nights and four days on that train. It was a long haul, believe me. But the ship, the *Manhattan*—it was a nice, beautiful ship. We were all together, all the athletes. Everybody knew everybody. It was lots of fun.

Media coverage of the '36 Olympics was exactly the opposite of 1932. Lotta coverage. Met a lotta great people. Lotta reporters. Not like today, though. No TV.

There was a grand total of six cyclists on the team, four on the road team, two for the track. Two from the North Hudson Bike Club, one from Chicago, one from California.

Once in Berlin, few athletes had full access, but we had to train and rode all over the city and the countryside. Nobody stopped us and asked anything. It was wide open. It's hard to say about what went on afterward with the Holocaust; the problem wasn't obvious to us. They already told them [the Jews] to leave, and the rich ones did. The poor ones, it wasn't so easy. There were no signs, no graffiti.

I did see [signs of] underground bunkers. They were preparing for war, oh yes. All the roads were dug up. Everything was going underground. We went out riding looking for planes, but we couldn't find them. They had put the hangers underground. It was real advanced, everything.

As for the people, they seemed free. Every night, beer gardens all over the place, they're all out there drinking beer and everything after work. Young people, old people. You couldn't tell they were living under the Nazis. Everybody was working. Germany was booming.

In the 100K road race [the first Olympic mass-start race, rather than a time trial], the first hill we come to, somebody goes down and takes 25 of us down. We fell at the bottom of the hill. Imagine getting started at the bottom of a hill. By the time we got up, the pack was far away. So we chased 'em. A guy fell in front of us and takes us down again. And we get up again and it was four of us chasing. We went down four times,

including one at the finish, too. Four spills. I finished way back.

We also rode the four-man team race at the track. Rode against the Netherlands. They shoot the gun, we went off, and we started to chase them. We went harder, and caught 'em and passed 'em. Then we slowed up. Since we won, the next day we went back to go against the other team, and got a shock: We were told we were disqualified for going too slow. We didn't have a fast enough time.

The international rules were based on time—but we didn't know that. In the US, you catch the team, and the race is over. When we caught the Netherlands team, we thought we were finished. We would have been way up there in the qualifications. But nobody knew.

When I came back from Germany, I got on a bike right away, within a week. The '40 and '44 Olympics were canceled due to the war. The 1940 Olympics was supposed to be in Japan, but Japan invades China and they call it off. But then they moved it to Finland, and Russia invades Finland. So that was called off.

I tried to qualify for the '48 Olympics, at age 34. I qualified for the state and even the sectional. At the sectional, I went down into a hole, broke my wheel, but then got a wheel off somebody and went out and caught the pack and qualified.

I was hurting so bad in the finals in Milwaukee, a 130-mile race. It had been a week since the sectional, and I wasn't healed [from the fall]; my ribs were separated. After 90 miles in Milwaukee, I went to the front, then quit. I couldn't breathe. Oh god, it was brutal! I thought I would heal. But ripped-up ribs take a long time to heal. At least I quit from the front.

After that, in '49, I quit for good. I got married. That ends the racing.

By then, in the races, I was getting the prize for the oldest rider. I wouldn't take it. At that time, they didn't have no Masters, or I'd have kept cycling. I rode a little bit after that, then I stopped for 30 years.

Retirement, Family Life, and Rebirth as a Legend

[SINIBALDI'S 48-YEAR-OLD SON *and frequent riding buddy, John Jr., interjects here*] *You didn't stop riding completely, Dad. I remember when we lived in Butler, New Jersey, my dad taking out a track bike off hooks in the garage, maybe once a month in the summer. Early in the morning—6:30 on a Saturday, we'd hear the garage door open. We'd still be in bed. He'd be back 8:30, 9 o'clock. Then he'd go out into the garden. Dad has two passions in life. He loves to ride and he loves to garden.*

He didn't talk about the old cycling days hardly at all to us kids. Dad didn't talk a lot growing up. I first heard the stories when I was 12, at Lenny Conditi's funeral in 1966. All the guys standing around. All the stories started with "Remember the time John was in the lead; remember the time chasing John; remember the time John won that; no matter what we did, when John showed up, we knew we'd all be racing for second." Even though we all knew Dad was in the Olympics, it wasn't until then that I recognized just how good my dad was. It wasn't until he retired, when I was an adult, that I began to really hear my dad's stories.

I KEPT IN shape by working in the shop—which was heavy work. Sheet metal is heavy; everything you lift is in the hundreds of pounds. Eventually I tried three, four different jobs and became a sheet metal mechanic. After all those years, I retired in 1975 getting $6 an hour. I was a top-paid man [said sarcastically].

At home, I worked in my garden. A huge garden in New Jersey. Did everything by hand. Turned all the dirt by hand.

When I retired and came down here to Florida in 1976, one day I took the bike out for the heck of it. That was the beginning; I went by a library and I saw a bunch of people standing there with bicycles. It was the St. Pete Bike Club. They said, "We go out every Sunday."

That's what I wanted to hear. I had somebody to go out with.

I was 62. Some of the club riders were pretty young, so it got a little rough in there. A few of the 20-year-olds were pretty fast. They rode me hard. But after a month or so, I kept getting better until I became the fastest rider.

I was the fastest rider of that club until I was 77. I could go out there and do almost 30 miles an hour. When I was 75, I lapped everyone at the Sunshine State Games criterium in the 65-plus and 55-plus age groups, and rode with the 45-year-olds. I won a $25 prime that year, but I was worried about accepting it because I was afraid they'd take away my amateur status.

Riding Secrets: Rest on Climbs, Stay Cool in Underwear

I RIDE FIVE days a week. I try to ride around 150 miles per week—about 30 miles each time. I take Mondays and Thursdays off. I gotta do my laundry, gotta hang the pots outside, gotta do shopping. I work harder now than when I was working. I don't get done till 7 o'clock at night, usually.

What do I think of Lance Armstrong? He's a good rider, no getting away from it. He's a type like I am: He rests when he's going uphill. That's when I do all my resting—uphill.

On the flat, everything goes pretty fast. But on the hills, everybody slows up. So that's when I'd rest. Three-quarters of the hill I'd rest, and the last quarter I'd take off. Armstrong didn't see me do it, but he got the same idea somehow [laughs]. When you can rest on the hills, believe me, you've got it.

As for gearing, I believe in leverage. I don't shift gears. I ride in the big ring, but I also ride with the big ring in the back [gears]. To have it in the small gear in the front and the small gear in the back—there's no leverage there.

I don't ride in a faster cadence than anyone else nowadays. It's a relaxing ride. I go 18 to 20 miles per hour. Maybe up to 25 mph, I can hang right there in the middle. I can still hit 30 mph in a sprint once in a while.

I definitely have declined, I can tell. Believe me, there are times when I feel older than 90.

A turning point was when I got slowed down by an accident when I was 77, my last crit. I broke my back, fractured several vertebrae. Took a long time to come back. While I was healing, I found out I had colon cancer. Luckily, I recuperated very quickly. In fact, I won another gold medal while on chemo at the national championships that year.

I don't do weights. Nothing. No other exercise besides cycling and gardening. I garden four to five hours a day, and it's like a combination weights and stretching routine. All by hand. I can stand straight up and touch the ground with my hands.

I ride a Kestrel [200SCI], and here's how I got it: I was going to do the '94 Race Across America 10 years ago on an over-70 team. My wife wasn't pleased about that. A week before the race, they said they didn't need me. But two months later, in the mail we get a brand-new Kestrel frame. Kestrel had sponsored the team for five riders. We hung a Campy record group on it. Probably put 7,000 to 8,000 miles a year on it for the last six to seven years. Probably got 50,000 miles on it. *[Note: The Kestrel was wrecked when Sinibaldi was hit by a car in April '04; now he rides a steel frame he had in his garage.]*

I use an old pair of Adidas cycling shoes, about 20 years old. Off the bike, I never wear shoes—just to weddings and funerals. Everything I do, I do barefoot. So my feet are wide. None of the cycling shoes fit. I got my Adidas for half-price because the guy couldn't sell 'em, they were so wide.

I use toe-clips like in the olden days. I like the pull-on straps. I wear a helmet. Didn't for a long time. It was compulsory to wear a leather hair net when I raced.

I used to ride those 100-mile races without drinking a drop of water. I don't sweat much. It takes me all day to finish a water bottle.

I have one secret: Wear a shirt under your jersey, no matter how hot it is, wool, anything. It'll get damp right away, and you will never use any sweat anymore. It'll keep you cool all summer, and you won't dehydrate. Like these runners that take everything off, the girls who have just a bra on, they dehydrate. They look dry. But they dehydrate, because the sun just dries them right up. If they were covered, they wouldn't have to drink.

Back when we rode a 100-mile race, who's going to give us water when we're riding from one city to another?

As a matter of fact, the old-timers all used a shirt under a shirt. When you see these guys today with a plastic jacket, they are dehydrating so fast. In other words, you go to Africa or Egypt, or any of these Arab countries, ask these guys to take that white shirt off—that sort of dress they wear—and they got a woolen shirt underneath it in the desert.

Diet Secrets: Soup, Veggies, Gardening, and No Restaurant Dinners

"WHAT DO YOU do that keeps you so young?" everyone asks me. It's what I don't do that's healthy. Not drinking, not smoking. I never smoked when I rode. I smoked a few cigarettes a day and a pipe a bit after I retired from bicycling for about 20 years. Then I quit in the '60s.

I'm a soup and vegetable man. Four or five different soups I make from scratch. A meat soup with ham. A vegetable soup. I have a 10-gallon pot. I throw in chickpeas in the water. Then rosemary. Garlic. Pepper and salt. On top, I put a half-inch of olive oil. Then I let it boil. It becomes a soup. It's beautiful.

I grow everything from peanuts to pineapples—three rows. In fact, I roast the peanuts myself and grind them into peanut butter. I make my own pasta, tomato soup. I grow cabbage, strawberries, kale, carrots, corn, parsley, cauliflower, onions, Swiss chard, parsley, fennel, rosemary, and one 50-foot double row of garlic. I have pecan trees. All on an oversized lot in St. Pete—a 50 by 90 plot.

I bake my own bread—8 to 10 loaves every couple weeks. Sometimes I make pizza from scratch when all the guys [from the bike club] come over here. I make my own pasta sauce and pasta.

My diet hasn't changed much over the years. Chicken. Liver. Whatever is on sale.

I don't eat too much meat, only when it's on sale. I eat fish when it's free. I won't pay for it. My Social Security is under $2,000 a year, so how can I buy it? I eat corned beef and eat it with cabbage and salad. I'll save the juice and use it three times. When the corned beef is left over, I'll make corned beef hash. Every once in a while—maybe twice a month—I'll have red meat, a hamburger. Not much chicken, either, really. The Atkins diet—all beef? No, no, that's bad. If you must eat beef, always make it well done, never rare. And don't eat anything fried.

I'm afraid to eat energy bars and gels. Any of that kind of food is something artificial; it doesn't sound right.

The best advice? Do all the right things. In other words, do all the things you hate to do, and do them right [laughs]. Do the things you say, "I don't wanna do this, I don't wanna do that." You find out that you live longer. It's important to eat the right things, and keep away from the restaurants a little bit. You're not gonna buy something you don't like at a restaurant; you're gonna buy something you like, and most of the time, it's not good for you.

We go to breakfast at the Gold Cup Coffee Shop three times a week with the club. Lot of the riders are overweight, but the stuff they order is unbelievable—fried eggs, fried hash, fried sausage. I eat a muffin. Or at home, a nice big bowl of oatmeal with raisins and milk. I have a tea on the side. I don't drink much coffee.

For lunch today I had a big cabbage soup, which had all the vegetables in it you can think of. And some chicken stock. For dessert, a slice of pineapple. Tonight, I may have an oversized bowl of oatmeal for dinner; that tastes good at night.

Don't eat a big meal before you go to bed at night, like these guys go out to eat at 7, 8 at night. You're not going to get rid of it; it's going to just sit there in their stomach.

And be busy. I've always got something to do. If I keep moving, I like it. If I sit down, no good.

The Best Memory in 90 Years

MY BEST RACE was a 100-mile race in New York in 1933. It was raining all the night before. I had wooden rims. I put shellac on the rims and used one brake. The race started at 5 in the morning. We had to take the ferry to the 59th Street Bridge. But when we got there, there's nobody there.

"They're all gone," someone said. "You're too late."

We got the highway number, ran to a garage station and got a can of grease, because it was raining hard. We greased up our whole legs to keep us warm in the rain—just like the people who swim across the English Channel.

We chased and chased and chased. We came to a 90-degree turn around a corner, and I applied the brake—it grabbed on and pulled right through the wheel. I jumped off the bike and bent the brakes out to make room for the [out-of-true] wheel, so I had no more brakes. Freewheel and no brakes. A 100-mile race!

Finally, after 70 miles, we caught the group. The last 30 miles it was up-and-down, up-and-down. We're going down a hill, and here we have another 90-degree turn; I had no brakes. So I jammed into the back of two riders; I grabbed one guy on one side and the other guy on the other, no hands on the handlebars, and make the turn.

I tell you, I got gray hairs that day. Maybe 15 miles from the finish, I took off, took two guys with me, and that was the end. I won it. It's late. No brakes. It's raining.

God, was I riding good that day!

6

BICYCLE SEX

Cycling and impotence: easy solutions to an (un-)hard problem

"[The] sex is out of this world. My wife jokes about my prowess." —Mike Miller, 53, 8,000-miles-per-year rider, August 2004 (Bike for Life, Chapter 12)

Nineteen percent of cyclists who had a weekly training distance of more than 400 kilometers (250 miles) complained of erectile dysfunction. —2001 study of 40 German cyclists by Dr. Frank Sommer

Selle SMP saddle

"When I'm not riding, I'm with Jody, providing her with endless sexual pleasure." — Dan Cain, 46, 20- to 30-hours-per-week mountain biker, September 2004 (Bike for Life, Chapter 12)

Frequent mountain biking may reduce fertility in men, according to an Austrian study. Of 55 avid mountain bikers who each rode at least 3,000 miles per year, an average of two hours per day, six days a week, nearly 90 percent had low sperm count and scrotal abnormalities, about three times the percentage of non-bikers with these problems. Researcher Dr. Ferdinand Frauscher, a urology-radiology specialist at University Hospital in Innsbruck,

suggests the cause is the frequent jolts and vibration caused by biking over rough terrain. —Presentation at Radiological Society of North America, December 2002

Riding a bike may substitute for Viagra in some men with weak heart muscles, according to Dr. Romualdo Belardinelli, director of the Lancisi Heart Institute in Ancona, Italy. "Cycling improves your sexual function," he said. Questionnaires given to 29 male heart patients and their sex partners showed the men who rode had better erections compared to the study's non-exercisers. —American Heart Association conference in Anaheim, California, November 12, 2001

"Men should never ride bicycles. Riding should be banned and outlawed. It is the most irrational form of exercise I could ever bring to discussion." —Dr. Irwin Goldstein, 1997

When you graph the impotency rates of cyclists against the general male population, cyclists were half as likely to suffer severe impotence and one-third as likely to suffer any form of impotence. —Charlie McCorkell, owner, Bicycle Habitat bike shop, New York City, at New York University School of Medicine Conference, December 2000

Fourteen of 15 members of the Marine Bicycle Patrol of the Long Beach Police Department, who each ride six hours a day, five days a week, complained of genital numbness during or after their rides. While none experienced impotence, Rigiscan erection monitoring devices measured a one-third reduction in erection quality and duration during sleep. The police were advised to study the feasibility of switching to noseless bike seats. —National Institute of Occupational Safety and Health, May 2001

Blood supply to the penises of healthy men, which fell by two-thirds from normal when they sat on a bike seat for three minutes, increased to 110 percent of normal levels when they pedaled in a standing-up position for a minute. —"Pressure During Cycling," BJU International, April 1999

A couple of cyclists once told me that they measured their rides in two ways: total miles ridden, and the degree of numbness in their crotch. Numbness was good, a barometer of a solid training session, and it usually un-numbed quickly, so why worry? Then came the 1997 article in Bicycling magazine, and things changed. People stopped riding, but some took a few precautions: a new saddle with a hole scooped out of it, a new bike fit, a habit of standing up more. Given what we know now, it's dumb to be numb.

🚲

It's a debate that still has legs, though the passion that the controversy once aroused has ebbed. "We don't see guys walking into our stores like we used to, all worried and inquiring about becoming impotent from cycling," said Mike Jacoubowsky, co-owner of Chain Reaction Bicycles of Redwood City and Los Altos, California. So does this mean men shouldn't be concerned about their plumbing? Does it mean that the famous (or infamous) 1997 article in *Bicycling* magazine that started the "cycling-causes-impotence" firestorm was wrong—or that its lessons have been forgotten?

What's the truth about the bicycle-impotency issue?

The truth is that we don't know what percentage of cyclists is impotent, but that it's probably higher than the percentage of runners and swimmers who are impotent. And yet it's certainly far lower than the percentage of the general population that is impotent. We do know that there is some undefined risk of impotency in cycling, but not for the vast majority of riders, as an alarmed cycling community came to believe after the aforementioned *Bicycling* article and subsequent airing of a similar story on ABC's *20/20* program. We do have a good idea of which bike riders are most at risk of impotency: ultra-distance riders who've logged 200-plus miles a week for years.

One such rider was the courageous 50-year-old *Bicycling* magazine editor who revealed his impotency in an essay in the magazine; he'd averaged 14,000 miles per year for seven years, much of it in the aerobar position while training for cross-state records and team Race Across America events.

That rider, who asked not to be named here, deserves our thanks. By personalizing the issue, he emboldened other cyclists to seek help and motivated the bike industry to do three things: **make safer bike seats, pay more attention to proper bike fit, and do a better job of teaching sex-safe riding technique.**

Bike for Life strongly advocates that those precautions, spelled out in detail later in this chapter, be observed by *all* cyclists, regardless of mileage. Here's why:

1. You never know. As you'll see below, although numbness indicates temporary (and generally non-damaging) obstruction of blood vessels and nerves, problems can arise as mega-miles add up over the years. But given variations in anatomy, riding style, and vascular resiliency, impotency has occasionally occurred in lower-mileage riders, too.

2. Taking precautions is cheap and easy. It's like putting on sunblock, said one man; the small inconvenience is worth the off-chance that it will stop skin cancer (impotency).

3. You're rewarded with super sex. Safe-sex cycling does more than preserve your sex life—it upgrades it. Numerous studies indicate that cycling, like all aerobic activity, stokes the libido, enhances endurance and power, and supercharges the duration and quality of sex.

ANATOMY OF A SQUISHED VESSEL

To understand why numbness and impotency occur in the first place, and why no cyclist should ignore it, let's go back to Anatomy 101: Sitting on a bike seat *improperly* can put unusual stresses on the perineum, the soft area between the base of the penis and the anus that houses the nerves and two main blood vessels responsible for an erection. When you sit straight up, as you do in a flat desk chair, your weight is focused on the pelvic bones known as "sit bones." But when you lean forward on the nose of a narrow bike saddle, your weight shifts forward and between these sit bones—directly on the delicate perineum.

"When a man sits on a bicycle seat, he's putting his entire body weight on the arteries that supplies the penis," said Dr. Irwin Goldstein, director of the Boston University Medical Center urology department and the featured player in the storied 1997 *Bicycling* article that broke the cycling-impotence connection. Although he'd studied bike-related impotency for years, Goldstein suddenly became the issue's "founding father" and an overnight media sensation. He was assailed by the bike industry as a scare-mongering, publicity-hungry opportunist who shamelessly preyed on male rider's fears. Unrepentant, he asserted that probably 100,000 male

cyclists in America had problems with impotence, that no one should ride a bike for more than three hours a week, and that the ideal bike saddle would be "shaped like a toilet seat."

This wasn't wild speculation, Goldstein explained, but a sober analysis of anatomy: From a study of 100 impotent patients, he had determined that it only took 11 percent of a man's body weight to compress the perineum arteries, causing a 66 percent average reduction in penile blood flow, when subjects were on a skinny bike saddle. Sit on those arteries enough times, compress them, rub them, flatten them out, and accumulate scar tissue in the artery walls, he explained, and eventually the arteries will become like a soft-drink straw you chew on: permanently narrowed and squished.

"For cyclists who put in many miles," he said, "it's a nightmarish situation."

How nightmarish? Try *Friday the 13th* grab-your-private-parts nightmarish. Just ask reporter Joe Lindsey, who visited Cologne, Germany, in April 2004 to write an update of the impotency issue for an article in *Bicycling's* January 2005 issue, "The Hard Truth." Lindsey was invited on the trip because an earlier article he'd written, about the damage done by the impact of mountain biking, had attracted the attention of Roger Minkow, who had gained fame as the designer of a popular anti-impotence saddle after reading the original 1997 *Bicycling* article. (Minkow was a Napa Valley doctor, ergonomics researcher, and spine-center founder who had also invented and successfully marketed lumbar-supportive airline pilot's seats—more on his story below.) Lindsey and Minkow traveled to the University of Cologne's Poliklinik for Urology to meet Dr. Frank Sommer, who would be conducting the first study to measure actual blood flow among cyclists while they pedaled.

Sommer, then 37, so respected that he was named the minister of health for the European Union earlier that year, had already conducted a

2001 study in *European Urology* that opened eyes: He found that 61 percent of 40 healthy German bike riders had numbness; worse, a fifth of those clocking over 400 kilometers per week complained of erectile dysfunction. He later surveyed 1,700 German cyclists and found similar problems.

Technically, Sommer explained, the problem is low penile oxygen retention, which causes increased collagen development. "That's very bad for the penis," he told me in a telephone interview on April 20, 2004. "Over the long term, you will lose elasticity. You will lose capacity of getting blood into the penis and holding it there. If you have sexual arousal, your erection won't be as good."

"Of course," he added, "this is a very long-term problem. This takes many, many years of riding before you find this problem." Mountain bikers are not immune, Sommer said, but for a different reason: trauma. "Shock waves to the perineum from impact can damage arterial vessels, which leads to restricted blood flow," he said.

In April 2004, Sommer became the first researcher to apply an oxygen-saturation measurement device to penile blood flow. He tested about 20 saddles on dozens of German amateur bike racers and triathletes. The results from his breakthrough study—in which Joe Lindsey was a participant—basically confirmed Goldstein's assertions and should serve as a wake-up call to riders who haven't yet gotten the message.

As Lindsey told *Bike for Life*, he had the ride of his life in Dr. Sommer's small, bare-bones lab—and it wasn't pleasant. In fact, it was unnerving. Yet, for some unexplained reason, his confession never made it into the magazine. Here's what Lindsey told me: "It was definitely a weird, funky situation. On the head of your penis, they taped a little centimeter-long capsule filled with water; it was the size of a watch battery. It measures oxygen saturation, which is directly correlated to blood flow. Sommer was the first to figure out this relationship.

"As you ride, a digital readout appears on a small screen in front of you. To get a good comparison, we were measured beforehand, while standing there, not on the bike. My raw number was 37, a measure of capillary density. Everyone's raw number is different, but whatever number you get is your 100 percent. All the subsequent on-the-bike numbers will be compared, in my case, to 37.

"The on-the-bike test is just seven minutes long. Which in itself is limiting, considering that cyclists ride a lot longer. After all, you never know what'll happen after an hour or eight hours.

"The first test was on my Fizik Alliante saddle, the one I've used almost every day for two years. Pedaling on the bike for a minute, my number drops off the f—ing cliff—to 6 (from 37)! I've lost 85 percent of my blood flow! [That wasn't so bad, actually. In his *Bicycling* story, Lindsey reported that another subject lost 95 percent of his blood flow.]

"Now I knew from watching a previous test subject that your number initially drops way off and then slowly comes back. Not all the way, but it tops out after about 4 minutes. Okay, cool, mine's coming back, we're on schedule, I thought. But after 4 minutes, I'm bummed. It didn't come back much—just to 10 or 12. I've still lost 70 percent of my blood flow!"

Lindsey was surprised to find that there was no correlation between comfort and blood flow. "I'm sitting there looking down at the seat I rode Montezuma's Revenge on because it is so comfortable—and I'm thinking, 'What's scary is that it *is* comfortable—and reducing my blood flow to a trickle!!'" he said.

There were several problems with Lindsey's test that he said might have skewed the results. "My set-up was wrong. The bike that they had there was too big for me and didn't have clipless pedals. Could it have affected the results? And Sommer, who administered the study, told me, 'Stay calm, don't affect the test by thinking about it.' But inside my head, I was thinking, 'That's crazy—I'm not thinking about *anything else!*'

"I was tested on three other saddles. They got progressively better. The last was best. I had 100 percent blood flow on the Specialized Body Geometry Road Pro saddle. Guess what I'm riding now?"

According to Lindsey, Sommer and Minkow ultimately concluded that no saddle can completely eliminate compression, and that numbness generally starts when there is 50 percent blood flow reduction for an hour or more. Minor blood flow reduction—10 to 20 percent—is no worry; that's about what you get sitting on an average desk chair.

MAKING A BETTER BIKE SEAT

Today, many manufacturers offer an "open-wedge" bike seat, which features a deep cut-out extending from the rear to the center or front of the saddle that is designed to eliminate the seat's contact area with the perineum. The paradox is that it owes its existence to Goldstein. On the one hand, he was attacked for his anti-biking message and research, which many cyclists thought seemed contrived and lacking in scientific rigor; yet on the other hand, his conclusions sparked a new growth industry in anatomically contoured seats.

"Dr. Goldstein is the man that we kind of love for what he did for our sales," said Paula Dyba, the marketing director of Terry Bicycles, which had been making bikes solely for women for nearly two decades when the impotency wave hit in 1997. Several years earlier, Terry had debuted the Liberator, a unique women's saddle with a hole cut out from it to relieve female chafing (see sidebar near end of chapter, "Women Cyclists and Sexual Dysfunction"). "The idea was comfort—nothing medical, just comfort," she said. "We got laughed at. Some people called it a 'toilet seat.' Then, surprisingly, we started getting calls—and orders from men."

"We couldn't claim that we stopped impotency—no saddle can," said Dyba. But we can claim comfort. We began working with the Italian seat maker Selle Italia to make a Liberator for male riders. The seat was designed to shift the rider's weight off the perineum, and has a long groove down its middle and is hollowed out in front. The seat became our number-one-selling product that year because of the hysteria over impotency. It grew the saddle business phenomenally. And sales stayed that way until 2003. Sales only dropped off because so many imitators have been coming into the market."

One of those imitators was Specialized's Body Geometry, the narrow saddle Minkow had developed, which had a V-shaped wedge cut from the rear. "I started riding a bike in 1997," Minkow said. Soon after that, he saw Joe Kita's article, "Are You at Risk?" the famous 1997 article in *Bicycling*: "Within three weeks," said Minkow, "I designed a bike seat with a cut-out wedge—which I thought was a big improvement over the hole in the Terry saddle, since men need the pressure relieved further back. I sent it to the *Bicycling* editor [with the impotency problem]. And soon after that, I got a call from Specialized's president, Mike Sinyard. 'I'd like you to help us,' he said."

"Sinyard is a visionary," said Minkow. "He smelled that this was a good opportunity.... There was resistance from all his people, but he said we need to do this. Sinyard backed the ergo-seat project even when his own dealers rejected it. They would send the product back."

In September 1998, a year after the original *Bicycling* impotency article, the magazine published a product review of the Specialized seat and gave it five chainrings, the best rating. Sales skyrocketed. Soon, Diamondback, Avocet, Serfas, and other companies started manufacturing seats designed to avoid compression of the perineum. Millions sold. Men were obviously not taking chances.

To further test its wedge seat, Specialized consulted with Dr. Robert Kessler, professor of urology at Stanford University Medical Center in

Palo Alto, California. In March 1999, Kessler recruited 25 cyclists, each of whom regularly rode at least six hours weekly and had suffered perineal pain, numbness, and erectile dysfunction. After they used the new wedge seat for a month, 14 of them experienced complete relief of their symptoms. Nine experienced almost complete relief, one had partial relief, and one indicated no change. Kessler presented his findings at the 1999 annual meeting of the American Urological Association.

Dr. Goldstein maintains that even open-wedge seats offer little assurance; he favors "wide, noseless seats that force you to actually sit, not to straddle, because the weight is borne on the ischial tuberosity and not on the perineum." Since this is an impractical solution for most cyclists (the nose is used for control and balance—riding without it would be like trying to drive a car using only your legs instead of the steering wheel), the open-wedge seat has emerged to grab a sizable chunk of the saddle market among concerned cyclists.

This isn't to say that the only option for diminishing numbness is to buy an expensive wedge saddle. The saddle that works best for you will depend on your anatomy, and everyone's is different. A few quick adjustments to your riding style and equipment (see next section) will help take care of that.

SEATLESS SEATS: THE NEW SUSPENSION SADDLES

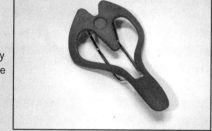

Infinity saddle

Short noses. No noses. Some with cut-out center sections. One shaped like the letter C, another like the number 8 turned sideways. The impotency issue spawned a cottage industry of imaginative pressure-relieving saddles over the years, with all the aforementioned styles reviewed in one of my *Los Angeles Times* gear columns in 2007. The one I've used on my road bike ever since is the Selle SMP, the beaked, bifurcated Italian masterpiece pictured earlier in this chapter. After riding the airy SMP, I've found that other seats make me feel like I'm being impaled on the tip of a spear.

Nothing came close to the SMP until January 2014, when I tested the most radical cut-out saddle I've ever seen: The Infinity, pictured here.

The Infinity is literally the edge of a saddle, with nothing but air in the middle. That's because inventor Vince Marcel, a chiropractor from El Segundo, California, decided that the only way to truly relieve pressure on everything *down there* was to remove the hard seat structure not just from under the soft, vulnerable-to-squishing, artery-dense perineum, but also from under the hard "sit bones" (at the base of the pelvis) that surround it.

A traditional saddle leaves the skin and the tissues around the sit bones swollen from the body-weight compression and side-to-side rubbing of each pedal stroke. "A seat with a hole or channel in it helps spare the perineum, but puts your weight squarely on the sit bones," said Marcel, a 51-year-old father of two and a budding Ironman triathlete. "You need a seat that will suspend the entire area. I realized that on the day that I was all black and blue down there after I rode 75 miles following six months of no riding. So I went back to my office and used my orthotic (foot) shaper to make a plaster-of-paris impression of my tush." With a facsimile of his delicate undercarriage in

(continues)

SEATLESS SEATS: THE NEW SUSPENSION SADDLES
(continued)

hand, he took a saddle and cut away almost everything.

The result—a striking, minimalist, air-conditioned work of art that depressurizes your entire at-risk zone—was dubbed Infinity by Marcel, and it was given a ringing endorsement on the world's toughest test track in June 2014: The 3,000-mile Race Across America.

Mike McClintock, an electrical contractor from Wooster, Ohio, who dropped out of the 2011 RAAM after 2,200 miles due to saddle sores, was so frightened of the same thing happening in 2014 that he did something considered heresy: used brand-new equipment on game day. Paranoid about her husband's tenderness tendency in the days leading into the race,

his wife Robyn scoured the Internet and found Infinity, which was not yet for sale. Marcel sent the 56-year-old McClintock a prototype, which he test-rode just once before the race. The result: a pain-free private area for 11 days, 20 hours, 27 minutes, good for sixth in the 50–59 age group. He was ecstatic.

"I had *no* saddle sores; *no* time off the bike tending to those sores, and *no* reduced speed due to not being able to get comfortable on the bike," said McClintock. "This saddle was not only instrumental in making my attempt successful—it may have been one of the primary reasons why I succeeded."

So, move over SMP. For all-around sit-bone comfort and sex-organ safety in a familiar, cycling-friendly form, suspended designs like the Infinity could well be the wave of the future.

BIKE FOR LIFE'S 12 ANTI-NUMBNESS TIPS

Does the right seat cure numb nuts?

Dr. Irwin Goldstein, the Boston University Medical Center urology department director who considers cycling a hazardous avocation, said cycling would be dangerous for male reproductive anatomy even with a foolproof seat, since you can still get injured by falling on the top tube. But Dr. Frank Sommer, the EU minister of health, who had raced bikes in his early 20s as a time trialist, believes that "cycling is a very healthy thing. But you have to do proper precautions to avoid any health hazard and sexual dysfunction. I think a good seat is very, very important. Nonetheless, for the sexual health, you also need good technique."

If you want to ride as much as you want, while being able to happily perform that other type of riding in bed, follow these 12 basic rules:

The Obvious One

1. Stand up! Getting off your butt is remarkably effective—the easiest, most effective antidote to erectile dysfunction (ED). Occasionally

rise out of the saddle. Stand for a one-minute interval every five minutes—even on a stationary bike. One study showed that this restored 110 percent of the blood flow to the undercarriage. The highest propensity for cycling-caused ED is among those riders who stay glued to the saddle hour after hour, consumed with achieving perfect aerodynamic form or lost in thought.

Type of Saddle

2. Firm, not soft. A hard saddle supports the sit bones while leaving the perineal area untouched. "I have some patients who like a soft, cushioned saddle very much," said Sommer, "but despite their comfort, they still have diminished blood flow. That's because the padding compresses as the rider's weight sinks into it, pushing very hard into the perineal area, reducing blood flow."

3. Concave, not dome-shaped. "A rounded shape that peaks in the middle is the absolute worst," said Sommer. "A flat or concave saddle stays out of your way."

Saddle Adjustments

4. Level the seat; do not tilt it up. All seats

instantly compress arteries and nerves when pointed up. Stick with horizontal, or just drop the nose a few degrees.

5. Lower the saddle to eliminate rocking. Rocking side-to-side means the saddle is too high and you are likely grinding across the perineum with your body weight. A check: Make sure your knees are not fully extended at the bottom of the pedal stroke.

Other Riding Techniques

6. Sit back. "If you sit back on the wide part of the saddle so that you are actually on the sit bones, the ischial tuberosity, you'll be fine," said Goldstein. "Of course, that's not the usual case. If you lean forward on a seat with a long, narrow nose, all bets are off. The narrower the saddle—and the more cut-outs—the smaller the surface area and the more pressure on the perineum."

7. Alter your riding position frequently on long rides. "This gives your penis a chance at good oxygenation," said Sommer. "If you are bending forward in the racing position, the blood flow is very, very, poor." If you start feeling numb, immediately change your position and give the aerobar a rest.

8. Use your legs as shock absorbers. While mountain biking over roots, train tracks, or curbs, stand out of the saddle and use your legs as shock absorbers. This minimizes harsh vibration and trauma to the penis and testicles.

Workout Tips

9. Strengthen your legs. "Although pro cyclists did not volunteer for my saddle test, I have made an assumption that their strong legs may help prevent numbness by lifting them up from the saddle," said Sommer. "Strong legs let you keep your whole weight off the saddle, and only use the saddle as a guide."

10. Stretch the hamstrings. Loose hamstrings allow you to sit back in the saddle easier and utilize your glutes.

Other Tips

11. Padded shorts and gloves. The padding cushions and spreads the contact area with the saddle, while bike gloves allow more weight to be put on the hands (and off the seat).

12. If in doubt, go recumbent. Recumbent bikes place the rider in an aerodynamic, feet-forward, lounge-chair position that is comfortable and causes virtually no blood loss. Because of the wide seat and full back support, there is no acute pressure on the pelvic region in recumbent riding.

CONCLUSION: THE RISK IS REAL

Several years ago, Dr. Goldstein and his colleagues at Boston University compared the rates of sexual and urinary dysfunction of 738 members of a bicycling club and 277 members of a running club who did not bicycle. They discovered that the level of moderate-to-complete impotence in cyclists was higher than in runners by a factor of 4 to 1.

Bikers, plain and simple, are the high-risk candidates within the general aerobic athletic population. That was Goldstein's most potent warning.

Goldstein, hailed by many in the bike industry for calling attention to the problem ("We've changed everything for the better because of him," said Minkow), remains unrepentant in the face of criticism by the bike industry that the issue is overblown.

"What is amazing about the bike industry," Goldstein told *Bike for Life*, "is that it's like the tobacco industry in how effectively the health risks are denied and hidden. The thought that you can have numbness and accept that in the hands and legs and wherever else you guys get numbness, and recognize that exists in the penis, and then be blind to the fact that the nerve and artery are within millimeters of each other. You can cause permanent injury to either of the structures' nerve or artery. It can happen at any one time in any one acute fall. So, I see it in non-bikers. I see it in weekend warriors. I see it in novice riders. I see it in kids riding for the first time. I see it in stationary bike riders. Any person who bears his weight on his perineum, puts his penis at risk. It is not complicated."

Goldstein's Boston urology clinic is a revolving door of concerned riders. "Our clinic sees many, many bike racers," he said. "I have so many patients who come here and say there can be no letters; there can be no notes taken. They tell me, 'If my sponsor ever found out I was here, I would lose my sponsorship. And that is my life.' The fear of being exposed is huge. Or even worse, we have all these men who go on these charity races like the Jimmy Fund in Massachusetts for children's research. Every year we get half a dozen men coming in the office with incidents following that ride. One fellow said, 'If someone would have told me the $2,000 I raised would mean taking this risk, I happily would have given it to them. But now I have impotence. It's not going away. I have numbness. It hurts. Why didn't anyone tell me this?'

"Luckily for a substantial number of people, the situation can go away. But not for everybody. There are permanent, irreversible erectile dysfunctions that happen. We have treatments. Viagra, Levitra, Cialis can help these men, and many do use it. They have diminished blood flow. They're just like a guy who has high blood pressure and diminished blood flow."

Besides Goldstein's anecdotal evidence, just how many riders actually visit his clinic? "Our clinic sees something like 80 men and 40 women a week," he responded in 2004. "It's about 3,500 men and 2,000 women a year."

And what percentage of them are bike riders?

"Let's look at a typical day of treating patients at my office," he suggested in response to that question. Back in 2004, he randomly chose the previous Friday, April 9, and began reading aloud entries from his appointment book:

ZD, a 68-year-old man with prostate cancer. He is not a biker.

RW, 44, biker, erectile dysfunction. Numbness, pain in penis, erection to hard 60 percent rigid, tenderness in Alcock's canal.

PW, 71, since hernia surgery erectile dysfunction.

SF, 27, sport soccer. . . . Likes bike riding but not exactly.

AL, 36, lifetime premature ejaculation. Mountain bike rider.

CP, 74, diabetes, hypertension, high cholesterol, smoking. Not biker.

ED, 42, England, bike rider thirty years. Decreased libido, decreased erections.

MB, 61, ED, five to six years incidence, always low libido. Heart disease, high cholesterol, depression. On antidepressive medication.

MS, 44, pain in penis after using penile enlargement device.

MW, 22, blunt trauma—fell on plastic bike seat.

RC, 54, neuropathy, disabled depression.

AC, 49, decreased libido, decreased erection.

Out of 12 patients, three were cyclists. At that rate, perhaps over 1,000 cyclists per year visit Goldstein for sex-related issues. Is cycling the cause of their problem? How many more across the country, out of 50 million Americans who ride for fitness, have problems?

No one has a clue. But with cycling participation numbers remaining stable, it seems that the vast majority of male cyclists either don't have the problem or prefer riding over fornicating. To millions, Goldstein's cure—abstention from the bike—is worse than the disease. Especially when less radical solutions are so rational and accessible.

A View from the Bike Shop

THE TYPE OF SADDLE IS OFTEN NOT THE MAIN VILLAIN. IT'S A COMBINATION OF TILT AND THE DROP FROM SEAT TO HANDLEBAR THAT MAKES THE DIFFERENCE.

BY MIKE JACOUBOWSKY

Much as we'd like to sell zillions of new saddles, in most cases the saddle itself is not the problem. It's more how one sits on the saddle that is at issue here, and it really doesn't matter whether you've got a $10 stock seat or the fanciest $100 aftermarket urologist-approved model. If you're not set up correctly on the bike, you're going to have potential for problems down the road.

The first place to start is the tilt, or angle, of the saddle. In almost no case is it a good idea to ride with a saddle that's tilted up at the front! This focuses the pressure on exactly the wrong areas. As you slide forward on the seat, you're essentially driving your most delicate parts (and the ones that could cause problems down the road) into the nose of the seat.

So do you want the seat "down" at the front? That's not a good idea either, because you're going to spend the whole ride pushing back from the handlebars, creating a lot of tension in your arms and shoulders. A level saddle is the best bet.

What if a "level" saddle causes discomfort? Then it's definitely time for a different saddle. You need to be able to distribute pressure across a wide area, and the only way you're going to be able to do this is if the saddle's level. If this gives you problems at the front of the saddle, then you might look into something with either a cut-out or soft layers of foam and/or gel in the appropriate location.

But there's more to it than just saddle tilt. If your seat is well above the level of the handlebar, then you're going to be rotating downward over the front of the saddle, once again bringing the wrong areas into hard contact with the seat. This, I believe, is the No. 1 reason for saddle-related male problems.

Specifically, note the difference in height between the top of the saddle and the top of the handlebar. For a smaller road bike (up to about 54

cm or so), try to keep this difference to 5 cm (2 inches) or less. For a mid-sized road bike (up to 58 cm), a difference of 6 cm (2.5 inches) is acceptable, and for larger bikes, try to avoid greater than an 8 cm difference (3 inches). The issue here is that, as the difference becomes too great, the rider is rotating his midsection downward over the front of the saddle, bringing undue pressure onto exactly the wrong areas. In my opinion, this is far more likely to cause a problem than a saddle!

Why would anyone want a stem so low that it might cause such trouble? Primarily for aerodynamics. Lower stem equals less torso and head up in the wind! Triathletes in particular go to great trouble trying to achieve the most aerodynamic position possible, and even serious recreational riders get into aerodynamics as well. But hear this, and hear this clearly. If your saddle/handlebar differential is beyond the recommendations above, or if you're feeling any discomfort in the saddle area, try raising the stem a bit. If this makes cycling more comfortable, your stem was low enough to potentially create serious problems down the road.

Something else to consider. The way you ride might make all the difference in the world. Most injuries don't occur instantly, but rather over a long period of exposure to whatever's causing the problem. If your riding style is such that you sit endlessly on the saddle and never stand up or stretch, you're much more likely to have problems. The best way to combat this is to regularly take a break from the grind and stand up for a bit, take a breather, stretch a bit, and then get back in the saddle. Wanna hear a secret? If you do this on a regular basis, before you start to experience a sore tail end, you'll go a lot farther without pain than you would otherwise. Anyone who has miles on a tandem knows this to be true! Even when you're feeling great, you still need to take breaks once in a while and you'll feel a whole lot better for a whole lot longer.

Cyclists most at risk are those living in flat areas, since it's unlikely they'd find many "natural"

(continues)

A VIEW FROM THE BIKE SHOP
(continued)

excuses to get out of the saddle and stand for a bit. On the other hand, those living in very hilly areas are more likely to find themselves alternating between sitting and standing as they climb.

But what about mountain bikes? Different issues here, since, in general, mountain bikers don't ride in such an aerodynamic (low) position on their bike, and the frequent need to stand up reduces the likelihood of problems caused by staying in the same position for long periods of time. More likely to cause problems on a mountain bike

would be impact with the top tube in the event of a crash—this can really hurt! Nevertheless, it's still possible that an overly aggressive riding position (such as that found with a tall rider on a small frame) could cause trouble.

Finally, it's all about common sense. If you're uncomfortable on your saddle for any reason, seek the advice of a competent shop or experienced cycling friend! And don't be quite so willing to sacrifice comfort in a quest for absolute speed.

Mike Jacoubowsky is co-owner of Chain Reaction Bicycles, Redwood City and Saratoga, California.

SADDLE NUMBNESS VS. IMPOTENCE

Bike for Life queried participants on several Internet cycling newsgroups for their views regarding saddle numbness and impotence. Here's a representative sampling of replies:

I have had considerable trouble with saddle comfort and numbness, particularly on long rides, and have tried almost all saddle types: standard flat, noseless, split, holes in the middle, you name it! All with little relief. The best seems to be a split V saddle made by Specialized. It has a wide V split from the back forward, and has a raised rear. The rear supports my sit bones; and when I push back on it, it raises the center of my bottom and relieves the pain. The only trouble is that this puts too much weight on my arms, and I can't sustain this for long (especially on my road bike; on the mountain bike, the more upright position helps produce a natural rearward force). I need to have a nose, and rest my mid on it for much of the ride; hence I hurt and go numb. I end up moving around a lot toward the end of a ride, and push back as much as possible.

Yes, I experience numbness any time I ride over

150 miles in a day; the numbness goes away in a day. No problems with impotence. No, I haven't seen a urologist. As for how I deal with saddle issues: Be one with the bike. My bicycle is adjusted perfectly to my body. My pedal stroke is so smooth, my body so motionless, because everything is just so, to the millimeter. An added benefit is that no matter how far I ride, I don't need Advil. Saddles are a very individual preference, as everyone fits their bike differently. I spend most of my time on long rides in aerobars, with the center of my crotch at the tip of my saddle. Thus, I use well-padded shorts (Performance Elite) and a saddle that's light but has a well-padded nose (Terry's Fly).

Except for the longest events (over 500 miles), generally no problems; over 500 miles, crotch and hand numbness. So far, impotence only has been a temporary condition. Haven't seen a urologist. Erection function is not what it used to be but not sure if it's cycling related or normal age/hormone condition. Saddles used: Brooks B-17 Champion Special (for over 500-mile events). Also have a bike with an Avocet O2-40 men's road model (the wide men's

(continues)

model). I use these seats because they work. I don't use chamois cream of any sort.

I am always struggling with comfort after 1.5 to 2 hours. But mostly in the sit-bones area (I'm 155 to 160 lbs.). I have tried many, many saddles. Cut-outs don't seem to make much difference. I've never had a lot of numbness problems, just here and there. On any quality saddle, it's been a non-issue. I seem to do best on a lightly, but softly, padded saddle, no cut-out needed, with slight curve to it. The Fizik Aliante seems best so far. The Arione, flatter and firmer, was awful. The supposedly great-for-private-area circulation, Specialized Body Geometry Pro, wasn't too bad, but padded thickly and too firmly for my rear end. I have had no issues with the private equipment's function. But

then, like I said, my issues tend to be with the duff/saddle connection, not up front. For example, the aero position is actually more comfy than a more upright one.

My saddle gives me numbness but only on time-trial efforts. Long rides no pain, no numbness. The numbness that I do have during time trials doesn't seem to affect me after I get off the bike.

Give up sex? Never. One thing does need to be mentioned on this issue that is often not addressed. If a man has an enlarged prostate for whatever reason, leading to pressure on the urethra and pudendal nerves, that will certainly make any saddle numbness and pain worse.

WOMEN CYCLISTS AND SEXUAL DYSFUNCTION

Women owe a huge debt to the bicycle. But, like men, they aren't immune from the wrath of the bike seat. Studies show that the majority of women also experience some genital pain and numbness. First, some history:

When the cycling craze first hit in the late nineteenth century, women saw this newfangled transportation device as a way to finally assert their independence and freedom to travel unhindered, without a chaperone. "Bicycling has done more to emancipate women than anything else in the world," said turn-of-the-century suffragist and women's rights leader Susan B. Anthony.

Not everyone agreed with this proto-feminist sentiment.

The medical profession was particularly alarmed by the prospect of women cyclists taking

to the streets. According to Ellen Garvey's book *The Adman in the Parlor, 1880 to 1910*, "Anti-bicycling doctors said it would be sexually stimulating—and that was dangerous to good Victorian women and to their marriage prospects. One doctor warned that the saddle could 'form a deep hammock-like concavity which would fit itself over the entire vulva and reach up in front, bring[ing] about constant friction over the clitoris and labia. The pressure would be much increased by stooping forward, and the warmth generated by vigorous exercise might further increase the feeling.' He reported the case of an 'overwrought, emaciated girl of 15 who stooped forward noticeably in riding, and whose actions strongly suggested the indulgence of masturbation.'"

If the bike was viewed as some kind of sex toy, then what did it say about women who liked to

(continues)

WOMEN CYCLISTS AND SEXUAL DYSFUNCTION
(continued)

bike? Were they loose, licentious, and sexually impure? Several bike manufacturers attempted to circumvent this overwrought and ill-formed perception by coming up with new types of saddles with crotchless designs. Furthermore, "manuals and catalogs instructed women to ride decorously: sitting upright (none of that pressing forward on the saddle), and not too fast," wrote Garvey. In 1880, the Cyclists' Touring Club of Great Britain, for example, admitted women as full members, but the club refused to encourage women's racing for several decades. The reasons cited for this stance: propriety and female physiology.

Now, over a century later, the issue of female physiology has resurfaced, but for a different reason: to investigate whether biking leads to declining sexual performance. Instead of causing sexual stimulation, medical researchers are now examining whether cycling leads to sexual dysfunction.

As you might expect, Dr. Irwin Goldstein of the Boston University Medical Center is front and center on the issue. "We now see anorgasmia—difficulty in having an orgasm—as the primary complaint of bicyclists," Goldstein told *Bike for Life*. "A lot of women who like horse riding have the same problem. Do other doctors make this connection? I'd have to say it's growing knowledge."

He's right, as several 2001 studies showed. The *Clinical Journal of Sports Medicine* (October 2001) reported that women cyclists experience vaginal numbness, inability to have climax, and limited blood flow to the clitoris. Another study, published in the *British Medical Journal* (2001), reported findings from research conducted at Brugmann University Hospital in Brussels, which looked at six women, ages 21 to 38, who had a unilateral chronic swelling of the *labium majus* after a few years of intensive bicycling at an average of 250 miles per week. "All six had typical unilateral lymphoedema, which was more severe after more intense and longer training. The position of

the bicycle saddle, the type of shorts worn, and the women's perineal hygiene were optimum. There was no family history of lymphoedema in any of the women, nor any common factor that might explain it," the researchers noted.

Obviously, riding 250 miles every week on a long-term basis is something very few women do, but what about the rest of the female riding population? How many miles, at what kind of intensity, or for how long does a woman cyclist need to ride before pelvic numbness, clitoral and labial lacerations, and even inability to reach orgasm start to arise?

It may not take much, according to a study reported in the November 2006 issue of the *Journal of Sexual Medicine*, which was directed by a pair of female professors at Yale University School of Medicine. Their study, "Genital Sensation and Sexual Function in Women Bicyclists and Runners: Are Your Feet Safer Than Your Seat?" found that the majority of female recreational cyclists they surveyed, who rode as little as 10 miles a week, experienced decreased genital sensation and more pain than other athletic women, such as runners. The researchers evaluated 48 cyclists and 22 runners with a median age of 33. According to the study, 62 percent of the female cyclists evaluated reported genital pain, numbness, and tingling, whereas the women runners evaluated did not experience any discomfort at all. The study found no correlation between miles or time in the saddle and genital numbness; all of the sexually active cyclists reported normal sexual function.

"It is clear that a majority of women cyclists had a history of genital numbness, tingling or pain," Marsha K. Guess, MD, lead author of the study along with Kathleen Connell, MD, told *Bicycle Industry and Retailer News* on January 1, 2007. "Additionally, when tested neurologically, this group of cyclists had decreases in their genital sensation compared to women runners," added Guess, who, like Connell, is an assistant professor of obstetrics and gynecology.

This was the first study to evaluate the effects

(continues)

WOMEN CYCLISTS AND SEXUAL DYSFUNCTION
(continued)

of prolonged or frequent cycling on the neurological and sexual functions of women. It was funded by the National Institute of Occupational Safety and Health (NIOSH) as part of its research on the reproductive health of bicycling police officers. Their studies had shown a clear correlation between riding and sexual erectile dysfunction among male officers. Since no similar studies had been done on female police officers, Guess and Connell were approached in 2004 and began conducting tests at that year's meeting of the International Police Mountain Bike Association in San Antonio.

The study continued in New York. Since there aren't many female cyclists with the New York Police Department, the researchers recruited competitive cyclists from Central Park. Volunteers were paid $50 each. The researchers used runners as controls.

The findings: "Women told us that they have numbness in their pelvic region if they ride too much," said Connell, with problems including chafing, numbness ("riders were saying 'we know we're "in the zone" when we're numb,'" she said), and chronic swelling on external genitalia—the labia. "Some women feel numb after two hours of riding because the pudendal artery—same as males' perineum artery—gets flattened. Many branches of the pudendal blood vessels go to the urethra, clitoris, and vagina. Putting proximal pressure there affects blood supply. For that reason, we think women police officers are more at risk, because they have 30 pounds of equipment strapped on them."

The researchers also looked at seat designs. "The cut-out seats with the hole are good for some women, not good for others," she said. "Why? The labia is very thin. It may fall into the hole."

If the cut-out seat doesn't work for all women, what does? What should women be concerned with? "A combination of things," Connell replied. "How a person rides—leaning forward or back. Tilting the nose down a bit helps. I'm guessing better-padded seats. It may come down to riding style and proper fit—seat, handlebar height."

One of the difficulties Connell's team faced was a natural reluctance by woman riders to discuss the subject. "There's still a taboo in women talking about this," she said. "Lots of Central Park riders didn't want to talk. They were embarrassed being approached by strangers asking about sexual function. Still, there is a paucity of data on this topic for women." Cyclists were asked to fill out a questionnaire and then ride in the lab while attached to a specially designed sensation-measuring device for the pudendal nerve.

Cycling-related sexual dysfunction in men is easy to evaluate. But determining whether numbness and/or a decrease in blood supply means that cycling may interfere with women cyclists' ability to enjoy sex and obtain orgasms is not as clear-cut. Would too much cycling turn the Big O into the Big No? "I was hoping we wouldn't find sexual dysfunction—just discomfort," said Connell, "and that's what happened." The findings indicated temporary damage. Connell said further study is needed to determine if long-term neurological injury and/or sexual dysfunction can result.

Missy Giove

THE PERPETUAL QUEST FOR A "NEW 100 PERCENT"

"Why are you so fast?" they'd ask. "I've got bigger ovaries than the other girls," she'd reply. A New Yorker to the core, Queens-born Melissa "Missy" Giove was always in your face and in a hurry: US Ski Team at 17; downhill mountain biker at 18; world champion at 21; first two-time World Cup season titlist (1997 and 1998); first three-time NORBA national champion downhiller (1999, 2000, 2001); first gold medalist at the first X Games; and first female pro athlete in any sport to wear a dead piranha on a necklace, sprinkle her dog's ashes in her bra, and confidently "out" herself as gay. Superlatives precede her name in every realm: most intense, most outrageous, most fearless. Her style was literally "go for broke"—nine torn MCLs, eight cracked ribs, five broken wrists, two broken tibias and fibulas, two fractured vertebrae, two broken kneecaps, five major concussions, a bruised lung, a ruptured spleen, and a whole lot more.

Before Giove retired from racing at 30 in 2003, her multicolored shaved/dreadlocked hairdos, brash four-letter-word-laced speech, and willingness to push the envelope as she racked up wins at 14 NORBA and 11 World Cup races helped her win a Reebok commercial, Letterman and Conan O'Brien appearances, more money than any other female rider, and more instant recognition than any off-roader of either sex. Belying rumors that a brain hemorrhage suffered at the 2001 World Cup in Vail had left her brain-damaged, the well-educated, articulate superstar sat down with Bike for Life in March 2004 at the International Health and Fitness show at the Las Vegas Convention Center and unveiled the next move in her career: master trainer for the Trixter X-Bike, an indoor "mountain bike" with a freewheel and rocking handlebars, maybe the most unusual take on classroom cycling since Spinning. Here's Missy "the Missile," who spits words like machine-gun fire, won a race the first time she rode a mountain bike, and knows only one speed—all out.

THAT PIRANHA WAS sort of my alter ego. I was always a crazy, full-blown athlete—rode motocross from age 11 to 16, played hockey, lacrosse, skied, mountain-biked in college—crazy sports that girls didn't always play often. And in my fish tank I had this piranha who I named Gonzo—because he was nuts. He would jump up out of his tank all the time. One day I came home and he had flopped out. I had a lid on it, but he popped it off. That wasn't normal for a fish. He was on the floor one day when I came home—all dried out, because I'd been away for three days. So I put him in the windowsill and dried him out, then punched a hole in him, strung some line through it, and put it around my neck. Gonzo became my warrior symbol, my reminder to be crazy. I'd ride fast and he'd be flopping behind me, tagging along. During hard times, he reminded me that I needed to go a little harder.

I wore Gonzo for a decade. Ten years. When he broke, I duct-taped him up. Finally, in 2000, a friend's cat made a meal out of him.

I got into biking in 1990 at 17 and used it as cross-training for skiing. I already had the downhill skills—and the guts. At UNH [University of New Hampshire, which she attended for one year], I was the national third-ranked J-1 downhill skier at age 17 and 18—which seems odd because I didn't really like the attitude of skiing and knew I didn't want to pursue that entirely.

I was introduced to cycling on a fluke. At my grandparents' in New York, I used to hang out with this Jewish family down the street. The son, Dave, was a friend of mine, but his brother had cerebral palsy and I would play Ping-Pong with him all the time. His dad appreciated it and said, "Hey, we want to give you something for being so nice." And I said, "Well, you don't have to give me anything for being nice. I really enjoy him." But he said there were some bikes up in the attic, including one that was his grandfather's bike. So I accepted the gift and went upstairs and picked out a road bike. I had a choice of a Barry Hoban or a sea-green Falcon. I didn't know anything about bikes. I liked the color of the Falcon. It was an English bike, a 12-speed. I rode that every day for training.

My first time on a mountain bike was in a race—the beginner category cross-country race at Mt. Snow, Vermont, later that year. My friend gave me a mountain bike to win a prize for him. "You ride every day; I want you to enter this race and win me a pair of Sidi shoes and pedals," he said. "I know you'll win."

So I went out there with no training, no number plate, no helmet. I wasn't registered, hadn't paid fees. I was a vagrant in army fatigues. In the race, I kinda went crazy, whipping around, weed-whacker lines. By the second lap they pinned a number plate on me, made me pay the fee, and put on a helmet. And I won.

When it was over, I was so happy. Mountain biking was awesome. I was really taxed. That day I found my "new 100 percent."

That has always been a key in my life, something I now preach to everyone in my talks: Find your new 100 percent—a challenge—every day. Age or circumstance does not matter. Every day, shoot for a new 100 percent, mentally, physiologically. You are only limited by your mind. Entering a new season, I would say, *last year was the maximum.* But you know what? I'll find a new 100 percent this year. I'll give myself better nutrition, more recovery. You will find a new 100 percent. But you've got to search for it. You've got to push.

So I found my new 100 percent in mountain biking. At first, I liked the idea of utilizing the fitness of mountain biking as cross-training for my skiing. But I jibed with mountain biking much more, attitude-wise, than skiing. It was more free rein. There wasn't as much tradition in it. And I was a nontraditional person. A little bit more extreme.

I was 18 when I won my first worlds—the junior mountain-bike championship at the first official worlds in 1990, Durango, Colorado. I entered the slalom and ended up second to Cindy Whitehead. So I entered another race at the same meet—and I ended up getting second to a pro.

I was still on a collegiate ski-racing scholarship. But after another season of mountain biking I realized I was skiing to bike, not biking to ski anymore. Biking is what I loved. So I dropped skiing and went full-time biking in '91. Soon, I started training specifically for the downhill.

Fame, Fortune, and "Coming Out" on Her Own

BY THE TIME I won the worlds in '94, I was more and more recognized, but I didn't personally recognize that I was famous. I'd talk to everybody as usual, and every once in a while they'd say, "Aren't you *that girl*?" That usually was cool, but occasionally it posed a problem. One time I was in a sex shop weeding through tapes or whatever when someone came up and said, "Aren't you that girl?" And I said, "No, I'm not," and very quickly got out of there. One time, I got arrested for skateboarding illegally, and, having no ID, just gave a different name—but the cops caught the lie because they recognized me. It's weird, but it seems like all of the highway patrol know who I am—and that's actually worked to my benefit. Many times I was speeding, or driving without ID or registration, when the cop who pulled me over said, "Aren't you her? Just get outta here now," without ticketing me.

Certainly, being gay added to it [the notoriety]. I had outed myself in the *Village Voice* in New York City [in 1992] at 19 years old—way before anyone else. In 1995, when the cover story of me in *Deneuve* [now *Curve*, a lesbian magazine] hit, it was a very big deal. That was before these TV shows featuring gays came out [including Ellen Degeneres, and *Will & Grace*]. It was more hidden. In fact, *Girlfriends* magazine just put me on the cover and named me "Athlete of the Decade" because Martina [Navratilova] and a lot of other athletes were outed, but they never came out—and I came out on my own. I was, "This is the way I am, you don't like it, oh well." It shouldn't have been an issue, but you know how society is.

Cannondale was a sponsor before I came out, but knew I was gay before they hired me. I'm definitely not going to hurrah them, "Wow, look at Cannondale—they hired a gay person." After all, I was the best in the world—why *wouldn't* they have hired me? I'm not going to give them any props for hiring somebody gay. But later on in my career, when the company changed hands [and dropped her sponsorship in 1999], I felt like I was discriminated against.

I'm not going to live a lie. I felt like if that's my lifestyle and that's how I chose to live, it's kind of like if you're a warrior and that's your oath, then stand by your oath. Not to mention, too, that it's

disrespectful to the person that you love, to hide somebody. Unless there's a true reason to do that—if it was going to jeopardize or harm somebody else, say, for instance, in a custody battle or something like that. Other than that, if you're not proud of who you are and what you're doing, then you shouldn't be doing it.

People who wanted to be my friend had to accept it because that was the reality. So you know what I got? I got a lot of the bullshit out of the way. People who really wanted to find out who I was for the right reason would talk to me, and the people that didn't eliminated themselves by not approaching me, because they were prejudiced. So in a certain sense I did myself a favor. At the same time, it's harder to live an alternative lifestyle—you definitely get a lack of support financially. I mean, if you're gay, kettcchh [sound of door slamming]. You hear about this issue all day long—she didn't get this, didn't get that, because she was gay. Well, you know, she also grosses $8 million a year in prize money, so it wasn't that bad.

There's a definite downside to taking a stand on anything. Like taking a stand on abortion—you'll get support from people who are for it, slammed by those against it. I'm not for abortion. But look at all the movie stars and singers like the Dixie Chicks who are catching slack for criticizing the war [in Iraq]. They are losing jobs because of it. There are financial repercussions for taking a stand. It's like declaring a religion. You say, "I'm a born-again Christian," and you're gonna get Catholics, saying, no, no, ours is better. You take a position and you are highly scrutinized, but at the same time you do get some support. I choose to focus on the positive and on the people who supported me and try to deflect the negativity.

Hopefully, my strength in taking a stance and showing people who I am will help other people, and not necessarily because they are gay. Over the years, I've done a lot of suicide prevention talks to gay youth. Maybe a couple less people would kill themselves because of the fact of their sexuality, over something they couldn't help and wasn't a choice. For some people it's a choice, but for most people it's not—they don't choose to live a harder lifestyle.

Fortunately, it's the 2000s now. It's a different place.

Crash Course in Fitness: Missy's 8 Rules

INJURIES CAME WITH the victories over the years, but you can't ride in fear. Some call it crashing—I call it R&D [research and development]. I was constantly breaking some of the things that were causing some of the crashes I was having. One time my handlebar snapped in a compression and I broke my collarbone. In 1994 I broke my pelvis in five, no, seven places. All compound fractures. Broke both my legs at one time. The list goes on. The worst was the brain hemorrhage at the worlds in 2001. The doctors told me not to ride again, but I came back in 2003 and qualified 13 seconds ahead of everyone at the first World Cup, then got a flat in the next round. I crashed, hit the shit out of my head, and tore my MCL [medial cruciate ligament] and PCL [posterior cruciate ligament] in the next race, but was back by midseason. Took a fourth at the Telluride World Cup and won the nationals in Durango in my last race. So I left on a winning note.

I could have probably kept going, winning races, and been on top of my game until however long I wanted to, really. I think I am that strong mentally an athlete that I could do it until my body would say, "No you can't." But it was really a choice of respecting the people in my life, around me, because if I was going to hit my head a lot, and hurt myself real bad again, then they're the ones who are going to have to be taking care of me. And I might not know what's going on. They're the ones who are left to pick the pieces up. And I thought that was kind of selfish, because I accomplished what I wanted to accomplish and had a lot of fun doing what I did.

I'd have crashed a lot more if I hadn't worked on my strength and flexibility and good nutrition. I did and still do a lot of core workouts, so I have maximum control over my limbs. I train in unstable environments, using trampolines and stability balls. Helps your kinesthetic sense to work on flipping, landing. With a more facilitated core and balance, you can actually pull yourself out of a lot more accidents. And if you do get hurt, you get better a lot faster.

I've spent lots of time in gyms rehabbing. But I was always in the gym two hours a day, five days a week. Starting at 15, I lifted weights—dry-land training for skiing. Downhill bike racing needs a lot more upper-body conditioning than regular cycling. Females especially, since we lack the muscle mass. I am naturally 120 pounds [5-foot-6], small for gravity sports. So I work my ass off to get 15 to 20 more pounds of muscle. I can bulk up to like 140. Downhillers have to do a skill every day—either motocross or downhill or jumps. After that I'd go hit the weight room two hours. Then my ride—two, two-and-a-half hours of intervals. Way different from a cross-country rider. They do the LSD, long slow distance. Just ride; no real strength or conditioning programs.

My experience made me a natural trainer. I love being a teacher. I've added academic training. A degree from the C.H.E.K. [Corrective Holistic Exercise Kinesiology] Institute in neurological training. I'm also officially a craniosacral therapist, from the Upledger Institute in Palm Beach Gardens, Florida.

If I had to give fitness rules to live by to someone getting older, I'd start with my old favorite:

No. 1: Find a challenge; find your new 100 percent every day.

No. 2: Quality, not quantity. Train smarter. When you're older, you can't hammer for a couple hours every day. So you do quality. An-hour-and-15 maybe every other day. Whatever is 100 percent.

No. 3: Balance stress and recovery in all aspects of your life. If you are always stressed out at work and you go home and work your ass off to lose body fat, you're imbalanced. Parts of your recovery are nutrition and sleep. Fall asleep by 11:30 p.m., or lose a lot of your neurological recovery and regeneration.

No. 4: Take responsibility for your own health. Everybody wants a quick answer and there is no quick answer. Don't necessarily rely just on doctors or trainers.

No. 5: Maximize workout time with functional fitness. Instead of dicking around for two hours in the gym, chatting it up, do more neurologically demanding exercises that mirror real-life movements. Rather than sitting in an ab machine, do physioball sit-ups with a medicine ball against the wall. Take the leg-press machine—Is there anything in the household that requires me to move while sitting in a chair? Better: Do a one-legged squat. It's functional, requires stability. It's functional fitness—good utilization of my time and energy. Do it indoors and take it outdoors. Taking a family ski vacation? Better be able to do squats—so train for them. Weights aren't necessary—do body-weight squats. Walk up and down the stairs while doing the laundry. Do step-up squats on a bench.

No. 6: Watch form. Bad biomechanics and bad form are going to alter joint mechanics.

No. 7: Work the core—front and back. With more of a facilitated functional core you'd be able to utilize your power better.

No. 8: Use your ass: "Most cyclists aren't making use of their glutes, but they are a must in downhilling, because you have to be explosive. Also, being a kinesiologist, I knew that strong glutes reduce back pain—cycling's No. 1 injury. I set my seat back and hit the weight room for butt-building exercises, including deadlifts, the one- and two-legged squats I mentioned earlier, plyometrics. Bottom line? You've got an ass—you may as well use it. [See Chapter 8 for more on the benefits of butt-centric riding.—ed.]

X-Biking into the Future

THE X-BIKE PEOPLE contacted me to be the celebrity endorser in 2002. Since you can rock its handlebars side to side and coast, it replicates what happens on a real bike a lot more. That means an all-body workout—shoulders, arms, core—that regular Spin bikes can't do. I was impressed.

So that's why I turned around and told them I wanted a bigger role. Wanted to train people, write training manuals, help design the program. I said I'm a high-performance kinesiologist; my thing is training and rehab. I was pre-med in college. After years of work, I got a degree from the C.H.E.K. Institute in 2002—a career move. When I got my brain hemorrhage, I decided to get some actual certification that I had been studying. Had my eye on retirement—not going to do downhill forever. I had to get started with other things.

I just kept shaking it in every direction I could. When you're into punk rock and have this image as a gonzo jock…I had to definitely prove what my intellectual property was worth. I said, "Look, this is what I think I can do for you. I know I can make you successful." I basically created a spot for myself. Got a three-year contract plus a six-year endorsement.

This is a perfect job for me. I love cycling. I love the gym. The X-Bike is both—a full-body workout, which I am already into because of downhilling. So I was a great advocate of the product from a personal and business level. I'm a stickler about form, and the ergonomics of this bike allow you to actually exercise in proper form. On bikes where the handlebars aren't moving, you can't move in a natural plane of motion. I think our bike is healthier in the short term and also in the long term. It trains your body to have the correct response. As a downhiller, my life depended on it! I had to train my transitionomics to kick in. Instead of going to my shoulder. I've already hit that tree.

So I love this product because it does all of that—multiplanes, proprioception, neurological training. I don't want to be limited by my equipment. This is for me. I would be involved no matter what they paid me.

Over the years, I turned down alcohol and tobacco sponsorships that could've made me a lot of money. I'd have made so much that I probably wouldn't have had to work again. But I was more idealistic. I contributed money to Team Amazon, which was dedicated to women who couldn't get sponsorship. I gave tips to girls who wanted to beat me. In my life, I've definitely stuck to my guns.

I don't miss the back-to-back races. I had a wonderful time. I got out from a full-time racing schedule at just the right moment for me—I left the sport when I was ready to move on to bigger, better things. The transition has been really smooth and easy. Besides, I still ride and motocross all the time. I'm a rider—I just like to ride.

I'll ride by myself on a Sunday, go downhill or dirt jump, just free-ride—tear down mountains with no line and no trails, jumping off cliffs. We're shooting Kink, a video all about dirt jumping and big air. Who knows if I get neurological problems or Parkinson's when I'm older? The brain is a mystery—you never know what'll happen. I'm not being stupid or trying to kill myself. I'm just having a good time. An accident's gonna happen, or it's not. It's a little bit of roulette, but I gotta live life.

Update

AFTER RETIRING FROM cycling in 2003, Missy Giove suffered some setbacks for a while as a result of her involvement in a multistate marijuana transport operation that ended in a bust by federal agents in 2009. Due to her cooperation with officials, she got off with six months' house arrest, five years' probation, and 500 hours of community service. She lives in Virginia Beach, Virginia, with her wife, Kristen, whom she wed in 2008. She works at a local bike shop.

7

BIKE FIT

Proper set-up is the foundation for comfort, power, and injury prevention.

At mile 100 I felt a twinge, but didn't have time to worry about it. At 200 miles it became pain, but I was in a groove and couldn't break my momentum. At mile 375, teeth clenched in agony as the needles under my kneecap pierced every pedal stroke, I checked into the turnaround point of the 1999 Paris-Brest-Paris, the quadrennial 750-mile randonnée from Paris to the Atlantic Ocean and back. And I didn't check out. For the first time in my life, I "abandoned" (as the French call it) a bike event. It was either that or risk permanent damage to my knee.

On the train back to Paris, I was struck by the irony: I was much fitter now than in 1991, when I completed P-B-P an hour under the cutoff in 88 hours and 55 minutes. But maybe I wasn't as fitted to my bike. Instead of using the bike and shoes I'd trained on for years and completed all the brevets (qualifiers) on, I'd come to France with all-new equipment I hadn't used before. Later, back home, checking it

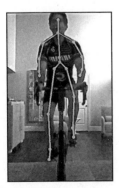

against the old gear, I found that the new bike's seat was set up an inch lower, the handlebars an inch higher, and that on my left shoe, the cleat was positioned back more toward the arch and slightly crooked. Roughly two inches of deviation from my correct position wrecked the event I'd trained two years for.

🚲

"I was suffering out there today," you might hear a cyclist say. "Suffer" is an odd and venerable term, strangely specific to cycling, that can have a range of meaning, good and bad. Your long-term cycling health may well depend upon how well you create the basic foundation that will make all of your suffering good suffering. That foundation is proper bike fit.

Usually, suffering is defined as good pain—when everything's working at full-speed efficiency, when your lungs are heaving and your legs are churning, and you're joining the company of the cycling gods as you push to the lactic-acid boundaries of your very being. In other words, good pain means high performance, when man and machine are indistinguishable, working as one, and you suffer from the joy of your muscles becoming fatigued by working at peak efficiency.

Bad pain and suffering, like my knee in P-B-P, indicates that something is wrong. Bad pain is when your knees, back, wrist, hip, hands, or crotch hurt; when your toes tingle; or when any combination of the above hurt; and you get the nagging feeling that you're working against yourself. Bad pain is a double whammy: bad pain = fatigue + unrelated pain + poor performance. Bad pain can have many causes, but often at its root is poor alignment. Ironically, there's a relatively easy fix for that: proper fit. But bad pain is too often tolerated, because it can be confused with good pain.

FITTING BASICS

"Strangely, people check common sense at the door when it comes to riding a bike," said Paul Levine, owner of New York–based Signature Cycles and the director of the famed Serotta International Cycling Institute (SICI). "There is a huge misconception among cyclists that there needs to be some level of discomfort for them to assume that they are riding well—that you actually need to be locked into a bad position. This is dead wrong. You should be comfortable on a bike. And comfortable means that your weight is distributed as evenly as possible over your back, butt, shoulders, arms, and hands so that no one muscle or joint is overly stressed."

In other words, a bike should fit you like a glove. It should bring about good posture. If it doesn't, if it isn't properly aligned with your body mechanics, you will not reach your peak performance, and you will waste energy on inefficient transfer of force from your muscles to the pedals. You won't be as stable, or breathe as well, or digest calories as well, as if you had a bike that fit so well that it allowed you to work at your optimal level. Without the right bike fit, you will expend precious energy compensating for the stress of your body, which is holding itself incorrectly on the bicycle, unnecessarily putting yourself at risk for aches and pains and injuries.

Over the past two decades, Levine has gained a reputation as the "Fit Guru," a name from which he recoils but will not deny. One of the most sought-after bike fitters in the country, he saw firsthand how changes in position caused changes in power output for several thousand riders while conducting SpinScan analyses for CompuTrainer in the 1990s. Now he's so busy giving $375 bike fits to wealthy buyers of $10,000 to $15,000 custom Seven, Parlee, Passoni, Guru, and Independent Fabrication bikes that he didn't have the time to schedule a *Bike for Life* interview for a week.

What does the right fit actually look like on a bike? If bike-fit seminars and magazine articles have left you bleary-eyed and befuddled with angles and percentages, consider this Levine advice, which *Bike for Life* considers the simplest, most understandable description of the proper overall posture on a bicycle.

The proper posture to have while seated on a bicycle is like sitting on a chair that you know is about to be pulled out from under you. This leaning forward, neutral spine position not only supports the weight of your torso with your quadriceps and hip flexors, but activates the core muscles that provide a stable platform for you to become more efficient. The neutral spine position rotates your pelvis forward, relaxes your shoulders, and opens up your air passages. It also puts you in the best position to produce power from your gluteus maximus—your butt.

Note: The butt is the cyclist's great ignored power source; tapping it gains you a stunning supply of mainstream power on par with that of the quads. To find out why, see Step 4 on page 154. In addition, a proper fit that activates your glutes can play a large role in reducing injuries to the back and knees (see Chapter 8 for butt and back strengthening exercises).

To understand the benefit of "sitting at the edge of the chair," consider what follows if the opposite occurs. If your pelvis is rotated backward, the pelvis essentially rolls up under your chest cavity—preventing the bottom of your lungs from fully expanding, rounding your spine, and pushing your shoulders farther from the handlebars. This position, in turn, tenses your shoulders, narrows your breastplate, and further restricts your airflow.

Cycling posture and alignment hinge on three connection points: seat, handlebars, and pedals. "If they are not all aligned together," said Levine, "the body tries to adapt, which leads to injuries and less power output."

Everyone is different, he said, and exact measurements are dependent upon comfort and a computerized power-output analysis, but certain basic rules apply across the board.

The Four-Step Fitting Approach

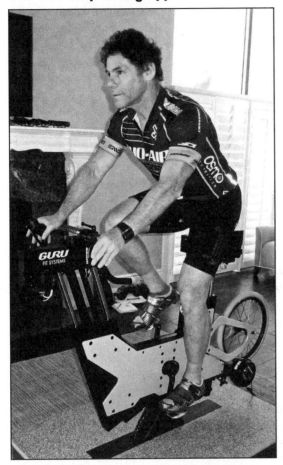

Ideal position: Foot level, with slight leg bend at the bottom of the stroke; hands on hoods, with upper arm at 90-degree angle to torso and slight bend at elbows to absorb shock.

Nothing about the Serotta fitting method used by Levine and others seems unconventional. The process isn't very different from what most other fitters (such as Victor Larivee, see sidebar, "The Bike-Fit Process") have been doing for years.

Step 1: Shoe/Pedal Interface:
Cleat at the Ball of the Foot

Clipless pedals, in widespread use among enthusiasts, increase efficiency by allowing the rider to make better use of the entire pedal circle, but they have also been blamed by many for the increased incidence of knee pain. The pain can be avoided with proper positioning of the cleat: It should be mounted directly under the ball of the foot and angled to match the rider's stride type. First, the ball of the foot: "People typically set the cleat of their clipless pedals too far back toward the heel—ultimately leading to numb foot, tingly toes, and inefficiency," said Levine. Nearly all bike fitters agree that maximum power is derived when the ball of the foot—the outermost protrusion on the inside of the foot—lines up with and pushes directly though the center-point of the pedal axle.

Not all fitters agree exactly where the ball is, however. Levine said this point is the second metatarsal phalange joint, while Andy Pruitt, director of the Boulder Center for Sports Medicine, said it is the first metatarsal. If you have lost your dog-eared copy of *Gray's Anatomy* and don't know a metatarsal from a metrosexual, heed the advice of Levine's fellow Serotta School practitioner Christopher Kautz, co-owner of PK Racing Technologies, who said if you must err on cleat placement, err toward the front of the shoe. Doing so gains you a mechanical advantage.

"The foot is a first-class lever arm for the calf muscle, and by locating the cleat forward, you effectively lengthen the lever and allow for more force production," Kautz said. In other words, a forward-placed cleat lets you push the pedal harder.

As for the angle of the cleat, common sense rules. Ride like you walk. If you walk pigeon-toed, point the bike shoes in; if you walk with toes pointed out, you'll ride the same way. Otherwise you will be fighting your body's natural movement and range of motion.

Step 2: Ideal Saddle Height:
Hips Don't Rock, Legs Don't Straighten

"When people come in to see me, their bike seat's all over the place," said Levine. "As a general rule, if it's too low, you'll get pain in the front of the knee. If it's too high, there's pain in the back of the knee. And if it's tilted back, you get serious back pain." Here's why:

A low saddle results in excessive bending of the knee at the top of the pedal stroke, causing the underside of the patella (kneecap) to jam into its tracking groove in the femur (thighbone). So instead of tracking smoothly in the groove, cartilage rubs on cartilage. But a saddle that's too high leads to knee pain on the back side of the leg, because the excessive reach stretches the hamstrings too much. It also leads to a loss of power, as the patella becomes a less effective fulcrum in the leg's lever system.

What's too high? There are many formulas, but the best one may be common sense, said Levine. If your hips start to rock slightly from side to side as you pedal, or your toes begin to point down, or you feel discomfort in your crotch, you're too high. Lower the saddle a few millimeters at a time until these symptoms disappear. From a profile view, your knee should have a slight bend at the bottom of the pedal stroke.

Step 3: Ideal Saddle Tilt and Fore-Aft
Position: Little to None, Slid Back

How much should you tilt your saddle?

All fitters recommend that the saddle should be nearly level—with no more than a 3 to 5 percent tilt up or down. A downward-tilted saddle (where the back is higher than the front) slides you forward, compromising handling and comfort. This tilt can irritate your crotch and put too much weight on your arms, hands, and front wheel. An upward-pointed saddle (with the front higher than the back) changes the curve of your lower back, putting you at risk of lumbar pain, and smashes up against the delicate blood vessels and nerves of the crotch,

increasing men's risk for numbness and possibly erectile dysfunction. The flexed lower-back position often leads to creep, a stretching of the ligaments that can lead to sudden instability and injury (see "Rules for Triathletes and Time Trialists" below). Another problem with flexed lower-back muscles, according to Chris Kautz, is that they turn off your gluteal muscles, forcing the quads to do more work. The right amount of tilt is ultimately determined by comfort and a computerized analysis that identifies maximum firing power.

As for the saddle's fore-aft position, beware of sliding it too far forward; the Serotta School says that will force the quads to do too much work. Here's the rule: At the 3 o'clock position on the crank circle, your foot should be horizontal. The reason: The foot can push straight down on the pedal at 3 o'clock, momentarily giving you maximum potential power. There is also a safety benefit: If your seat is too far backward or forward, it tilts your foot and can lead to injuries and chronic pain, according to Andy Pruitt.

Describing the process used to find correct fore-aft positioning is rather technical, so skip to Step 4 when your eyes glaze over. All fitters make use of a plumb line (a string with a weighted end) to check that there is a vertical line-up between the knee and the pedal axle. Traditionally, the plumb line is dropped from the tibia tuberosity, the bump below the knee, but Serotta fitters believe that the unnamed soft hollow just behind the kneecap on the lateral side better indicates the true function of the knee joint. Pruitt said if all that is too complicated; just drop the plumb from the front of the kneecap.

Step 4: Upper Body Position:
Comfort Is King

Handlebar height is the least "scientific" part of the fitting process, according to Levine, because it's all about one thing: being as comfortable as possible in a variety of positions for a couple of hours at a time.

"A lot of people tell me that they've never been comfortable on a bike, and that's a shame," said Levine. "Unfortunately, that's because recreational riders often imitate professional cyclists, whose handlebars are typically set very low for aerodynamics. The pros have a high tolerance for pain; regular people don't." In other words, Levine said forget rules and forget aerodynamics; upper body comfort is king. Handlebars that are too low are the biggest cause of back pain. Don't copy other people.

"An indicator of poor bike fit for a road bike is when you can't comfortably ride in any of the handlebar positions, including the drops," said Levine. "It usually means the handlebar/headtube is too low and/or the stem and top tube are too long for you." Road bike handlebars are designed to allow the rider to take advantage of many positions, allowing the use of different muscle groups and aerodynamic positions. Not surprisingly, the most common request asked of bike shops by bike buyers, whether they are newbies with $300 hybrids or veterans plunking down thousands for exotic custom machines, is this: Raise the handlebars.

You simply shouldn't be riding in pain or in a stretched-out position that hurts your hands. You shouldn't be riding humpbacked. You shouldn't get numb hands—suffered by 20 percent of riders. You shouldn't look like a silhouette of the letter "C." You should be riding with a neutral spine.

One problem often leads to another: To reduce pressure on the hands, people automatically roll the pelvis forward, causing the neck to hyperextend. The spine is considered neutral when the muscles around it are relaxed, not in tension. Levine said that when a bike takes you out of neutral, it's because the handlebars are in the wrong position—usually too far away and too low.

Q: *How high should the handlebars be raised?*
A: *Higher* ...

"A good start for recreational riders is to match seat height and handlebar height," said Levine.

"Performance riders can drop the handlebars 3 to 4 centimeters [about $1\frac{1}{8}$ inches to $1\frac{5}{8}$ inches]." In practical terms, the handlebars should be high enough so that a road bike rider can ride most of the time on the hoods (the rubber covering the top of the brakes) with arms in a shock-absorbing position. For most people, that's a revelation. "You should ride 80 percent of the time on the hoods, 15 percent on the top of the bar, and 5 percent on the drops," said Levine. The hoods are very practical; from there, you can shift, brake, and instantly jump into the classic out-of-the-saddle climbing position. Biomechanically, the hoods are the most comfortable, natural place for riders to put their hands, because doing so reduces the risk of carpal tunnel syndrome and puts the wrists in a neutral "handshake" position: thumbs pointing forward, wrists turned vertically.

In this position, said Levine, you should not be riding with straight arms. The upper arm should be at a 90-degree angle to the torso, with a slight bend to the elbow and the wrists not hyperextended. "The bend helps turn your elbow into a shock absorber; without it, the shock runs all the way up to your shoulders and neck," he said.

...but not too high.

Although high handlebars are a good thing, too-high handlebars are not. "The 'comfort' fit that brings your back almost perpendicular to the ground is okay for casual, flatland riding, like at the shore, but it'll cost you power and discomfort, especially in the hills," said Levine. Here's why: The largest muscle group used for cycling is the gluteus maximus, the butt, and it is not called into action until the hip is flexed at an angle of 45 degrees or less. Very high handlebars do not allow this.

Example: Sit with your back straight up in a chair (at a 90-degree angle), then try to stand out of the chair and notice what direction your back moves. It moves about 45 degrees to your hips for the gluteus maximus to activate and raise you out of the chair. "Pretty cool, huh?" said Levine. "Now try getting up without leaning forward.

It's extremely difficult. Welcome to the 'comfort' position. Try climbing hills in this position, and your wrists and neck start to hurt."

The reason for this, he explained, is that you can't stop your body from naturally wanting to lean forward as you climb, just like getting out of the chair. However, since the handlebars are too high and close to your chest, your leaning body puts excessive weight on your wrists. This is why a too-high bar is as bad as a too-low bar.

Q: What about mountain bikes and hybrids?

A: The same handlebar rules apply on flat-bar bikes, including cruisers. Your elbows should be naturally bent outward, serving as shock absorbers. To lessen the potential of carpal tunnel syndrome, nearly all fitters recommend that you add bar-ends—short, 90-degree-angle handlebar extensions that, like hoods on a road bike's drop bars, provide a comfortable "handshake" riding position. Platform grips, pioneered by Ergon, are designed with a flat shelf that the heel of your hand rests on, also preventing wrist hyperextension and numbness.

Q: What adjustments should older riders make?

A: Get more flexible. Remember that flexibility—the range of motion of your hamstrings, hip flexors, external hip rotators, and back—also plays a major role in handlebar placement. Paul Levine likes to use the example of two identical twins: a flexible one who does yoga and can bend over with his legs straight and put his palms on the floor, and a couch potato who can only reach his knees. The flexible twin will need a longer top tube or stem and can ride in a lower, more aero position; his stiff brother will need a shorter top tube, a shorter stem with a positive rise, and/or a headtube extension.

Aging has a similar effect. An adult's inevitable loss of flexibility after age 35 forces him or her upright. Given the vast increase in the number of older riders today, it is no surprise that one of the hottest new bike categories is the comfort road bike, which is characterized by a taller headtube and a softer seat. Formerly limited to custom bikes, particularly from Serotta, taller front ends are now showing up on production bikes like the Specialized Roubaix line. Personally championed by Specialized founder Mike Sinyard (see interview on page 276), these bikes include a number of novel, shock-absorbing inserts throughout the frame, specifically placed to add comfort for older riders.

Q: How wide should my handlebars be?

A: Match handlebars to shoulder width is the accepted rule. Don't go wider; it's not aerodynamic (it increases the rider's frontal surface area) and encourages a sagging between the shoulder blades. In the long run, this will lead to neck and shoulder pain. Bars that are too narrow can lead to more nervous steering, and hence to loss of comfort. But they do not inhibit breathing, as many think. That's good news for those who use aerobars for aerodynamic positioning, such as triathletes, time trialists, and even bike tourists.

Rules for Triathletes and Time Trialists: Watch Your Back

Brace yourself for the world's simplest triathlon advice: Don't stretch out. Wind-tunnel tests prove that being narrow on a set of aerobars is more important to aerodynamics than being low. Being too low hurts performance, because it encourages a humped back, not the flat back that gives the glutes a solid platform from which to fire. More importantly, a low position is uncomfortable and harmful to your back.

"It is not surprising that there is a much higher incidence of herniated disks among time trialists and triathletes," said Dr. Pam Wilson, a Duke University biomechanist and bike-position researcher who treats many cyclists and runners, teaches clinics with seven-time national champion Karen Livingston, and consults frequently with Levine. "Beware the curved, humpback position you get when stretched out on low handlebars. The hump causes 'creep' hysteresis, a permanent lengthening of the spinal ligament that breaks down the integrity of the bonds."

Avoiding creep, which has long been an issue among people who sit at a desk all day, is easy on a bike: Adjust your aerobar armrests as high and as far back as possible. Your upper arms should be almost vertical, with your elbows lined up just ahead of your shoulders.

Two warning signs of poor bike fit for a triathlon bike are: (1) the inability to maintain the aero position throughout the ride without straining your neck, lower back, or shoulders; and (2) sitting on the nose of the saddle and constantly readjusting your position. Remember, the goal is to stay in the aero position! All the work you do to get an aero position doesn't do any good if you're not in it. Again, keep in mind that the optimal time-trial position is probably not the most aero one, but the one that finds the best balance of aerodynamics, power, and efficiency.

Despite the relatively straightforward rules about handlebars and comfort, a final comment is in order: the bike industry doesn't make raising or adjusting handlebar height easy. Although pre-1990 bikes came with threaded steerer tubes and "gooseneck" stems that could be easily raised by loosening a quill, they were replaced by fixed-length systems that don't adjust. Today, you must buy a new "riser" stem, or acquire a whole new bike, like those from Giant's compact road-bike line, that come standard with adjustable stems. Don't be surprised if you have to go back to the bike shop several times to get your handlebar height issue resolved most comfortably.

Good Fit, Good Riding

Poor bike fit is like having a tire out of alignment on your car: You don't get a smooth ride, and you start seeing unusual wear patterns after a while—aching knees, back, neck, butt, and feet. A proper bike fit is the absolute first step you need to take to assure more comfort and power, reduce fatigue, and gain precise handling. If you buy a new bike, get a fit. If you feel pain on your old bike, get a fit. If you've never gotten a fit, get a fit. Because until you do, you won't be riding as efficiently as you could be, and you may waste time and money trying to remedy your aches and pains.

THE BIKE FIT PROCESS
TWO HOURS WITH A FITTING MASTER

"I'm going to give you an extra 15 miles tomorrow," boasted jumpsuit-clad Victor Larivee, beaming with the conviction of an Old World craftsman. Any cycling aficionado knows that proper bike fit aids performance, minimizes injuries, and can counter biomechanical inefficiencies, but few seem as, well . . . *fitting* as Victor.

Seating his subject in a platform-mounted shoeshine-type chair, Larivee strips off a sock and begins probing and poking the bare foot, beginning yet another of the two-hour fitting sessions he performs over a hundred times a year at his small Bicycle Workshop bike store, an institution in Santa Monica, California, for the past 30 years. Some Westside bike shops offer fitting services, but few can match the sheer number of contraptions

Larivee uses to make sure his customers ride in the most efficient and stress-free biomechanical position possible. "Hey, a lot of 'em know how to do this, but not enough to make a science out of it," he said. "Remember, I do this for a living."

The 15 extra miles Larivee promises come from finding the rider's neutral position on the bike. "Everything I'm about to do will simply be duplicating your natural gait—that's your neutral position. It's where you're most efficient," he explained. Does that mean that if you walk like a duck, you should also ride like a duck? "Yeah—that's right. I like that," he smiled, dedicated teacher to eager student.

CUSTOM-MOLDED ORTHOTIC

Larivee starts off a fitting by making a custom heat-molded Superfeet brand orthotic of each

(continues)

THE BIKE FIT PROCESS *(continued)*

foot, both of which are worn inside cycling shoes. "This stabilizes the foot, giving you more power," explains Larivee. In a static situation like cycling, where the feet themselves aren't moving, a foot will automatically collapse on the downstroke, dissipating your energy. The orthotic keeps the foot arched and aligned in its own neutral position—putting 100 percent of your power through the pedal. Also, it maintains the neutral position by allowing the natural tilt of the rider's feet.

CLEAT POSITIONED SO YOU PEDAL THROUGH THE BALL OF THE FOOT

Next, Larivee slips a cycling shoe on the foot, pokes a rod tipped with wet paint through a hole in the shoe, and performs one of the most critical tasks in a fitting—finding the ball of the foot. "The ideal situation in cycling is to have the center of the knee driving straight through the ball of the foot, which then should drive directly through the pedal spindle," he explains. Larivee redrills holes and moves the cleat fore and aft until it is over the ball of the foot. Then, to make sure the knee is directly over the ball of the foot, he uses a plumb line to position the saddle back or forward.

MATCHING LEG LENGTHS

Next, the rider lies on his back and Larivee measures the legs from the top of the thighbone (femur) to the heel. If one is any more than a half-inch longer than the other, he builds up the bottom of the cleat to make up the difference. Normally, there is no surprise involved here. "People know when they're that far off."

NEUTRAL ROTATIONAL ALIGNMENT

At this point, orthotic in shoe and cleat in place, the rider goes to his own bike, which has been placed on a stationary trainer. Larivee hauls out a small, square steel box with two rods—one red, one white—sticking out of its side. This is a RAD, or Rotational Alignment Device. The angle of the cleat is adjusted until the two RAD rods stay parallel through several rotations. At that point, the pedal stroke matches the rider's natural walking gait—the long sought-after neutral position.

PROPER SEAT HEIGHT

While the rotational alignment is being done, Larivee is also adjusting the seat. Using a pivoting ruler called a "gagiometer," he either raises or lowers the seat to give the leg a slight bend at the knee—about 150 degrees—in the bottom pedal position. This position is not only the most efficient one for riding, but also puts the least amount of stress on the knees.

COMFORTABLE HANDLEBAR HEIGHT

The final step is the least scientific. Larivee adjusts the handlebar stem for the best comfort of the individual rider. "This is the only time I let your brain tell me what to do—not your body," said Larivee. As a general rule, performance riders ride with their handlebars parallel to or just below the seat height. Riders with shorter torsos—especially women—can use a longer stem to keep them from having to reach too far.

The fitting just described took the fast-working Larivee about two hours. He charges $159 for a fitting and $109 for the Superfeet orthotic molding. Cleat fitting is $25. "People who've been sent by other shops never complain about the price," he said, "but the people who call up on their own freak out. They have no idea of what's involved."

Incidentally, Larivee's fits have gotten faster over the years. "More older people are riding today, which is why back pain is the biggest complaint I hear—bigger than knee pain," he said. "If the guy who comes in for a fit is 35 or older, I won't just raise the handlebars. I'll say, 'You want to ride faster than you've ever ridden—with no back pain ever again? Try a recumbent.'"

Then he points to his showroom. The inventory at the Bicycle Workshop, once composed entirely of exotic foreign road-racing bikes, is now 90 percent recumbents. "One ride and they're sold," said Larivee. "But that doesn't mean a 'bent [recumbent] rider doesn't need a bike fit. Although the upper body gets a break, his feet, legs, and knees are just as at-risk."

CASE STUDY: THE FIT GOT HIM FITTER

Javier Saralegui used to dread the 54-mile ride from Bridgehampton, New York, to the tip of Long Island and back with his brother-in-law, Melchior Stahl. "I'd come back from the ride and feel like my neck was broken, like someone took a two-by-four to it," said the president of the online group of Univision, the Spanish-language network. Then, one day in 2003, he saw the Serotta Legend titanium bike in an *Outside* magazine article entitled "The Best Toys in the World." He called the company and was told, "Go see Levine."

"It changed my life," said the father of three, 44 at the time.

Levine asked Saralegui his goals, where he rides, what surfaces he rides on. He put him on rollers and on a CompuTrainer, analyzed his form, and put him on the fit cycle. He made him stretch for half an hour. After four hours, Levine looked at him. "You say you want to be superfit, to ride with your brother-in-law, but I don't know how serious you are," Levine said.

"This is an animal sport, and I'm going to give you an animal bike. I'm going to give you a Ferrari; what you had before [a LeMond] was sporting goods."

Then Levine looked Saralegui in the eye. "But it isn't the bike," he said.

Saralegui did start stretching, as Levine advised. In fact, he started taking Pilates. He got more flexible, and began riding with his heel lower, too. But at first he would have argued that it was the bike.

"Suddenly, everything was 100 percent different," he said. "I'm a different rider. No neck pain at all. Less fatigue. Now I use a lot less energy to go the same distance. Today, I just did a 54-miler and don't even feel it; in the past, I'd be in the Jacuzzi and telling you to call back. Right now, if you were to say, 'Let's go for a 20-mile spin,' I'd say, 'Let's do it.'

"The new bike doubled my mileage, upped my comfort, upped my power. I don't cramp up anymore. The Napeek stretch, where you're in the drops for a half-hour against 25- to 30-mph headwinds, doesn't kill me anymore. Going to Montauk used to be a once-a-summer ride. Now it's once a week. I don't even see it as being a hard ride. Now I lead my brother-in-law. I ride all day with my heart rate between 155 and 170 beats; before, I couldn't hold it for more than a few minutes. Look at the real numbers on my CompuTrainer: it used to be 160 to 170 watts for a 90-minute ride; now it's 190 to 200. On the road, I ride now at 24 to 25 mph, compared to 18 to 19 before. The next level above me are guys who don't have jobs."

"The new bike gave me a new sense of power," said Saralegui. "For the first time, I feel myself using the glute, a huge muscle. Another big thing: the calf works more.

"I'm manic. I started tennis 10 years ago and now I'm an 'A' player. I started surfing a few years ago and I'm good at that, too. But I've always been into cycling—just not like this."

Saralegui's fit took four hours and cost $500. The bike was upward of $7,000. In the decade since, he has bought more fancy, super-expensive bikes from Signature Cycles. "But maybe Levine was right," he said. "It's flexibility. It's motivation. It's the fit, the efficiency. It's not the bike."

Gary Fisher

THE JOY OF BEING MR. MOUNTAIN BIKE

There may be no one who embodies the sport and culture of mountain biking as completely as Gary Fisher. He is a bike maker, an athlete, a promoter, and, most importantly, a pioneer. He was there at the creation, and, along with early business partner Charlie Kelly, gave the world the first company to produce and sell mountain bikes exclusively—as well as the name "mountain bike"—earning both of them lifetime "Founding Father" status.

With a knack for innovation and marketing savvy, Fisher pioneered the use of the unicrown fork, oversized headsets, suspension forks on production bikes, long-top-tube/short-stem cockpits, and oversized wheels with 29-inch tires. As an athlete, he's been a top road racer, cyclocrosser, and age-group mountain biker. He's raced the Coors Classic road race, set the record at the fabled "Repack" downhill race on Mt. Tamalpais, and, as he's aged, pushed the envelope by winning Masters offroad championships, tandem off-road races, and monumentally difficult events, including the 400-mile, eight-day TransAlp Challenge stage race across the Alps. In 1988, he was among the first inductees into the inaugural Mountain Bike Hall of Fame. Outside magazine named him one of the 50 most influential outdoorsmen of the 1980s.

Fisher saw hard times—including a failing business—but it all turned into a dream lifestyle when bike industry behemoth Trek bought his trademark in 1993 and turned "Gary Fisher" into a mainstream brand. For over a decade, Fisher has had what many think is the best job in the bike business. He travels to cycling events around the world, exerts influence as a board member of social programs like Trips for Kids (which takes poor urban kids mountain biking), and spends his days riding and thinking of new ideas for the bikes that bear his name. All the while, he remains superfit and endlessly creative, and, as he told me in his original Bike for Life interview in March 2004, he feels decades younger than his chronological age. That came in handy as Fisher became a father again in 2004 at age 53. He'd added a few more kids by the time we spoke again a decade later.

LOTS OF PEOPLE say that they don't have a chance to ride, but I think people allow themselves to be worked into a place where they can't ride.

There's more to cycling than exercise and the fitness benefits. Just lately my girlfriend [now wife], Amanda, and I have had a lot of fun riding "town" bikes [low-tech, relaxed-geometry cruisers] around. We take them shopping. And along the way, we do this thing where we try to find the most arcane way to get from Point A to Point B.

Take the trip from Fairfax to San Anselmo [in Marin County, California]. Normally you come down Center Boulevard. Well, we go off and try to find another route on one side of the valley and find a different route back on the other side. Sometimes we find ourselves walking the bikes up some staircases and down others, just because they connect a couple of streets together. Every time, we end up going to all these places we've never been before—just to get to the grocery store about a mile and a half away. It's the serpentine route, and no one else is on it.

The sense of discovery is one of the things that makes me happy, and there is no better way to find a new place than on a bike. They're the get-off point. Besides not having to find a parking place, I love the instant gratification. The being in the now—taking the back routes, spending more time together, having fun. A lot of it is like, do you like what you are doing, here and now?

I started road racing when I was 12, in 1962, and cyclocross a couple years later. I was attracted to it because there were older guys doing it, 15-, 17-year-olds who were working at the San Mateo Bike Shop in San Mateo. I couldn't quite hang with them. I was small for my age, one of the smallest kids in school. I wasn't even 98 pounds; I was 89 pounds when I was in eighth grade. As a freshman at Burlingame High School, there was one kid smaller than me. But from the first ride those older guys couldn't get rid of me. I kept following them. Then they said, "Well, OK. We'll let you come."

You've got to realize that it was so different then. There were a thousand registered race riders in the whole USA. And there were 50 or so in Northern California. Every time you saw somebody on a bike who wasn't a kid on the sidewalk or was obviously someone convicted of a DUI [and therefore had no license to drive a car], you went up to 'em and asked who they were, where they were from, and if you could ride with them. There were that few riders.

So we all stuck together—and we stood out. When I was in seventh grade, some girls from school saw me and said, "You farmer!"

That was a big put-down back then. The first six months, all I heard was, "Look at this farmer. With his little girl socks, little black wool shorts, and funny-looking jersey."

I thought about the total injustice of it. All these things that I was wearing had a reason. So I didn't care that much. Because I had my own pace, my own world. The style was accepted by my peers.

It's ironic now that kids that age accept it, even like it, to some degree. My son has even come around. He's 16 now. But for years, he'd say: "Lose the Lycra, Dad."

A Mountain Bike and an Image Change

I DIDN'T KNOW mountain biking was going to be big at first. In the beginning, I thought, this is for athletes. This is really tough. This is really cool. But there's only a few people that are into something this hard-core. Then I remember this guy, Bob Burrows—a local fireman, not in particularly good cardiovascular shape, older, in his 40s. In about 1975, I made him a clunker—you know, the old cruiser frame, precursor to the mountain bike, cobbled together with all old, found objects for parts. And I thought to myself, here is another bike that will wind up in a garage or just ridden around the neighborhood.

Well, I was so wrong.

We took Burrows out on a ride. He took forever to make the climb. But at the end of the ride, his eyes were so big and he was just so...new. It just changed him. Right there. It really surprised me, how much he liked it. And that was it.

Then I knew—this was going to be really big. This was going to go somewhere, by hook or by crook. Because people would do it. The percentage of 'em that said, "This is incredible. I'm gonna do this all the time and then follow through with it," was amazing. Amazingly high.

They loved the thrill so much, they were willing to get the fitness. So Burrows's bike didn't stay in the garage. He kept it out. And he rode it a lot.

What if your doctor prescribed cycling and your insurance company co-paid it?

Why not? Hell, they do it with all these other stupid things. And who says it helps you or not? But I KNOW cycling helps. There's nobody that rides a bike that doesn't get better.

I worked some for Rodale Press in the late '70s, writing bike reviews for *Bicycling* magazine. In 1979, I went back to Emmaus, Pennsylvania, and there were people in the office who would give me hard-ass because I rode my bike the six blocks from where *Bicycling* was to the main headquarters. They'd ask me, "Can't you rent a car?"

Can you believe that? That's insane. But if you think about it, it was typical for the times. Back in the '70s and '60s, people were in the mindset of "the bicycle is a primitive device."

So, in 20 years, everything's changed. We were at the bike messenger championships a few years ago in San Francisco. It was the coolest thing you could go to. Here I am, riding through Broadway Tunnel in a critical mass with all these people on a Friday night. There were 3,000 riders. And I was thinking, cycling has gone from being totally uncool to being totally cool.

Aging Ungracefully

I'M 53, BUT I feel like I'm in my 20s.

That's because I can get on my bike and do what I do. It's still the same. I'm not as strong or as fast as I used to be. But that's just the sheer speed. All the same actions are there: standing up out of the saddle, powering through this, climbing in certain gears. The act of being able to do this is really important. I've been in places where I wasn't able to do that, like when I broke my wrist last summer [2003] and I had to spend three straight months at home.

The incident happened a couple of miles from home. I was riding with insolence. I was just too full of myself.

I was alone. I'd ridden to the top of Mt. Tam on July 5. I found out that morning that the UCI was going to change the 29 rule. [In 2001, Fisher had introduced a mountain bike with fast, huge 700c wheels and 29-inch tires and had been lobbying to get it legalized for racing.] I'd been to see the UCI on June 13 at their headquarters just outside of Geneva, Switzerland, and sat in on a mountain bike commission meeting and presented my case. It went very well. I was really surprised at how cordial and logical they seemed in their approach.

I had gone there six months earlier. I knew the rules: make a face visit. That's what I did the first time and said, "When can we talk about this?" That's all I said. I didn't bug 'em. I know how to do these things. That's the nice thing about getting older. You've been through every scenario. And I've made most mistakes maybe once. Maybe twice. I've learned a lot over the years. That's how you do it with people like that—a face visit.

I didn't know what was going to happen. People all around were telling me, "Oh, you can't deal with those guys. They won't do what ya wanna do. They'll just ignore you." And it didn't turn out that way. I found out, by email on July 5 in the morning, that they okayed it. They had changed the rules.

So I was full of myself. I rode by myself to the top of Mt. Tamalpais. It felt great. And I'd just been to Crested Butte the entire week before, for the Mountain Bike Hall of Fame. There was a big party and a big reopening of their museum. I went riding all the time. You know? Nine thousand-, 10,000-, 11,000-foot elevations with a bunch of hard-cores and just going crazy. Perfect. Didn't fall. Didn't hurt myself. Didn't even get a flat. And then I come home and I ride up to the top of Tam. On the descent I was looser and faster, and faster and looser. Just ripping through everything. Because I know every square inch. This one section near the bottom I felt, I'm just going to wind it out in the biggest gear. I think I was going about 35 and my front wheel was going through a rut. Nice sculptured little rut, and I let the front wheel get outta grip. The bars flipped around and I'm stepping off the bike at about 35 and saying: This...is...stupid!

And I just rolled around. I looked up at my right hand and said, "Oh, my beautiful wrist!" It was in a Z-shape.

But it turned out to be a beautiful experience. I just laid back; suddenly there was another cyclist there, another Mt. Tam regular. She went down and got Matt, the ranger in the mountain district and an avid mountain biker. He came up and said, "Gary, what are we gonna do?" "Little ice, please," I said, "And get an ambulance down to the parking lot." And they did that. And the ambulance driver was Helena Drum, who's a road racer that I used to ride with.

That's what getting old does—you know everybody in your neighborhood. She says, "Gary, are you allergic to morphine?" When I get to the hospital they say, "Don't worry. We know who you are. We have all your medical insurance stuff online. Don't worry."

And it was fine. I stayed home for three months. It was the first time I stayed home in like 20 years. That went through the summer.

It's the worst injury I've had mountain biking, but it won't stop me. A big part of staying young is staying at-risk—despite being cautious to some degree. People will say, "You're really fast." But that's not all. I'm also really cautious. It's like both times I rode the TransAlp Challenge; I finished it, but didn't crash once.

I'll ride within myself and ride fast. But I'll ride within what I know I have confidence I can do.

Part of it is that, you know, as you get older, healing and recovery slow down. In lieu of a cast, they put a couple of long screws into the biggest bone on my hand and the big bone on my forehand, then held them together with a Robo Cop–like device that goes from one to the other. Now if I was a young punk, they'd have taken

that off in five and a half, six weeks. But it took eight to grow back.

I see all the signs of growing old. I can't recover like I used to. I'll stay tired longer. My muscle growth won't be as fast. Overall I don't have that total energy output. Take my heart rate: I can get it up to about 177. In the old days I could take it to about 200. When I was a kid, I had that much more burst power. And recovery has changed for me. I could ride harder more often back then. No doubt. For a competition over 100 miles, what used to take two days off to recover from now takes five.

But there are fitness advantages at this age. When I'm well-rested, I can go really steady, really hard. In fact, I think the way I'm fit now allows me to perform better than what I could do in my 20s. That's because I've been able to really prepare myself correctly and feed myself during the ride. I'm a better coach to myself than I ever was before.

I can still bolt from the get-go, but I've gotta get a good warm-up beforehand. When you rode the TransAlp, you didn't have time for a huge warm-up. You'd start and it'd be cold for a while. There'd be a lot of bumping around at the front. It was crazy.

In one sense, though, riding when you get older is easier. For me, easier to win.

I was a good rider when I was young. I rode Category 1 for ten years, and would be in the top 10 in Northern California, and maybe the top 100 in the nation. But my age started to become an advantage when I got into my 40s, because there are fewer guys that do it, that ride hard, and have avoided injuries.

Taking on New Challenges

MOUNTAIN BIKING IS tough. Guys stay away from it because they are worried about hurting themselves. Yes, the risk of injury is there. But that's back to what I said about youth, about continuing to push it.

It is really helpful to give yourself a challenge

and a chance to ride with people who are just a little bit better than you; sometimes, radically better than you. Just to see how people are doing it, to keep up the urge to master something. Some things, like mountain biking, you've got to master to a certain extent to enjoy. You master the bike—the same brand tire, your position, get it all dialed. If you're changing equipment all the time, it's a little more difficult to master it. And you master riding technique. You've got to work on it a lot so you can have it embedded into your memory and you can do things automatically. There's a real simple pattern to improving: You look for a weakness. Identify it. And then start to do something that works on that weakness.

It's like when I swim, which I started to do during the time I had the wrist injury. It was the hardest thing I've ever done. Amazingly, I'm not really efficient with my legs. So I gotta make sure I do a lot of paddleboards. It's like if I'm having a lot of trouble with a trail drop-off or something, I'll go back and do the same one over and over and over again. In a little tiny lap pool. I'll just go and do it again and again and again. Very soon you get very familiar and you do it. Not to overpush it, not to be obsessive about it, but to the point where you give yourself a chance. Finally you get it and you step on. I will always do that. I do it with surfing, which I got hooked on in Australia at the Olympics four years ago. It's hard to do something brand-new, that I'm a beginner at. It's the process of learning and relearning and doing it over.

I didn't really plan on having all this—the success, the notoriety. A lot was luck—like Trek reviving the brand name when my company was dead (in 1993). I never tended to look off too far into the future, to make myself promises, because I think that's a big source of disappointment. However, I could never imagine not being able to use my body. My philosophy has always been "Use it or lose it." That's why you have to continue to do things, and then go back and redo them again. It's like swimming again. Even

though I had taken lessons when I was four and five years old, my body had grown, changed, and forgotten how to do it. Your body adapts to whatever lifestyle you go to. If you neglect a part of it—i.e., don't use it—you'll lose it. I'd lost my ability to breathe properly above water, to move properly and coordinate all these things together. That's where I brought it back.

It's important to try different things and push new challenges. For years, I'd only ridden a bike and done a little yoga. It's good for me to get off into some different things. The bike, though, is the cornerstone. I don't know of any tool that elicits such amazing physical things out of a person. And it has such tonic qualities. Some people might think of it as a torture rack, and it can be at times. But it does something to the body that helps you recover and perform better. It's a really special thing that way.

I've gotten a lot more active in advocacy in the last 10 years. I'm lucky I'm able to do something as simple as just show up someplace and help somebody. That's unbelievable to me. I'm on the board of Trips for Kids, which takes inner-city kids on rides. I'll be at about four events a year in the Bay Area, and I'm going to start doing some more chapters. The kids don't know me, but they have seen the name on the bikes. They know nothing about cycling heroes, and nothing about Olympic athletes or anything like that. But they know what they like. Once, when I brought along [two-time gold-medal mountain biker and longtime Fisher endorsee] Paola Pezzo, all dressed in gold, with a totally gold-plated bike, they just went ape! They didn't know who she was, but they just knew she was important. It was hilarious. A world-class photo-op. [Amanda] was more of a commuter in the city and bike activist. That's how I met her. She's got it going naturally. We got a couple of commuter bikes—a Breezer for her and a Dutch bike for me. It's a real Dutch bike. Single speed. Fifty pounds. Old school. Brand-new. And it's so much fun.

You should see her; my god, she's a good rider. But she can't hoist her bike and walk up stairs too easily right now. She's six months pregnant. We're going to have a new kid. A boy. I'll be a new father at age 53. [Gary's son Miles was born on May 14, 2004.] Now I gotta keep it going like that 90-year-old guy [see the interview of John Sinibaldi at the end of Chapter 5].

Advice: Ride Often, Eat Better, Think Young

WHEN I WAS young, I read the CONI Blue Book, a cycling manual originally published in Italy. It was like the bike racer's bible and it still rings true to me. It had a section in there about having joy and youthfulness in your riding. It said things like that you've gotta have that flair—like bike racers should have a fast car, not a slow car, just because of the feeling of it. And a racing cyclist should feel youth in their training. It was a way of saying don't overtrain. And don't lose that youthful feeling. As you get older, keep a balance. Ride every day, ride hard once in a while, but keep it fun.

I'm lucky. I have an unusual job situation. At the end of the day, my sponsor won't fire me, no matter how I do in the race. For me it's ride, smile, and finish. I don't have to win. But when I want to, I have the time to train almost full-time—20 to 25 hours a week plus time to recover. For fitness, though, just riding every day, even if it's only like half an hour, makes a huge difference. After I broke my wrist and couldn't ride for three months, I rode in a celebrity chase race in San Francisco. Whoa! It hit me so hard. Not having stressed my body on a fairly regular basis, I was hurting bad. I think, as a rule, you need to do whatever it takes to do a good and hard ride at least once a week—maybe three times a week if you want to get better. Then make the time to recover between. On just a small amount of riding, I can maintain an amazing amount of my strength.

I am much more careful than I used to be. In my late 20s, I had a pretty good quality diet, but I could eat as much as I wanted. As I got older, I stayed away from dairy, which shrunk my gut, and ate the things I could digest thoroughly and relatively easily. I'll eat a huge salad or something that doesn't have much dressing—just olive oil and some lemon or something. And a ton of organic vegetables and a little of some kind of protein. You know, now I almost do the Atkins diet. But then when I'm actually on the bike, I'll have three-quarters carbohydrate and one-quarter protein. And then try to stay away from the carbs after the recovery. I always try to get drinks and foods where you get a little bit of protein in there.

To keep a balance as you get older, I think of three areas: building yourself up in one aspect—requiring some intense workouts and a fair amount of time; maintaining—daily riding and once-a-week stress; then there are new skills—the one that is a lot of fun. I'm learning to swim. I'm learning to surf. I wanna go back and ride a fixed-gear bike at the velodrome. There are things within the sport that you used to do and you need to pick up again. Then there are brand-new things. I want to go up to Whistler and do the free-ride park more.

If you don't mountain bike, try it. Those new physical experiences will keep you a kid at heart.

Update

THE PAST DECADE has been a wild ride for Fisher, who was 63 when I called him in January 2014. He got married to another woman 20 years his junior; he produced two kids, then 9 and 6; he got out of shape and back in shape; he watched his brainchild, the 29er, take over the mountain bike world; he watched his namesake Gary Fisher brand become so successful that it was subsumed by parent company Trek; and he remains the company's celebrity spokesman and formal "product executive," jetting off to festivals, races, and product brainstorming sessions around the world. He was most excited by the recent return of his long-lost sense of smell, which he'd missed since 1979 when he was in a bad bike crash while wearing a thin leather hair-net helmet. The accident had cracked his skull, put him in the hospital for 10 days, and oddly left him smell-disabled. "It's a whole new world," he said. "Now, I can tell the difference between the aroma of wine and roses again."

Fisher was almost as excited about bicycle advocacy—getting more people, especially kids, to ride bikes—as he was about smelling the roses. "We make our money from the sports side of it, the MAMIL (Middle Aged Male in Lycra), but the handwriting is on the wall: The market is headed to people in their 20s, teens, kids, cyclo-cross, bike polo on tennis courts, using the bike as transportation, as a lifestyle. The bike fits the economy. The old paradigm of go-to-college/get-a-job/buy-a-big-house-and-car is no more. Many people move back home with no job and $100,000 in debt from student loans. So they pull the old bike out of the garage. The bike never lies to them. The bike fits their needs."

Physically, Fisher was still in very good shape. Although he said he'd gained weight and stopped riding during his tempestuous previous relationship, he had trained hard for three months and had done a sub-five-hour century in 2013. "It hurt, I tell you. I ride fewer miles, and need more recovery now. I think the best way to go now is to go hard a couple times a week for a few months, then take it easy for a few months to recover." He does not lift weights, but does some casual daily stretching, yoga, and core work, and he gets his strength work in by climbing the 58 steps to his third-story apartment and "hangin' out with my little kids." He reduced his red meat consumption, added more oatmeal, and goes out for an occasional hammerfest with a group of local 1970s and 1980s racers "with intense egos."

The bottom line? "I'm tough," he said. "I work hard because I don't want to feel like shit. I still feel like I'm in my 30s."

8

PREHAB

How stretching, weights, butt-centric pedaling, and lateral glute strengthening can prevent and rehab cycling's two biggest injuries: "cyclist's knee" and "biker's back"

July 26, 2000, Day 5, TransAlp Challenge: "Vhy do you alvays do zat at ze checkpoints?" asks a German mountain biker. He's curious as to why my partner, Rich White, and I are tossing a Frisbee back and forth at Forcella Ambrizzola, elevation 7,000 feet, the highest stop on this grueling eight-day, 400-mile race across the Alps.

"It's a natural way to stretch and strengthen your core," explains Rich. "Since cycling is a linear activity—that is, you move forward with virtually no twisting movements—your back is the first thing to go. It gets weak, stiff, and subject to strains. Throwing a Frisbee requires a transverse motion that works your abs and the muscles around your spine, protecting you from a bad back."

I'm dumbstruck. For years, I'd viewed Rich simply as a witty bike-shop manager, not a quasi–physical therapist. Throwing a Frisbee actually helps to cure "biker's back," one of the most widespread maladies in the bike world? Crazy, but...logical. And to think: All this time, I thought we were just having fun.

🚲

May 4, 2002, Day 3, TransGabriel Challenge: Rich and I have just finished our hardest-ever ride, a self-mapped, 125-mile mountain bike expedition across

the length of the San Gabriel Mountains. We think we might be the first bikers to have conquered the fabled "Roof of L.A.," the immense wilderness just north of Los Angeles where motorcyclists scream around isolated mountain roads and serial killers dump bodies. Our route had 25,000 feet of climbing and only two remote water spigots. We each lugged camping gear and 3 gallons of water in 60-pound trailers.

I trained hard for the TransGabriel, which we designed as a training ride for the first-ever Trans-Rockies Challenge in Canada in August. Every weekend for months, I climbed hills for hours. My bike fit was perfect. But at ride's end, my knees ached; two weeks later, I dropped out of a double century at mile 96, hobbled by clicking/scraping sounds and excruciating pain. Something was wrong; this was no mere muscle strain. I stopped riding. I canceled on the TransRockies. Six months later, I had an operation on a torn meniscus. Two years later, my bad knee still wasn't right and the good one hurt.

Back in 2000, I was the first person to complete the TransAlp and La Ruta in the same year. I felt indestructible. But by early 2004, after physical therapy and a dozen doctor visits, I could barely ride, or run, or sometimes even walk.

Cycling is famously easy on knees, yet knee injuries dog the sport, due to poor bike fit and overuse. The former zapped me at Paris-Brest-Paris in 1999; the latter got me at the TransGabriel in 2002, when I'd been in shape, but hadn't trained pulling a 60-pound trailer, like Rich had. Moral of the story? It's not just "Use it or lose it." It's "Overuse it and lose it," too.

One works too little, the other too much. Those reasons, and more, are why physical therapists say that the back and the knees, respectively, are the two biggest problem areas for cyclists.

"Knee pain has been the Number 1 problem in cycling for years, but back pain is catching up fast as the cycling population ages," said Andy Pruitt, director of the renowned Boulder Center for Sports Medicine in Boulder, Colorado. Studies have shown knee injuries to be the most common overuse injuries evaluated in sports medicine centers, and can occur in over half of the participants at endurance events.

Generally, "cyclist's knee" arises from too much of a good thing. The knee becomes a victim of its own success—cycling is so fun and challenging that sometimes you can't help but overdo it. Pedaling a bike, normally so benign an activity that cycling is the preferred rehab therapy for knee injuries from other sports, can be a source of injury through sheer repetition. Since an average cyclist can turn the cranks 5,000 times an hour (around 83 rpm), the smallest amount of misalignment, whether anatomic-, technique-, or equipment-related, can lead to dysfunction, impaired performance, and pain. Moreover, even with perfect alignment, cycling's efficiency and ease on your body encourages overdoing it. On the flip side, "biker's back" is the result of inactivity—first, of the sedentary lifestyle that keeps modern humans, athletic or not, seated most of their lives, and second, by the standard cycling position, in which the spine stays hunched over and virtually immobile. Underworked and stretched-out, back muscles become too weak to do their job of maintaining your posture, and they spasm in pain.

As you saw in Chapter 7, proper fit can eliminate many knee and back problems. But fit is only a necessary first step, on its own not enough to reverse the misalignment caused by years of accumulated injuries, age-related muscle decay and inflexibility, ingrained bad habits of form, over- and underdevelopment of certain muscles, plain old overuse, and off-the-bike inactivity. In other words, if you have a history of training improperly on the bike, and your body is weak, tight, out of balance, and generally neglected off the bike, you're a ticking time bomb. Just one ride too hard and too soon, and the nagging twinges you've shrugged off for years could explode in knee and back pain bad enough to keep you off the road for weeks, months, or longer.

To make sure that doesn't happen, to roll through your 60s, 70s, and 80s on a bike saddle, not a wheelchair, this chapter watches your back with several detailed, straightforward programs of on- and off-the-bike stretching and strengthening that can restore a natural, balanced posture. To protect your knees, it provides a commonsense "overtraining-avoidance" checklist, recommends specific stretches and weight-lifting plans to keep the knee on track, advocates basic joint-building supplements, and preaches self-discipline to monitor and throttle back training loads. It also suggests that you relearn the way you ride—specifically, pushing the pedals on a vertical line like pistons in an engine (so the knee doesn't move sideways). Helping that cause is butt-centric pedaling (in which you push the pedals more with those giant, ignored powerhouses, the glutes, than with the quads).

Bottom line: The prevention and rehabilitation of cycling injuries are two sides of the same coin, which is why we call this chapter "Prehab." For long-term cycling health—and surprisingly potent gains in performance—you can't start it too soon.

SECTION 1: CYCLIST'S KNEE

Some people call it "cyclist's knee." Some call it "the overuse syndrome." Doctors officially call it patellofemoral pain, a burning sensation that occurs between and around the patella (kneecap) and the femur (thighbone). But the most succinct explanation of cycling's most common malady that I've ever heard came from Greg Stokell, a longtime manager of the old SuperGo bike shop in Santa Monica, California: "macho-itis."

"No matter the terrain or the wind or how out of shape they are, these people say, 'Pain isn't gonna stop me—I'm not gonna downshift,'" Stokell would say. "And their connective tissue screams, 'No!'"

In theory, cycling is not hazardous to your knees. One reason that the sport has grown so popular over the past 40 years is that it improves fitness in a "joint-friendly" manner (i.e., without the repetitive, 5 to 6 Gs of joint-impact forces associated with running). Overall, cycling is considered to be much less injury producing than running, and many runners substitute cycling for running workouts in order to give their legs a break and recover more completely between running sessions. "Knees don't have to be a problem in cycling. In fact, it's so stress-free that we put people from other sports into cycling for rehabilitation," said Gail Weldon, a Los Angeles physical therapist.

Nonetheless, knee pain happens in cycling. "And when it does, it indicates that you are doing something wrong," said Weldon. "That's why any problem a cyclist has with his knees was probably avoidable—and generally fixable. Even hill climbing is no problem—as long as you have the strength and conditioning."

That's it in a nutshell: If a proper bike fit, and, to a lesser degree, proper training and technique (Chapters 1 and 2), don't help you avoid knee pain or rehab it, you're probably overdoing it. "Overuse" injuries result when the chosen volume or intensity of training causes damage to tissues that are not adequately repaired during a training cycle. Cyclists feel the pain if they ride too long, too fast, too steep, or too soon without a sufficient warm-up or training base. That's why overuse injuries are especially prevalent early in the season, after months of winter inactivity. "They haven't done anything at all, then they go on a full-day ride on a Sunday," said Beverly Hills chiropractor Russell Cohen. "And we see them in the office on Monday."

Hard-core racers are no different from average Joes. "Most injuries I see are from competitive cyclists who come back too soon," said Jim Beazell, PhD, former chief physical therapist and professor at the University of Virginia–HealthSouth physical therapy clinic in Charlottesville, and an avid cyclist. "These people are too gonzo—they ride 100 miles the first weekend without training." That tendency has been encouraged by the growth of ultra-endurance events, cross-state road rides, 24-hour mountain biking, and 200-mile gravel road races over the past couple decades.

Cyclist's knee doesn't discriminate by age. Older bodies and joints aren't as strong, flexible, and well-lubricated as they were 15 or 20 years before, so they get hurt if they aren't warmed up enough or given enough recovery time. Yet youthful vigor can create problems, too. Although younger riders tend to be stronger and more flexible, they get hurt because they go harder and longer.

Conclusion: Beware overuse. Ride too hard, too steep, too far, or too fast, and something's gotta give. Often, what will give is the weakest link: the knee.

Why Knees Are at Risk in Cycling

The knee is one of the body's most vulnerable joints, and extra-heavy demands can overwhelm it. Acting as part hinge and part pulley, the knee extends and flexes the leg by functioning as a juncture of our biggest bones and muscles: the thighbone (femur), the kneecap (patella), and the shinbone (tibia), as well as the smaller bone of the shin (fibula); the quadriceps and other muscles of the thigh; the hamstrings (the muscle group running down the back of the upper leg); and the calf muscles. All of these are strapped together by a crisscrossing latticework of tendons, ligaments, and cartilage.

"The knee is a relatively unstable connection in which bones can be easily displaced, which is why it has the most stress and abuse potential of any area of the body during athletics," explains Peter Duong, PhD, an anatomy instructor at Indiana State University. "Even though bicycling, unlike running, is a non-weight-bearing activity and has little lateral motion, it generates forces in the area between the kneecap and thighbone that can actually amount to several times the body weight."

For a cyclist, knee pain is most often manifested in two different conditions: *patellar tendinitis* and *chondromalacia*. The most common is the former, which refers to a strain of the tendons, the tough fibers that attach the quadriceps to the kneecap and the hamstrings to the shinbone. Tendinitis is painful, but quickly and easily fixed with rest.

Chondromalacia, burning pain that occurs between the patella and the femur, occurs less frequently than tendinitis, but it's far more serious. For some rather complex reasons (to be described below), including extreme training, poor alignment, and natural overdevelopment of one side of the thigh muscle, the kneecap can get pulled off its track during the leg extension, tearing up some cartilage in the process. Initial patellofemoral pain can be severe, but often occurs after cycling rather than during the ride. Further agitated, it can become chondromalacia, a painful, almost audible grating sensation with every stroke that cannot be completely rehabilitated. Chondro is permanent damage, and it usually leads to arthritis. It is to be avoided at all costs.

Below, more details about chondro and tendinitis, and a plan to deal with them.

Patellar Tendinitis
Patellar tendinitis, the most common cycling

knee injury, is the inflammation of the tendon structure that surrounds the kneecap and connects the thigh's quadriceps muscles to the lower leg. When the tendons are repeatedly stretched beyond their capability, they become inflamed and enlarged by microtears that heal as scars. The swelling causes them to move with increased friction and pain. According to Andy Pruitt, patellar tendinitis shows up as a burning pain in the front of the knee, below the kneecap, while pedaling or walking up or down stairs. It hurts to the touch and may, he said, "squeak like a rusty hinge."

The reason that tendinitis occurs in cyclists' knees at all, despite cycling being a low-impact activity, has to do with the knee's essential functionality in movement. The patella is designed both to protect the knee from a direct blow and to create a fulcrum that increases the mechanical efficiency of the quads, which are the prime movers in cycling (for those who haven't yet tapped the power of the butt muscles, see "Butt Power," later in this chapter). The contraction of the quads and tendons pushes the pedals down. Seems simple, right? But usually only the tendons get strained, not the muscles. That's because tendons have a poor blood supply, so they don't strengthen as fast as the muscles. Since the muscles don't get tougher faster, there is a tendency to push them beyond the tendons' ability to cope, resulting in pain in the tendons and within the knee joint.

Of course, fitness is relative; what's too hard for your tendons in March may not be what's too hard for them in July, when you're better trained. As you'll see below, knowing where you stand fitness-wise is a key to staying injury-free.

CAUSES AND SOLUTIONS
Most of the time, tendinitis is caused by a training volume and/or intensity that is too high for under-conditioned and under-strengthened tendons. But other issues also play a role. To help avoid tendinitis, we've outlined its causes and effects in the table below.

TENDINITIS AVOIDANCE/RECOVERY PLAN

Cause of the Problem	Solution
A. Lack of conditioning	Off-season weight training; SAID principle (gradual buildup; see below); periodized training plan; 10-percent-increase rule
B. Sudden, overly hard efforts	10-minute warm-up; spin in low gears
C. Under-lubrication of the joint	Same as above
D. Cold weather	Knickers and tights; gradual warm-up
E. Tight hamstrings	Stretch before, during, and after rides; massage afterward
F. Too-low seat	Raise seat

A. CAUSE: *Lack of conditioning.*

Tendons will strengthen over time; you can't rush them. They'll get overwhelmed without time for conditioning. Since they become stronger more slowly than muscles on account of their poor blood supply, assume that they are getting hurt if your muscles are starting to hurt. Beware of increasing your mileage drastically and/or using gears that are too high. And if they do get hurt, remember that they take longer to repair and heal than muscles do.

SOLUTION 1: *Weight-train in the off-season.*

Strengthen your knees and the quadriceps muscle before you begin serious training with leg presses, squats, bench step-ups, bicycle leg swings, knee extensions, hamstring curls, stair climbing, and very small amounts of cycling against high resistance. Weight-maintained tendons will not fatigue as quickly as untrained tendons when the riding begins. (See the "Lift Weights" section of Chapter 1.)

SOLUTION 2: *Use the SAID principle, maintain an off-season base, and start gradually.*

For decades, athletic trainers have sworn by the SAID principle—Specific Adaptation to Impose Demand. "Tissue and ligaments actually get

stronger with stressful activity," explained Jim Beazell. "That response is there in your body. If you don't abuse it—meaning adding more stress gradually—you'll be okay."

Starting slowly strengthens most structures involved in cycling: muscles, tendons, and ligaments—everything except bones (see Chapter 9). Once body structures are strengthened, they can handle high training loads.

"We didn't have many injuries at this level because all the connective tissue had been strengthened," said former US national team coach Dan Birkholz. "Once in a while, we'd get a little tendinitis when a guy hadn't been working out for a while, then would jump back in too quick."

Generally, cycling trainers promote a 10 percent rule: Don't increase the duration or intensity of a cyclist's training by more than 10 percent a week. Some trainers and physical therapists are even more conservative, recommending maximum weekly increases of only 5 percent. "That's why it's important to keep some sort of base in the off-season," said Jenny Stone, a former USCF athletic trainer. "You won't have so far to come back."

Ultimately, the most foolproof tendinitis-avoidance method may be to follow a periodized training program like the one described in Chapter 1. Periodization, honed by Eastern bloc strength coaches in the Cold War era and now a staple for all types of athletic training, carefully stair-steps athletes up to performance peaks through successive four-week training blocks. In a methodical sequence, it focuses on incrementally building strength, endurance, and speed, preparing the body to handle larger loads without injury.

Incidentally, the "gradual increase" rule also goes for terrain. Start off your training on flatter surfaces first. Don't do a 50-mile cross-country trip through the mountains right away. Don't pull an 80-pound trailer over steep hills for 125 miles if you've never ridden with one before!

B. CAUSE: *Sudden hard efforts and impact.*

According to Pruitt, tendinitis can appear with sudden, high-stress actions, including hard sprinting, big-gear climbing, and off-bike activities such as hard leg presses, squats, or jumping.

SOLUTION: *Do a 10-minute warm-up with low-gear spinning.*

Apply the "start slowly" rule to the beginning of every ride, not just the beginning of the season. A good analogy is starting a car. Any mechanic will tell you that you "shock" your engine and reduce its life by instantly zooming away when the ignition is turned; any motor will last longer if you let it warm up for 60 seconds in the driveway, allowing it to coat its pistons and other moving parts in a soothing oil bath before hitting the freeway. An easy 5- to 10-minute warm-up in lower gears does the same thing for your body, calmly priming your capillaries to open up and begin distributing blood throughout the muscles and the heart to increase their workload. The result: You don't go anaerobic, your knees smoothly transition into action, and your tendons don't get stressed.

C. CAUSE: *Under-lubrication of the joint.*

Muscles and tendons aren't the only things that are ill-prepared for sudden increases in stress; you can also exceed your body's ability to lubricate the joint itself. To keep the bones sliding easily against each other without rubbing, the knees manufacture their own lubricant, called synovial fluid. Like any manufacturing plant, the synovial membranes scale down production during periods of inactivity. That's why, if you lay off all winter and then go all-out on the first day of spring, your knee will be under-lubed.

"If the biomechanics of the rider are okay, the problem is one of overstressing the structures in your joint," said Beazell. "It's like the bearing surfaces in an axle: If they're not greased or lubed, they'll break down. Same thing in a joint." Beyond the fact that the joint itself can suffer significant injury without lubrication, the tendon must work harder to overcome the added friction in the joint.

SOLUTION: *Ride in low gears and spin.*

Rapidly pedaling in lower gears puts much less stress on the joints than slowly pushing large gears. Big-gear pushing exacerbates all other problems. Spinners generally don't get much patellofemoral pain.

D. CAUSE: *Cold weather.*

Riding in the cold without adequate covering also restricts lubrication. Blood vessels constrict in the cold, shunting blood and oxygen away from surface areas—like the knees—to the vital organs. All knee structures, including the synovial membranes that lubricate the knee, will be undernourished. That's why the knees ache after a cold day.

SOLUTION: *Cover up.*

Ride in knickers or full-length tights to keep the knees' joint-lubrication mechanism warm enough to maintain flow to tendons and muscles. Doing so even makes riding in the dead of winter knee-safe. "There's no such thing as bad weather—only bad clothing," said fabled Minneapolis bike messenger Gene Oberpriller, who for years rode every winter day, in temperatures as low as 40 degrees below zero, with a 70-below windchill. Oberpriller is to cold-weather bike clothing what Imelda Marcos is to shoes. Of course, it takes him 20 minutes to put his clothes on. In the winter, he wears fleece-lined tights over his regular padded cycling shorts, making them easy to strip off when it warms up. And when the cold is combined with a stiff wind, Oberpriller slows down. "Windchill increases exponentially," he said. "Stay under 22 mph or in your middle chainring."

E. CAUSE: *Tight hamstrings.*

The range of motion of the leg on the downstroke is limited when the hamstrings are tight, compressing the knee. The hamstrings, actually three separate muscles at the back of the leg which connect the pelvis to the back of the knee, serve to bend the knee—the opposite function of the quads. If the hamstring muscles are tight, the quads and tendons have to work harder to straighten the leg on the downstroke. (Note: Tight hamstrings also have highly negative effects on the back and all-over bike fit. See Chapter 7 and the "Back" section later in this chapter.)

SOLUTION 1: *Stretch hamstrings before, after, and during the ride.*

Stretching should be an integral part of cycling. Before a ride (cold stretching, contrary to some reports, is completely safe), it prepares your body by getting nutrient- and oxygen-packed blood flowing to all parts of the muscles and tendons. Spend additional time stretching in the morning, as muscles tighten during sleep. They are naturally more stretched-out in the afternoon or evening due to daylong movement. Stretching after a workout helps to restore ("warm down") the body to its normal state by re-elongating exercise-tightened muscles and blood vessels. Stretching speeds the inflow of blood—and the outflow of exercise waste products, such as lactic acid.

What is the correct way to stretch the hamstrings? According to physical therapist Bob Forster, whose Phase IV High Performance Center in Santa Monica, California, specializes in cycling, triathlon, and running training, all stretches are safest if performed on the ground. Sit with your left leg outstretched and the right bent so that the bottom of the foot is wedged against the upper inside of the left thigh. Slowly reach for your outstretched toes and lower your upper body by bending at the waist, keeping the back as straight as possible. Don't move fast; that will stimulate the muscle to tighten up. Also, don't hold the stretch for more than five seconds; that leads to permanent elongation, which is not the goal here. Do this stretch several times, then switch legs.

Note: Avoid the old-fashioned hurdler's stretch, in which the foot of the bent leg is placed straight back under the glutes. That puts too much pressure on the knee. (For a full range of stretches, see Chapter 4.)

Ideally, cyclists should stretch not only before and after riding, but while they ride, as muscles and tendons tighten. But you don't need to get off the bike. If you just climbed a hill, for example, you can stretch in the downhill and the flats. Here's how: While coasting, stand and press the heel of the lower leg down, then arch your pelvis toward the handlebar.

SOLUTION 2: *Get a massage.*

Often overlooked, sports massage, like stretching, loosens and rearranges muscle sheathing and helps to bring oxygenated blood back into your muscles.

F. CAUSE: *Too-low seat.*

Riding too low or too far forward in relation to the pedals is how millions of recreational cyclists unwittingly simulate overtraining. A low seating position causes the knee to flex more, generating more stress and causing the quadriceps tendon to rub against the thighbone. It forces the rider to push the pedal at a less efficient angle and to work the tendons and quads too hard.

SOLUTION: *(Surprise!) Raise the seat.*

Sit high enough on the bike to give only a slight bend to the knee at the bottom of the pedal stroke—about a 150-degree angle. This is the most efficient, least stressful position.

What to Do Once Tendinitis Strikes

1. Back off. There's no need to stop training completely, but at the first sign of tendinitis (i.e., pain and swelling) you must shift into "active rest." Cut your mileage by 50 percent, pedal easily, avoid hills, and eliminate all interval training. Coordinate your "active rest" with icing, stretching, restrengthening, and perhaps ultrasound and anti-inflammatory medications. Of cyclists with patellofemoral pain, most symptoms were alleviated by the use of those simple, traditional treatments. Warning: Do not immediately return to the same training load as before; that will probably bring the pain right back again.

2. Ice the area. "Ice is the miracle treatment," said physical therapist Bob Forster. "It blocks pain and reduces many aspects of an injury, including spasms, inflammation, and swelling." How ice works may surprise you. Although pain is a good thing—it is a protective mechanism that creates increased muscle tension that limits movement—the swelling that comes with it can do more harm than good, especially for an athlete who needs to recover fast.

"Swelling occurs when the body dumps a large quantity of water in the area, which has the unfortunate effect of stopping blood flow," explained Forster. "So we have to out-think the body—and limit the inflammatory response by immediately applying ice to minimize the swelling. This causes an initial vasoconstriction, which pushes out fluids." When the ice is removed after 20 to 30 minutes, the veins open up, the flow is reversed, and the body sends blood, not water, flooding back to the area.

Andy Pruitt recommends that a two-step icing process be used three times per day until the tendon feels healed. He said to place crushed ice or small cubes in a resealable plastic bag and place it on top of a washcloth laid across the affected tendon. The cloth protects the skin from damage. After 15 to 20 minutes, remove the ice pack for half an hour, then reapply. You can also rub raw ice on the affected area with a gentle massage motion, but you must stop after about 5 minutes, when the skin gets numb. Pruitt said you may speed the tendon's recovery by performing cross-friction massage (rubbing across the tendon fibers with your thumb for 10 minutes) before reapplying the ice.

3. Get whirlpool treatments. Whirlpools bring more blood to the injured tendon by vasodilating and massaging the tissues, while the microstimulation speeds the healing of injured tissue.

4. Modify your activity. Early in the season, limit situations that put extreme stress on your tendons, such as squatting, lunging, leg presses, and stair climbing.

5. Continue stretching. Stretching will not disrupt healing if it's limited to the pain-free range of motion, said Forster.

6. Take aspirin. To relieve the inflammation, most physical therapists recommend aspirin, taken at a rate of six or eight each day spaced according to package instructions.

7. Use heat and cover. Before riding, increase blood flow to the area by applying products such as Ben-Gay or Icy Hot, said Pruitt. Then shield the injured tendon from cold winds with leg warmers or a coating of petroleum jelly.

Chondromalacia and Lateral Tracking

Chondromalacia is bad news. The word comes from the Greek words for cartilage (*chondro*), bad (*mal*), and softening (*acia*). It refers to the shredding, softening, and wearing away of the cartilage on the underside of the kneecap that occurs when the kneecap is not centered in the groove at the bottom of the femur and scrapes against the lateral side of the groove. Felt as a burning sensation between the patella and the femur, chondromalacia occurs less frequently than tendinitis, but it's far more disabling, often leading to serious structural damage or arthritis. Tendinitis responds to rest, but the tissue damaged in chondromalacia doesn't quite return to normal—ever.

One look under a microscope explains why. "In a normal knee, the kneecap should slide on your thighbone as smoothly as two ice cubes against each other," said Beazell. "That's because the patella is surrounded by shiny, super-smooth hyaline cartilage, which is meant for gliding. But with chondromalacia, the cartilage gets frayed. In its bad stage it looks like kelp hanging off the back of the kneecap."

Chondromalacia is painful; extending or flexing your knee may include a grating or crunching sensation that can sound like the crackle of Rice Krispies and feel as painful as being raked by shards of broken glass. It especially hurts when you're pushing big gears, or climbing or descending stairs, and may feel achy and stiff after you've been sitting. If you feel any symptoms resembling these, don't wait for later. Chondro is difficult to rehab and portends a future of arthritis.

Why Chondro Happens:
Lateral Tracking of the Kneecap

If "Know thyself" is the key to self-enlightenment, "Know thy anatomy" may be the key to understanding and preventing chondromalacia. The hyaline cartilage that Beazell mentioned gets torn up when the kneecap doesn't track evenly where it should: in the groove at the end of the thighbone, which is formed by its two ball-shaped knobs (the same shape you see on a chicken drumstick bone). Although the front of the kneecap is flat, the back part—the part you don't see from the outside—is V-shaped, so it can slide

smoothly in the thighbone's groove throughout all ranges of a kneebend.

Two groups of muscles are involved in moving the knee: the quadriceps, found on the front of the thigh, which straightens the leg and extends the knee as it flexes; and the hamstrings, on the back of the thigh, which bend the knee back as it flexes. In bicycling, the quads push the pedal down while the hamstrings pull the pedal up.

The quadriceps ("four-head") is actually made up of four separate muscles that all begin at different points ("heads") on the hip and attach together at the bottom of the thighbone at the knee. When the four muscles contract, the patella is pulled up and the knee straightens out. If you hold your leg out straight and flex your thigh, you may be able to see three of the quad muscles—the *vastus lateralis*, on the lateral (outside) of the leg, the *vastus medialis* on the medial ("middle" of body, or inner) thigh, and the *rectus femoris* in the middle. You can't see the *vastus intermedialis*, which is underneath the other three, around the femur.

The problem, "lateral tracking," occurs when the kneecap comes out of the groove on the lateral (outside) side of the leg. This has the same effect on your knee as a car tire that is out of alignment: It wears the cartilage out in one spot.

When the kneecap is out of its track, all the pressure of the cyclist's pedal stroke is focused on only one small part of the kneecap, instead of being distributed evenly and painlessly over the entire kneecap surface. The cartilage is scraped at that point and chondromalacia begins.

Runners, because of the weight-bearing pounding their knees take, have far more trouble with chondromalacia than cyclists do (so much so that it's commonly known as "runner's knee"). But what bicycling lacks in quality of stress, it often makes up for in quantity. "Cyclists spin at a fast rate," said Beazell. "Eighty-rpm bicycling legs are extending and flexing twice as fast as a guy running a four-minute mile—and you can ride at 80 rpm for hours." As a result, biomechanically imbalanced cyclists can put a little bit of stress on a specific area of cartilage repeatedly for a long period of time—maybe 10,000 revolutions on an average three-hour, 40-mile ride. The problem may not surface at low riding levels. "A lot of people can get away with a little biomechanical inefficiency at lower workout levels," Beazell adds. "But when you increase in intensity, it really shows up."

Getting Your Knee Back in the Groove: A Four-Step Strategy for Treating Chondromalacia

Ask any physical therapist about "curing" chondromalacia, and you'll get a look of resignation and a variety of answers, none of them good. You can fix the problem, limit the damage, and even rebuild the knee a bit. But the truth is that once chondro strikes, the knee will never be as good as it used to be.

"That's because the hyaline cartilage (that was ruined) replaces itself with a lesser grade of cartilage," said Beazell. "It fills in with fibrocartilage, which isn't as good—and can be ruined even easier." Surgery is iffy, and radical pain-reduction methods that attempt to smooth the frayed cartilage through arthroscopic "patella shaving" surgery, or rapid-flexing, tissue-sanding isokinetic exercises (such as on Cybex machines), are poorly regarded by many physical therapists and often considered ineffective. (The latter are particularly dangerous for people with high blood pressure and other heart-related problems.)

In spite of its poor prognosis for full recovery, chondromalacia doesn't have to be a lifelong curse that stops you from riding. Here are four steps you can take to try to get your kneecap back in its groove and tracking properly, stop further damage, and get back to pain-free riding as soon as possible:

Step 1: *Get a proper bike fit and gear down.*

Since chondromalacia is considered an overuse injury, the first stage of its rehab sounds a lot like the strategy for tendinitis: Stop riding, correct your position, and resume riding at a radically reduced level. In the short run, rest will stop further damage from occurring and allow for some healing. You can fix harmful, inefficient biomechanics through correct bike fit, paying particular attention to seat height, said Pruitt. (Too low, and it puts shearing force on the back of the kneecap; raise it to the point where you start rocking, then lower it just enough to stop the motion.) Then avoid or gear down your training to the point where you can ride with no pain, and gradually ramp it back up. Because the kneecap cartilage is left permanently weaker after chondromalacia, the rider should be careful to spin in lower gears in all future riding. "It doesn't mean you'll have to hitchhike up hills or ride in a 42x19 [an easy gear ratio] for the rest of your life," said Beazell. "Just be smart in your training—and keep aware of the SAID principle."

Step 2: *Correct the kneecap position by strengthening and stretching.*

If a better fit doesn't work, it indicates that your lateral tracking is caused by biomechanical problems that can be rooted in two areas: (1) physiological abnormalities, such as leg-length differences; and/or (2) imbalanced muscular development, such as an overdeveloped vastus lateralis, a product of imperfect genetics or poor form. Whatever the causes, quickly take deliberate steps to address them in order to reposition the kneecap back toward the center. Bad biomechanics accelerate knee destruction. The knee is a complex joint that is under constant assault from microstresses between the kneecap and the thighbone that are present in nearly everyone. But the more imbalanced a person's biomechanics and muscular development, the shorter the time period before cartilage irritation arises. Your solutions will be found in a fitter's toolbox and in the weight room, via strengthening relatively weaker muscles and stretching the stronger ones.

1. Address physiological abnormalities.

A good bike fit will take care of bicycle and equipment settings (saddle height, cleat position, cleat type, and shoe type) and abnormal fore-foot and rear-foot alignment. But what about something natural, like leg-length discrepancies, excessive feet pronation (duck feet) or supination (pigeon-toed), flat feet, bowlegs, or knock-knees?

"Any of those may cause problems, but over a quarter-inch difference is a red flag," said Victor Larivee, a Santa Monica bike fitter. "A cyclist puts stress on his joints when he doesn't ride in his 'neutral position,' or natural gait, and leg-length differences beyond a quarter-inch are not considered neutral."

Solution: Use artificial means to raise the short leg to match the other one, such as shims under the cleat, a lift on the pedal, or platform shoes.

2. Strengthen the inside thigh muscle (VMO) and stretch the outside leg muscle (VL) and the iliotibial (IT) band.

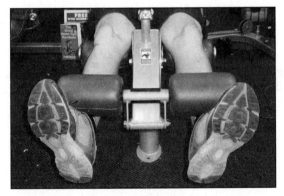

Leg extension: To help pull an off-track kneecap back to the center, strengthen the VMO on the leg-extension machine. During this movement, tilt your feet and legs to the outside, as pictured. Do them one-legged frequently to check and fix unequal quad strengths.

Some researchers believe that the motion of cycling—a straight-ahead leg movement rather than the centered, in-line footprint of running

and walking—has a natural tendency to cause an imbalance in the thigh muscles, which can cause lateral tracking of the kneecap. This imbalance is the overdevelopment of the muscle on the outside of the thigh compared to the one on the inside. Bike racers are famous for having huge quadriceps, the group of four muscles on the front of the thigh that extend/straighten the leg, but cycling apparently causes the one on the outside, the vastus lateralis (VL), to become much bigger and stronger than the one on the inner, or medial, front of the thigh, the vastus medialis (VMO; technically the muscle is called the vastus medialis oblique).

According to a study completed for the book *Physiology in Bicycling*, a seminal overview coproduced by a prestigious Danish sports-research institute and USA Cycling, the VL and the gluteus maximus (the large buttock muscle) are heavily involved in pushing the pedals down at peak force, but the VMO is not. That is understandable: Put your fingers on the VMO as you sit on a chair and straighten your leg; it does not flex (stiffen) almost until the leg straightens, which *should never occur* in the pedal stroke. Although the study was made on track racers, the researchers found a similar recruitment pattern in recreational riders.

Why is this a potential problem? The overdeveloped VL, now relatively stronger than the VMO, can exert a strong pull on the kneecap that can tug at it laterally. You know the rest: When the difference in strengths between the VL and the VMO is great, the kneecap can be yanked sideways, lateral tracking begins, and the underside of the kneecap begins scraping valuable cartilage away from itself and the end of the femur. Does this mean that a lateral tracking of the patella is unavoidable in cycling? Not necessarily. "After all," asked Beazell, "if the lateralis always got stronger than the medialis, then why is it that every Tour de France rider doesn't have a patella lateral-tracking problem?" Why some biomechanically sound cyclists get lateral tracking of the kneecap and others don't isn't clear. Natural overdevelopment of the VL in cycling is a fact; concluding that this causes knee pain isn't always accurate.

Still, if you have problems with your knees, many agree that it couldn't hurt to do two things to stabilize the kneecap: Strengthen the inside muscle of your quad, the VMO, to pull the kneecap back into line, and stretch the outside of your leg, which can help to loosen its outside pull on the kneecap.

A. Build up the vastus medialis, the inner-thigh quad muscle. Get familiar with the leg-extension machine, because you'll be using it a lot to prehab and rehab lateral-tracking problems. During the exercise, keep your toes pointed out to the sides as if you had duck feet, then complete the exercise to full extension. Bring the bar straight up with your leg at full extension. This exercise works the entire quad, but specifically targets the VMO. Like the pedal stroke itself, standard leg extensions don't fully extend the leg, somewhat ignoring the VMO. Lift heavy weights with low reps to build strength and size.

B. Loosen up the lateral pull on your kneecap by stretching the VL and IT band.

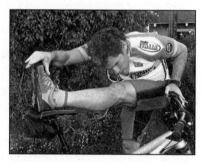

Opposite hand-foot crossover: This IT/quad stretch loosens the lateral pull on the kneecap.

VL Stretches

1. Standing quad stretch: Stand on one leg, grab the opposite foot or ankle from behind, and pull it up toward the butt. Put your knees together and push your hips forward. Hold on to something until you can balance freestanding.

2. Prone quad stretch: Lying on the ground, facedown, pull one foot up behind your butt, and slowly raise your leg off the ground.

3. Kneeling quad stretch: Kneel on one knee with the shin of that leg resting flat on the ground behind you. The other leg is out in front, bent at the knee at a 90-degree angle, shin perpendicular to the floor, with your foot flat on the ground. From here, push your hips forward to feel a stretch in the quad of the kneeling leg.

4. Side quad stretch: In this stretch you lie on your side with the bottom arm outstretched past your head, with knees together, as if you were doing a standing stretch that is turned horizontal. Then pull your top leg behind your butt and push your hips forward.

5. Tensor fascia lata stretch: Lie on your back with knees bent and arms out wide. Cross your legs and use the top leg to push the bottom leg over to the side. Take your legs over until your opposite shoulder starts to come off the floor; you should feel the stretch on the outer thigh and hip area.

IT Band Stretches

Some think that a tight iliotibial band is more responsible for lateral tracking of the kneecap than an overdeveloped VL. (I personally found that IT band stretches provided immediate relief for my lateral tracking problems.) The IT band is a wide sheath of tough, fibrous connective tissue extending on the outer side of the thigh from the front of the pelvis's iliac bone (the crest of the hip) to the top of the lower leg's tibia bone just below the knee. Flexible only at the hip, it feels like the thick, old-fashioned leather belt on which barbers sharpen their blades.

1. Crossover bend: Stand erect, move the left foot to the right of the right foot, thrust the left hip out sideways, and tilt your upper body to the right. If you can't balance, extend your left arm against a wall or chair or other stable object. You'll feel the IT band stretch from the hip all the way down the length of the thigh to the knee.

2. _The lazy leg stretch:_ Lie on your right side at the very edge of your mattress so that your butt is almost falling off the edge (as you are facing the middle of the bed). Let your top leg (left) fall behind you and over the edge of the bed. Let the weight of your leg stretch your hip. Repeat o[n] the other side.

3. _Hanging crossover:_ Lie on the floor on [your] back with your body in a T shape, with arms spread wide and legs straight forward. Then lift your left leg up one foot and move it sideways over the right leg, until it is suspended at a right angle. All the time, keep your arms outstretched and back as flat on the ground as possible. Let gravity pull it down toward the ground; hold for a minute. Repeat on the other side.

4. _Roller massage:_ Lying sideways on the floor, roll back and forth over a 6-inch-diameter Therapy Foam Roller (about $20 at fitness stores) from hip to knee. "It'll hurt at first," said Bruce Hendler, owner of the AthletiCamps cycling school in Davis, California. "But there is no better way to loosen up the IT band—especially as it gets more rigid down toward the knee. It's a cheap private massage." Hendler believes the majority of knee problems, from tendinitis to lateral tracking, are related to tight IT bands.

3. _Stretch tight adductors._

In June 2004, I served as a test subject for a motion-capture experiment conducted by Christopher M. Powers, PhD, a physical therapist and director of the Musculoskeletal Biomechanics Research Laboratory at the University of Southern California Medical Center in Los Angeles. The test led him to speculate that tight adductors (the upper-inner-thigh muscles, which pull the leg toward the midline of the body) and/or weak external rotators and abductors (gluteus minimus and medius, which pull the leg away from the midline) may lead to knee-cartilage

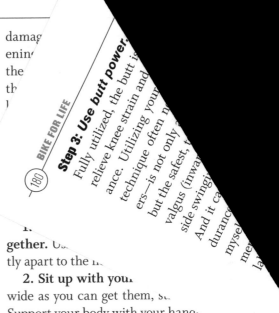

damag[e]
enin[g]
the
th[
]

Fully utilized, the butt i[s] relieve knee strain and ance. Utilizing you[r] technique often n ers—is not only but the safest, t valgus (inwa side swingi And it c duranc mysel me la

[
]
gether. U[s]
tly apart to the [n]

2. Sit up with you[r] wide as you can get them, s[t] Support your body with your hand[s]

Abductor Strengthening

1. Crabwalks: With a rubber stretch band around your knees, do side-to-side crab walks for 1 minute, increasing to 5 minutes over time.

2. Abductor machine: Start by sitting forward on the seat with the pads spaced so that your knees are close together. Spread the pads out with your legs for a count of 5 seconds, doing as many reps as possible. Increase the hold time to 10 seconds when 5 becomes too easy.

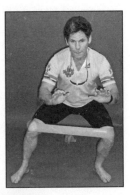

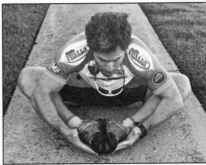

Stretch-band crab walk aids vertical pedal stroke by strengthening weak gluteus medius and minimus muscles.

Adductor stretch

a powerhouse that will
increase speed and endur-
glutes during pedaling—a
t even used by the best rid-
superb way to generate power,
o. Glute-centric riding eliminates
d knee bend) and excessive side-to-
ng of the knee during the downstroke.
clearly give you more power and en-
, as studies have documented. I saw it for
during my own motion-capture experi-
t with Dr. Powers at the USC biomechanics
. My heart rate didn't change as the watts rose
when I powered through my glutes and straightened my knee through the pedal stroke. More on
this in a minute; first, some background.

Many racers almost seem to touch the top
tube with their knees as they ride, pushing inward to get leverage as they set up their downstroke. Some believe that riding with the knees
angled inward is aerodynamic. Pictures of the
pros in such a position inspire amateurs to ride
the same way, effecting a figure-eight motion
from the hip down when viewed from the front.
But pedaling this way is not a good idea. It is inefficient and can lead to injuries.

"Valgus—an inward bend of the knee—increases lateral force on the kneecap and is
known to lead to knee injuries," said Dr. Powers.
"The knee should stay in the same plane during
the pedal stroke, like a piston in an engine."

In fact, the proof that valgus leads to injuries is
well documented. One study found "excessive
side-to-side swinging of the knee during downstroke in more than 80 percent of cyclists with patellofemoral pain." The late Ed Burke, PhD, a
prodigious ultra-cycling participant and University
of Colorado researcher, who wrote extensively on
cycling biomechanics, found that of "cyclists with
no patellofemoral pain, most had a linear pattern
of downstroke, with little mediolateral deviation."

Another nail in the "valgus-is-bad" coffin is
the common knowledge that women have a

natural valgus, and that it makes them more pre-
disposed than men to lateral tracking problems
and chondromalacia. Wide hips cause the thighs
to bend in, the knees to come together, and the
lower leg to bow out, creating the valgus syndrome and a lateral pull on the patella.

A cure for valgus in male riders and narrow-
hipped women is both simple and complex: Use
butt power—a full utilization of your gluteal
muscles while riding. An accurate fitting that
aligns hips, knees, and ankles theoretically eliminates valgus and puts the rider in an efficient
position that yields more power. Specifically,
this correct position—a hip-flexor angle under
45 degrees—forces you to make more use of the
huge, powerful gluteus maximus muscles, which
are routinely underutilized in cycling.

"After a fit, so many people call me and say,
'Wow, I can feel my glutes working—I've never
climbed a hill so fast," said Pam Wilson, a biomechanist who provides the EMG studies used by
Paul Levine of Signature Cycles (featured in Chapter 7). "When you aren't fit correctly, the glutes are
turned off and you focus too much on your quads."

Everyone, regardless of injury, should use a
glute-centric pedaling technique; it yields reduced valgus, more efficiency, and less potential
for injuries. But achieving that ideal form requires more than a perfect bike fit; it requires a
change of mindset. You have to change your
thinking from quad-centric to glute-centric.

The importance of the butt in maximizing
power through the pedal stroke (and the opportunity cost of ignoring it) is what led me to participate in the "time-in-motion biomechanics
mapping" research with Dr. Powers at his USC lab.
That's a fancy way of saying that he turned me into
a cartoon movie. When I arrived at his lab with my
regular road bike in June 2004, he attached a
dozen light-reflecting diodes to the clothing on my
legs and back. His computer program then converted those points of light into an onscreen, moving, stick-figure version of me. Then,
experimenting with different pedal strokes, such

as initiating power for a few minutes with a normal quad-centric contraction and then consciously switching to a butt-centric stroke initiated from the hips, we overlaid the various cartoon images and synched those with their respective heart-rate and power data. Here's what we noticed:

⥤ A butt-centric pedal stroke resulted in less valgus, flatter back, less quad fatigue and perceived exertion, and same power at same heart rate, probably meaning better staying power and endurance.

The seated pedaling, focusing through the butt muscles, rather than the quads, instantly caused striking changes in my biomechanics, muscle usage, joint stress, and pedaling efficiency; reduced valgus and side-to-side rocking; and kept my back flat instead of bowed (therefore reducing the risk of back pain). The butt-centric riding not only promised long-term reduced knee and back pain, Powers said, but also appeared to provide a more solid platform for push-off, based on my CompuScan results. Those results showed that my glute-centric riding had nearly the identical wattage and heart-rate levels as my quad-centric riding, but with *less perceived exertion.* As the gluteal muscles became conditioned to the new motion, we found that my endurance (ability to maintain the same power over time without a rise in heart rate) increased. My own anecdotal on-the-road riding experiences over the years have made me a butt-centric believer.

The bottom line: The butt is a knee-saving powerhouse that will allow you to ride stronger longer. Ignore it at your own risk. Tapping it will require you to do something hard: Completely rethink your riding technique, focusing on initiating the pedal stroke with the butt muscles before you engage the quads. But by doing so, you will ride with a better, more piston-like form; spread the workload over more muscles; and protect your knees *and* your back from injury. Reeducating yourself may be the most difficult aspect of butt-centric riding. But it is too beneficial to ignore, especially if you want to be riding a bike to year (and mile) 100 and beyond.

BUTT INTO TENNIS
WHY CYCLISTS NEED ITS IMPACT, HAND-EYE COORDINATION, TWISTING, AND SIDE-TO-SIDE MOTION, ALL OF WHICH CYCLING LACKS

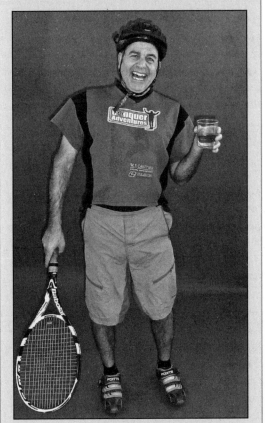

John Kennedy . . . is probably fitter than you.

John Kennedy—a 59-year-old resident of Irvine, California, who sells magic tricks for a living—is a robust 5-foot-7, 162-pounder with big shoulders, a 35-inch waist, meaty thighs, and a wry sense of humor. He's also a bon vivant who loves to cook and throw parties. A self-described "bowlegged, pigeon-toed nerd"

(continues)

BUTT INTO TENNIS *(continued)*

who never did anything athletic in his life until he started mountain biking in his early 40s, Kennedy today can climb and descend the most extreme trails. Most significantly, he keeps improving—even though he's pushing 60 and only rides once a week. On top of that, he never gets hurt, and never has a backache or a hurt knee. Is it because he lifts weights, or cross-trains with running, or does Pilates or yoga?

"Hell, no—I only do fun stuff," he said. "It's the Scotch." (Kennedy drinks Chivas Regal at the rate of about a bottle a week. Riding OC trails with him most Sunday mornings for the past 12 years, I notice he emits a distinct Scotch-scented vapor trail.)

"Okay, it's the tennis," Kennedy finally admits. "Four times a week, two hours at a time. I'm convinced that the tennis helps my cycling and the cycling helps my tennis. The aerobics of cycling helps my stamina on the court; I can wear out younger people. And the hand-eye coordination and quick reaction time of tennis improves my bike-handling skills."

Tennis does even more than that for cyclists, say the experts. It gives you a long list of benefits: ground-force impact that keeps bones strong and fights osteoporosis, which cycling can actually cause (see Chapter 9); upper body strength and agility; improved posture; and twisting movements that work the transverse abdominal muscles and the multifidus muscles that attach to the spinal column and support the lower back—all of which cycling ignores. And, in a huge boon to on-the-bike performance, off-the-bike-health, and knee safety, tennis blasts the butt muscles—all three of them, the well-known gluteus maximus and its under-the-radar siblings, the gluteus medius and gluteus minimus.

"The medius and minimus move your thighs outward from the hips, providing the hips' lateral stability and control, and keep your knee tracking in a straight line, not collapsing to the inside," said Kevin Jardine, a Toronto-based physical therapist,

chiropractor, and acupuncturist who has worked with the Canadian Olympic Team and Team BMC, winner of the 2013 Tours of California and Colorado. Although well-functioning medius and minimus muscles are essential, they get out of shape in modern life, he said. They get no work at all while we're sitting in a desk chair all day, deteriorate quickly with aging, and get worked very little in straight-ahead movements like cycling and running, ironically leading to problems in those very sports—especially knee pain.

"When we traced cyclists' knee pain back to its source, we found that weak gluteus medius and minimus muscles are often unable to hold the leg in line, allowing the thigh to rotate and cave inward toward the top tube," Jardine said. "The old wives' tale that the knee should graze the top tube is dead wrong. The knees should not cave in—that creates torsion, and all kinds of damage can result. They need to be properly aligned—moving straight up and down and symmetrical."

To keep the knees aligned, Jardine developed a series of easy body-weight exercises designed to get the rider's medius and minimus activated before a race or time trial. It takes just a couple of minutes to do 20 reps of each exercise. "This will not pre-fatigue the riders, but get their neuromuscular pathways—the connection between muscles and brain—activated and firing," he said. "All my BMC and Olympic riders do most of them."

Jardine would not reveal his entire exercise regimen (that's for his own book), but said that the No. 1 medius-minimus exercise is the stretch-band side step (the crab walk, pictured on page 179)—where both legs are inside a big stretch band and you move one foot to the other like a tennis or basketball player shuffling from side to side. Jardine noted that "100 percent of people—not just cyclists—should be doing sidesteps with a band, or playing tennis, like your friend Kennedy."

As mentioned, the core twisting muscles (the transverse abdominus on the stomach and the multifidus on the lower back) get weak and

(continues)

BUTT INTO TENNIS *(continued)*

atrophy from under-work in cycling and life. "That leads to back problems and pain, so the brain eventually shuts them off," said Jardine. "This is the concept of neuroplasticity, where the nervous system learns and the brain stops communicating with muscles that hurt. What we need to do is keep these muscles 'on'—reconnecting the brain and body together with skill-based movements to get the system back on line."

These skill-based movements focus on the smaller stabilizer muscles, because they deteriorate—that is, are shut off by the brain—faster than the big muscles. That's because the body can't afford to shut down the prime movers. The trouble with that, Jardine explained, is that big muscles

are less precise than small ones, and like a bull in a china shop, they make joints shear and compress, eventually causing structural damage.

So the key to designing exercises that prevent those ravages and fill in the gaps of limited-motion activities like cycling is to include skill. Hence tennis, racquetball, squash, basketball, soccer, boxing, skating—sports with lateral motion and twisting.

Conclusion: "Tennis is a great sport for fitness—a perfect activity to combine physical activity and mental function," said Jardine. "It creates neurogenesis [grows new brain cells] and hits all the stabilizer muscles of the glute and core that cyclists need. If you don't have time for it, use stretch-band sidesteps."

CASE STUDY: WHEN THE BUTT GOES BAD

I personally know what happens when your gluteal stabilizer muscles fail. In August 2012, when I returned from a 4,000-mile driving trip with my son from Sydney, Australia, to the Great Barrier Reef and back, I could not walk without deep pain in my butt, thighs, and back that would bring me to the edge of tears. Several people at the Interbike show in Las Vegas that September, seeing me hobble and grimace at one-quarter of my normal speed, stopped to ask what was wrong with me.

A couple of days later, it took physical therapist Christine Gore about 30 seconds of pushing and pulling to figure it out: my glutes were profoundly weak.

"By the looks of your legs, you're a cyclist or runner, right?" said Gore. "Those activities do not work the butt well." When I told her that I'd spent the past August sitting in a car in Australia for eight hours a day, that I hadn't played any racquet sports or skated for several years, that I do lots of squats but no lateral butt exercises at the gym, that I was 56 years old (beware baby boomers: unused muscles deteriorate very rapidly after 50), I'd answered my own question.

I thought my dedicated swim-bike-run-Cross-Fit workout blend made me fit, but the lack of twisting and lateral-motion activities had left me with big weak spots. The long drive in Oz blew those holes wide open.

My butt was so weak that Christine had to start me off on the thinnest possible stretch band. She prescribed the same sidesteps that Kevin Jardine spoke of above as well as a dozen more exercises in a 90-minute routine. Within three sessions, the pain was reduced about 20 percent. I was 50 percent fixed in a month, 100 percent in two. Now, occasional twinges remind me when I haven't done my sidesteps and wall-sits (page 194) for a few days. Now I use the thickest stretch band and go out of my way to blast my butt frontways and sideways whenever possible, even flexing it side to side as I sit at my desk and drive my car. I also religiously work the leg curl, hip abductor, and hip rotation machines at the gym and play tennis once a week.

Ironically, I'd written a big story for *Bicycling* magazine in 2004 that promoted utilizing the butt, and I talked extensively about the performance

(continues)

Step 4: *Try joint-building supplements like glucosamine and chondroitin—but don't expect much.*

"People over 35 should baste themselves in the stuff," said Andy Pruitt in the November 2003 issue of *Bicycling* magazine. He was talking about glucosamine and chondroitin, the pair of supplements viewed by some over the past three decades as miracle joint-builders and arthritis fighters. Go to big, long rides, like the Davis Double or the Terrible Two, or Paris-Brest-Paris, and you'll hear riders swearing by G&C. They're both natural substances found in cartilage, the hard connective tissue that pads joints and coats the ends of the bones that meet there. Cartilage, like bone, is living tissue—always wearing out and reforming. Glucosamine is an amino acid that is a precursor to a molecule called a "glycosaminoglycan," which may be used in the formation and repair of cartilage. Chondroitin sulfate is a complex carbohydrate that is thought to help cartilage retain water and resiliency. Are they the real deal? Do they actually help build and protect your joints?

Before 2006, some limited studies had shown a benefit from G&C, sometimes dramatic, but all were deemed too small to be regarded as legitimate. The first large-scale study that everyone was waiting for was published in 2006 in the *New England Journal of Medicine*; it reported the results of a $12.5 million randomized clinical trial funded by the National Institutes of Health that tested G&C's effectivenesss. Using a sample of 1,583 people, researchers gave each test subject either glucosamine, chondroitin, a combination of the two, an anti-inflammatory drug, or a placebo. The results were a blow to those who'd responded to Andy Pruitt's clarion call: The study's authors reported "no significant difference in pain relief between glucosamine, chondroitin, a combination of the two and placebo."

There was some benefit for a few patients who had moderate to severe arthritis pain in a knee: 79 percent had a 20 percent or greater reduction in pain, versus 54 percent for the placebo. But because the number of patients in that subgroup was small, even that conclusion was not definitive, according to the study.

The upshot: Most patients who took G&C were no better off than those who took a placebo. X-rays showed no improvement on the structure of the joint or slowdown in the progression of joint deterioration. That leaves us with the same two osteoarthritis relievers that we started with: weight loss (which relieves pressure on the joint) and exercise (which lubricates the joint). Neither strategy can repair your joints, however, and in the end, G&C are cheap; a couple months' worth will cost you $30 at Costco. Taking them may keep you more psychologically in tune with maintaining a diet and exercise program.

Step 5: *Go under the knife.*

Surgery is a last-ditch option if the four steps described above fail to get the kneecap tracking correctly, but it's far from a sure thing. Surgical procedures for lateral tracking include the following:

1. Lateral retinacular release: This arthroscopy involves the cutting of all the lateral structures from the patellar tendon to within the muscle fibers of the vastus lateralis. Results: fairly good if done in conjunction with a postoperative rehabilitation program.

2. Dynamic realignment: Realignment counteracts the lateral pull by strengthening the medial pull of the VMO through transfers of muscles or tendons. Results: iffy, and rehab is quite slow.

3. Arthroscopic lavage: This simple procedure, also known as "washing out the knee," can have a profoundly positive effect on knee pain. Potentially, it can remove small particles of cartilage that produce synovitis.

SECTION II: BIKER'S BACK

A *Cycling News* item from July 8, 2004: "*McGee Packs It In:* Bradley McGee of Fdjeux.com abandoned during today's stage of the Tour de France. The Australian rider had been having a very good year, and was a favorite to take the prologue, but he's been suffering from back problems since the Tour started, problems he blamed on planting some olive trees at his new home."

🚲

Since the modern bicycle was perfected in the late 1800s, the No. 1 complaint from bike riders has been knee pain. "But there's been a paradigm shift in the last decade or so," said Andy Pruitt of the Boulder Center for Sports Medicine. "With the aging of the cycling population, back pain is now rivaling knee pain."

At a meeting with a bike manufacturer in 2002, Pruitt brought in a chart showing that the growth curves of two cycling trends now meet: baby boomers and high performance. His point: Forever-young boomers are still pushing the big ring, but they're also pushing 50. And that means they are subject to some of the same middle-age medical conditions that dog their non-cycling peers. Topping the charts: back pain.

The fact that back pain is now No. 1 is no surprise, considering that it's America's equal-opportunity affliction, similarly affecting blue- and white-collar workers, athletes and couch potatoes, Colnago connoisseurs and Huffy-puffers. Endemic in our sedentary society, back pain leads three-quarters of the population to seek medical attention at least once in their lives, and up to 10 million people to miss work every day. Back pain is undoubtedly exacerbated by cycling, which keeps your body seated and your back bent over, humped, stretched out, virtually frozen in place, and, in the words of John Howard, "stuck in a strange semi-fetal crouch found nowhere else in the athletic world."

The result: The key support beam at the bedrock of your body's stability is weak, tight, and ready to blow. When it does, you have been officially introduced to the condition known as "biker's back"—pain in the muscles along the spine, pain in the area just above the pelvis, and pain between the shoulder blades.

Howard reports that more than half of the students at his cycling school complain about biker's back. He personally understands the pain; he's had it ever since he began riding in an aerobar tuck in the late 1980s.

The seeds of biker's back, however, were sewn not the day you bolted an aerobar to your new high-performance carbon-fiber dream machine, but about the time your dad bought you your first $39 two-wheeler from the local hardware store. Yet the bike itself wasn't the problem; going to kindergarten and sitting all day was.

"Your postural decline starts at age five, when you stop running around all day and begin slumping, hunched over a desk," said Patrick Mummy, whose Symmetry Pain Relief Clinic in San Diego has developed a reputation for curing near-hopeless back-pain cases. A lifetime of sitting—while doing homework, driving, cycling, and surfing the net—stoops the shoulders, shortens the hip flexors, draws the butt in, and flattens the lower back. The result, said Mummy, is a constricted position that squeezes your lungs and intestines and both weakens the lower back and makes it work harder. By age 35 or 40, this weakened posture may lead to the dull agony or debilitating flare-ups of biker's back.

Back pain is no mystery if you understand the lower back's anatomy, consisting of five lumbar vertebrae separated by discs of hard cartilage, each with a soft, watery center called a *nucleus pulposus*. The spinal cord ends in this region, and exiting between the bones and the discs are a series of nerve roots that can become compressed and inflamed through degenerative changes in the structures. When the body is bent forward and the spine rounded (the opposite of its normal concave profile), the back wall of each disc stretches and its front wall contracts. This pushes the soft nucleus pulposus toward the back wall of the disc, where sudden twisting and turning motions over time can tear, rupture, or "herniate" it. When that happens, the nucleus pulposus can rupture through these tears, irritating or pinching the nerve roots when they emerge between the vertebrae, thus causing low back or leg pain.

Cyclists shouldn't ignore biker's back. It's a fact: A nonrecumbent racing bike forces riders into a bent-back position that can harm discs, already at risk by years of sitting. Failure to adopt lifestyle changes, alter your bike position, and follow a regimen of specific strengthening and stretching exercises can end a cycling career and lead to irreparable damage to the lower back.

The incidence of biker's back is even driving product changes in the bike industry. For years, custom builders such as Serotta have been swamped with orders for bikes with taller headtubes and higher handlebars, which allow aging enthusiasts to ride with a more erect torso. Specialized got wind of the trend and in the fall of 2003 introduced the Roubaix, a high-end production road bike that, like the pricier Serottas, featured a taller headtube. Adding to the comfort, the Roubaix included "Zertz" elastomer shock absorbers in the frame, seatpost, and fork.

Of course, riding more erect on a new bike that will cost you thousands is not the only way to fight biker's back. At most, new hardware is the first step of an evolving plan that includes strengthening your back and core muscles and making other surrounding muscles more limber; eventually, that will allow you to resume or maintain a high-performance riding position without back strain. Here are the details of the *Bike for Life* "banish biker's back" plan:

How to Banish Biker's Back
1. Raise the front end.
Beware the low handlebars of triathletes and time trialists. Beware the curved round hump in your back. From a performance standpoint, it does not provide a good core-stabilizing anchor. And from a biker's back standpoint, the hump is terrible for the spine. It causes spinal creep, or hysteresis, a permanent lengthening of the posterior spinal ligament, hastening a breakdown of the integrity of the bonds that hold the vertebrae together. It is not surprising that there is a much higher incidence of herniated discs among time trialists and triathletes than among normal cyclists.

The quickest and least expensive way to get immediate relief from biker's back is to simply raise the handlebars of your existing bike, either by rotating the bar upward, raising the stem, or buying a taller stem. An adjustable stem may be ideal, allowing you to exactly dial in the most comfortable height as you develop improved strength and flexibility over time. The added height, which you can also achieve by buying a bike with a shorter top tube and/or taller stem, will minimize the unhealthy convex curve of your back and the pressure it puts on your discs.

At the same time, be aware that an upright position can compromise your power. As discussed in Chapter 7, the Serotta Fit School believes that an angle greater than 45 degrees between a cyclist's back and seated hips will not activate the glute, which will cost you power and increase knee strain. That's why an adjustable stem is a good hardware choice; you can lower the handlebar height as you use some of the following tips to become more limber.

2. Straighten out your body first.

"What good is it," asked Patrick Mummy, "to stretch and build big, beautiful muscles on top of a bent 'frame'?" His Symmetry Pain Control clinic uses a number of unique exercises to straighten out your body. (For a detailed all-body Symmetry posture plan, see sidebar, "How to De-slump Your Posture" on page 191.)

3. Address leg-length differences.

Pruitt reports that laboratory studies have shown that leg-length inequality is the most common cause of back pain in cyclists. For those with a difference of 5 millimeters (mm) or less, Pruitt moves the cleat on the short-leg side forward by 1 to 2 mm. If the difference is 6 mm or more, he recommends that you have a shoe-repair shop place a shim between the shoe sole and the cleat.

4. Stretch hamstrings, hip flexors, and glutes.

When the three aforementioned muscle groups tighten with age, they cause a number of secondary problems: The quadriceps are forced to push harder to extend the leg, tiring them and stressing the knee joint, and the difficulty in bending at the waist puts pressure on the back to bow. A humped back is bad; it can squeeze the discs.

Fortunately, tightness is one aspect of aging that is easily reversed. Do not start a ride without stretching; even cold-stretching is safe, according to physical therapist Bob Forster. Occasionally stand up to stretch while on the bike, and especially stretch after the ride, when the muscle is warm and the sheath that surrounds it is malleable. Here are two stretches cyclists should do a lot:

1. Hamstrings stretch: Lie on your back with your knees bent. Grab one foot with your hands and pull the leg straight up. Then straighten the knee as much as you can, stretching the hamstring.

2. Hip flexor stretch: Kneel with one foot forward, keeping the front knee at a right angle and the other leg behind your hips. Keep your upper body upright. Tilt your pelvis back, tucking in your stomach and squeezing your glutes. You should feel the stretch strongly in your hip flexor.

3. Toe-touch hamstring and calf stretch. Never do a standing toe-touch. Warning: Bending over and touching your fingers to the ground causes a stretching of the back ligaments, which can lead to injuries. But using the toe-touch to stretch your hamstrings and calves is safe done from the ground, which avoids adding tension. Keep your head up, and focus on bending at the waist and keeping the back flat.

5. Strengthen core muscles.

Blame a lifetime of sitting for tightening the lower back's spinal erector muscles and weakening the transverse abdominus, the deep abdominal muscles that draw the belly button to the spine. Strengthening and stretching these can improve posture and reduce back pain.

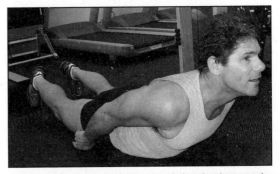

Back extensions are a simple, safe low-back strengthener. Also do bridges and cable ab twists.

1. Back extensions: The spinal erectors line each side of the spinal column. These muscles become weak and tight through lack of use, especially if your only athletic activity is cycling. They strengthen quickly with back extensions, which can be performed anywhere by lying belly-down, keeping hands at your side or clasped behind your neck, and simply raising your head and upper back off the floor for several seconds.

Warning: Beware of the feet-anchored back extension stations at the gym. Their leverage may overstress the small spinal erectors, expecially when done while holding weights.

2. Transverse abdominus (TA): To work these stomach muscles, which are used in twisting motions, stand with your knees bent and light dumbbells at chest level. Then, in the air in front of you, draw a sideways figure eight, dropping and raising your arms as your torso flexes slightly side to side.

6. Activate and strengthen the glutes.

Those glutes again. You already know from the "cyclist's knee" section above and the preceding chapter that the underestimated, underutilized butt muscles become major contributors to cycling power when you have a proper fit. But you may not realize that this power derives from the key role that the three gluteal muscles (gluteus maximus, medius, and minimus) play in extending the trunk and helping you maintain an upright posture, and thus in preventing back pain. my biomechanical experiment with USC's Dr. Christopher Powers showed, initiating the pedal's power stroke with the glutes not only lessens valgus (the inward drift of the knee while pedaling) and enhances core stability (minimizing side-to-side rocking), but also effectively straightens the back. Glute-focused pedaling clearly lessens the hump that characterizes quadriceps-focused pedaling. For that reason, insufficient recruitment and strengthening of the gluteus maximus may increase the risk of back injury.

Several exercises can improve the gluteus maximus's ability to support the extension of the spine:

1. Bridges: Lying on your back with your knees bent, draw in the lower abdominals and thrust the butt off the floor, lifting the hips until the knees, hips, and chest are in line. Hold this position for 10 seconds, squeezing the glutes and lower abs to support the bridge position. Do 10 reps. Over time, build up to 2 reps of 60 seconds each, then try a one-legged bridge, straightening one knee to lift that leg up into the air.

2. Wood chops and kettlebell swings: This is a dynamic exercise where the glutes must work to extend the trunk from a flexed position. Standing with feet shoulder-width apart with knees slightly bent, hold a weight in both hands above your head (10 to 15 pounds for men, 5 to 10 pounds for women) and act as if you were wielding an ax to chop wood. Bend forward while bringing the weight down between your legs, keeping your back flat. Do not bend the knees further as you move your torso forward. At the bottom, draw in your abdominals and squeeze your glutes for support before returning upright to the starting position. Straighten up in the correct sequence: straighten your lower back first, then bring your shoulders up, and finally lift the weight above your head. It is similar to a kettle-bell swing, though in the latter there is a lower knee bend and an upright back. Begin with two to three sets of 10 reps each, building up to 20 reps.

3. Hip flexor stretch: Because inflexible hip flexors can cause an excessive pelvic tilt, which inhibits the gluteus maximus, they must be stretched (see 4, above).

4. Wall sit: See this do-anywhere butt blaster on page 194.

Additional Back-Saving Tips
7. Change position.

Move around on the bike often to take pressure

off your back. On long rides, change hand positions and stand up for one minute out of every five. Stretch out, scooch here and there. Standard road bars allow many different positions—drops, hoods, top of the bar. For the same reason, bar-ends on mountain bikes are a good thing. On long climbs, slide around from the front to the middle to the back of the saddle.

8. Go swimming.

In several ways, swimming is almost a perfect cross-training counterpart to cycling, because it fills in the latter's deficiencies. Where cycling bends you over and generally leaves you stiff, swimming stretches you out and makes you flexible. Where cycling is all legs and linear, a swimmer's upper body delivers 70 percent of his or her power, and the pronounced hip-twist on every stroke works the core ab, transverse abs, and back muscles that are ignored on a bike. Swimming travels well, unlike bikes, so packing a pair of goggles helps a bike-less cyclist maintain cardiovascular conditioning on the road. Of course, you may want to pack a pair of running shoes, too. The first sentence says "almost" because swimming, like cycling, lacks the weight-bearing and impact benefits that help to build bone. You'll need running and weight lifting for that.

9. Do pull-ups.

The huge lat muscles frame and stabilize the entire back. Pull-ups and lat-pull machines work them. Don't be intimidated if you can't do one at first; you'll get strong fast. Start with assistance bands and an inexpensive doorjamb bar. You'll build up to 10 or 12 pull-ups in no time.

10. Do push-ups.

A good set of push-ups a couple times a day can help save your back, according to Julie Bookspan, MD, a Philadelphia orthopedist who has helped the US military develop back-friendly exercise programs. The key is keeping a straight back. Perfect form in a push-up is the same as perfect upright posture. Bad form—too much arch—can resemble bad posture. Good push-ups train you to hold a good posture in life, cutting the risk of back pain.

In fact, push-ups are better for your back than bench presses, according to Michael Clark, a Certified Strength and Conditioning Specialist, physical therapist, and president of the National Academy of Sports Medicine, because they build your entire muscular support system. In particular, push-ups develop scapular and rotator-cuff muscles that stabilize your shoulders far more than presses do.

Finally, do push-ups during your bike rides. Besides building your back, they'll warm you up on a cold morning, revive you after a long 7-Eleven break, and shake off a chill while waiting for slower partners at the top of long hill climbs.

11. Protect your back all day.

Incorporate back-friendly behavior into your normal life. For instance, don't bend over to lift something up; squat and use your legs. Drive a lot? Strengthen your core muscles while seated in your car with this "red light" ab workout, invented by Carol Ross, a Venice, California, chiropractor: When you come to a red light, hold your abs to a count of three. Do it at every red traffic or tail light, and soon you will be giving your body a subconscious cue: When it sees red, your stomach contracts. "One of my clients told me that he contracts when he sees his boss's red tie," said Ross. "He also said that one girl in red thought he was making a pass at her."

Jim Beazell takes Ross's tummy tightening a notch further, recommending that you tuck your abdomen anytime you sit or stand. Positioning is important, too. "Try sitting with your knees lower than your hips," he said. "This will straighten up your spine."

12. Consider a recumbent.

"Instead of fussing over tall, back-friendly handlebars and glute-strengthening exercises, just test ride a recumbent," said Victor Larivee. "You won't go back to your old bike." Larivee converted his Bicycle Workshop in Santa Monica, California, from racing bikes to 'bents two decades ago, when the baby boomers began hitting 40. Comfort (i.e., relief from back pain) brings them in, but aerodynamics make them believers. Recumbents own many bicycle speed records; as it turns out, a well-fit 'bent puts riders in the ideal glute-centric position for generating power. Your back—and other parts of your body—will thank you.

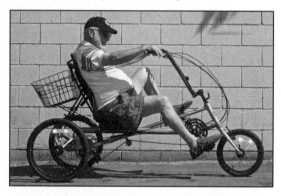

When all else fails, remember that recumbents are famously easy on the back.

13. Go dancing.

A 2004 study in the *British Journal of Sports Medicine* suggests that dance training may help athletes alleviate back pain. Swedish researchers had 16 elite cross-country skiers take dance classes 6 hours a week for 12 weeks, while 10 skiers served as controls. The dance exercises included ballet, modern dance, and jazz, with the aim of improving balance, coordination, muscle flexibility, and agility. After three months, the dancing skiers showed improved spinal flexibility, better posture, and greater range of motion in their hips. And while the dancing didn't necessarily make them better skiers, four of the six who had previous back problems said their backs no longer hurt following the three months of training.

13. Play tennis.

As my mountain-biking buddy John Kennedy illustrates (see "Butt into Tennis," page 181), the squatted, side-to-side motion of tennis is a superb transverse ab strengthener, developing the tight but flexible midsection girdle that armors the back against injury. The squatted position and lateral motion also make it a tremendous butt builder, specifically working the always-neglected, but very important, abductor muscles, the gluteus medius and minimus. The abductors are key to giving you a piston-like, un-valgus pedal stroke that does not fall inward and supports a flat back.

15. Finally, throw a Frisbee.

The introductory anecdote at the start of this chapter was no joke. You may have used a Frisbee as a food tray, a makeshift sand shovel at the beach, or a water tray for a thirsty dog. So why is it so farfetched to find that the famous flying disc can save your lumbar discs? Tossing a Frisbee opens your cycling-collapsed chest, twists your inactivated cycling trunk, works your unused transverse abs, and loosens your stiff back—the perfect antidote to long hours in the saddle.

EPILOGUE

A year before the first edition of this book was published, I was seriously worried that my left knee was permanently disabled. By the time the book was printed, due to the advice in this chapter, I was back to normal and pain-free, and have remained so for the decade since.

Following a January 2004 X-ray, which showed that my kneecaps were visibly pulled to the lateral side, a doctor immediately wanted to perform a lateral-release surgery on the left knee, which I refused. Fearful of being sliced up without exploring noninvasive remedies, I was quite motivated to make myself a guinea pig for this chapter, and I have religiously tested much of the advice offered here.

I stretch my IT bands several times every day and during every ride, hit the leg-extension machine to work my VMO muscles at least twice a week. I begin every ride slowly, in lower gears, getting the synovial lubrication flowing in my knees. Talking with fit experts such as Paul Levine, and spending a morning with Dr. Chris Powers, drove home the importance of butt-centric pedaling. Powering through my glutes keeps my legs lined up from hip through knee through ball-of-the-foot. I go out of my way to get in some tennis—even solo against a concrete wall of the high-school gym—once a week.

It worked. At that low point in January 2004, I literally couldn't walk 10 feet without feeling my kneecaps scraping as they slipped out of their groove. But I was running and riding normally eight months later, and nine months later I rode 11.5 pain-free hours in one day at the Furnace Creek 508.

When I feel pain, inevitably it is because I've neglected to stretch my IT band for weeks, and therefore have not relaxed the pressure, forcing my kneecaps into lateral tracking. The pain immediately goes away when I get off the bike and stretch the ITs for a minute.

Stretching the ITs joins a growing list of exercises I'm afraid not to do. As you get older and learn more about how your aging body works, you see that it takes more work to keep it functioning. That why I now religiously do back extensions and hit all the glute muscles—maximus, medius, minimus—with side-to-side stretch-band crab walks, deep squats and thrusters, kettle-bell swings, and tennis. I use Symmetry posture exercises every other day to warm up for the strength work and to counteract the long hours in front of my computer screen. For me, "prehab" isn't just a clever word. It's what I need to do to keep riding my bike.

HOW TO DE-SLUMP YOUR POSTURE
SYMMETRY'S UNIQUE EXERCISES WILL STRAIGHTEN OUT YOUR CROOKED BODY AND FIX YOUR BACK

If you've got a bad back, and you don't have a major weight problem, chances are that poor posture is the cause. "The slumping and hunching that first becomes noticeable in your 30s causes poor athletic performance, restricts your breathing and digestion, and is the basis of most injuries and joint diseases, like arthritis," said Patrick Mummy, president of Symmetry, a unique pain-relief clinic with offices in Sacramento and San Diego (www.symmetryforhealth.com). "And cycling makes it worse; it reinforces a bad habit." Fortunately, like misaligned wheels on a car, bad posture is fixable. Symmetry, a leader in the relatively new field of postural therapy, prescribes custom stretching and strengthening exercises that are designed to get your posture back to where it was when you and your back were bombproof: age five.

"Chest out and proud. Butt high and back. Shoulders square. Body balanced front-to-back, side-to-side. This is perfect, symmetrical posture—and it starts to degrade the day you go to kindergarten and begin sitting at a desk all day," said Mummy.

Being crouched forward to write and type hunches the shoulders forward. It angles the pelvis up, changing its natural forward tilt of 10 degrees to something closer to zero, or level. The result: The hip flexors shorten, the back is pulled into flexion, and the lower back muscles are overworked and strained. Eventually, most sedentary adults develop what Mummy calls the "Suck 'n Tuck": butt drawn in, belly pushed up, shoulders stooped forward, diaphragm collapsed, and lower back flattened—a backache-ridden, constricted position that squeezes your lungs and intestines.

Over the years, good posture is further corrupted by leg-length discrepancies, accumulated injuries, right- or left-hand dominance, and repetitive motion activities such as hitting a tennis ball (which can cause a side-to-side torso tilt that puts one shoulder higher than the other). "Then add sports activities that train you to be imbalanced," said Mummy. "A common one is overemphasis on

(continues)

How to De-slump Your Posture *(continued)*

chest presses over pulls in the weight room. Another big one is cycling.

"Over time, your body mimics the activity. Whereas basketball or soccer uses your body functionally in its natural state, with your pelvis as the center of gravity, cycling removes the pelvis from the equation. Leaning forward to the handlebars, your back is now the center of gravity, the tie-in between the upper and lower body. Cycling trains you to take the shape of a C; so off the bike, your back struggles to keep you upright."

According to Symmetry, undoing the damage isn't as simple as going to a chiropractor for an "adjustment" that temporarily pushes a vertebra this way or that; for cyclists, it requires a complete overhaul of your body's misaligned and out-of-balance muscles as well as daily exercises before, during, and after your ride.

The process at Symmetry, which I've personally gone through, begins with two full-length photographs of your body—straight ahead and profile. After noting your points of deviation from the ideal form of a five-year-old (shoulders and hips should not be tilted, and head, shoulder, hips, knees, and ankles should be in a vertical line), Mummy prescribes a series of stretching and strengthening exercises that will restore the balance. The exercises are not easy and don't involve lifting weights (Mummy is against pumping iron until you've straightened your posture; to do otherwise is akin to "building a Ferrari on a bent chassis," he said). Some people see immediate improvement; others take months. Asked to provide exercises for this book, Mummy initially hesitated; he designs exercise regimens specific to individuals. But eventually he did agree that a series of general exercises, described below, can help anyone at risk for a bad back, including all cyclists.

"Hypothetically, do them before, during, and after you ride" he said, "But especially before. You brush your teeth at the beginning of the day. You need to start any activity in a balanced body position."

SYMMETRY POSTURE FIXERS

While Symmetry designs custom posture rehab programs, Mummy believes a generic anti–Suck 'n' Tuck strategy can go a long way toward eliminating biker's back. The strategy will stretch the hip flexors to restore the correct pelvic tilt, reposition the shoulders back, and equalize the hips to restore bilateral symmetry. At 1 to 2 minutes each, the eight exercises below should take 10 to 15 minutes to complete. Perform them at home or in the gym in the order given and as often as possible, especially before any weight training or aerobic exercise:

1. STATIC FLOOR
Purpose: Relaxes and evens the spine and spiny erector muscles to prepare for exercise.

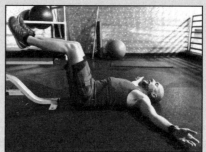

Static floor

How to: Lie on your back, calves flat on the seat of a chair, with your thighs perpendicular to the floor, arms out to the sides, palms up. Sink into the floor and breathe through the diaphragm. Tighten your abs for one second at end of each exhalation.

2. CROSSOVER (PIRIFORMIS STRETCH)
Purpose: Removes pelvis elevations, untwists the hips (evens right-left bias), and indirectly repositions the shoulders.

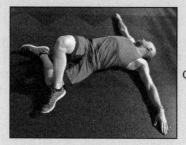

Crossover

(continues)

HOW TO DE-SLUMP YOUR POSTURE *(continued)*

How to: Lie on your back with your arms out to the sides, knees bent, and left foot on the floor. Cross the right ankle to the left knee and rotate the right foot and left knee to the floor as one unit until the right foot is flat on the floor. Look in the opposite direction and press your right knee slightly away, feeling the stretch on the outside of the right hip. Hold for one minute. Repeat in the opposite direction.

3. CATS AND DOGS

Purpose: Restores natural tilt to the pelvis by aligning it with the spine.

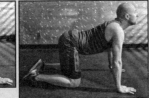

Cats and Dogs

How to: Starting on your hands and knees, pull your chin to your chest while pushing your lower back up toward the ceiling, then look up toward the ceiling and allow your back to sway and the shoulder blades to pull back and together. Keep a constant, smooth motion, not allowing your body to move forward or backward. Repeat 10 times.

4. ARM CIRCLES

Purpose: Strengthens the shoulder girdle and repositions the shoulder blade back.

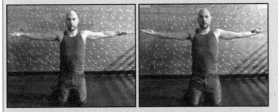

Arm circles, palms down   Arm circles, palms up

How to: While kneeling on the floor, raise your arms straight out from your sides as you squeeze your shoulder blades together. With the palms facing down, rotate your arms in six-inch circles; then switch to palms facing up.

5. SHOULDER ROTATIONS

Purpose: Stretches and repositions the shoulders.

Shoulder rotations, positions 1 and 2

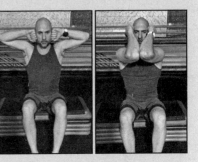

How to: Sit in a chair with your feet on the floor and your knees bent at a 90-degree angle; your hips should be rolled forward to create an arch in the lower back. Place your knuckles on your temples, pivot your arms inward until the elbows touch, and then raise your arms up if you can.

6. SITTING TORSO TWIST

Purpose: Gives the back a transverse stretch.

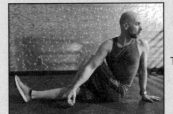

Torso twist

How to: Sit on the floor with your legs straight and your hands behind your back. Bend your left knee so that your left foot is positioned on the outside of your right knee. Place the right elbow on the left knee. Sit up as tall as possible by arching your lower back. Pull your left shoulder back and twist your torso, looking back over your left shoulder.

7. TRIANGLE POSE

Purpose: Lengthens and unkinks the torso.
How to: Stand against a wall with your right foot perpendicular to the wall, and rotate the left foot so

(continues)

How to De-slump Your Posture *(continued)*

that it is perpendicular to the right and three inches away from the wall. Take a large step sideways out with the left leg, keeping the foot three inches from the wall. Holding your arms horizontally at your sides, tighten your quads and keep both your glutes and your shoulders on the wall as you rotate and lower the upper body from the waist toward the left foot. Slide down until the right glute starts to come off the wall, hold that position, and stretch your right arm directly above you in a vertical position.

8. OVERHEAD EXTENSION

Purpose: Repositions the shoulders.

How to: Standing with your fingers interlaced, push your palms up and away from your body toward the sky until they are straight. Pinch your shoulder blades together, look straight up, feel the arch in your lower back, and hold.

9. EXTENDED FLOOR POSITION

Purpose: Dramatically tilts the pelvis forward and pulls the shoulders back by putting the spine in "traction."

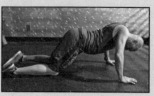

Extended floor

How to: From the "Cats and Dogs" position, walk your hands forward four to six inches and place your elbows where your hands were, putting your hips in front of the knees. Let your back sway, your shoulder blades collapse together, and your head drop. Hold this position one to two minutes.

10. WALL SIT

Purpose: Lowers the body's center of gravity back to the pelvis and changes the posture from a bow to a straight line; strengthens the pelvic muscles and quads to help them hold your spine and legs together as one unit.

How to: With your lower back pressed firmly against a wall, slowly walk your feet away and slide down until your knees are bent at a 90-degree angle. Keep your weight on your heels. Increase the length of time you can hold this stretch to 60 seconds. Repeat five times and do two or three sets.

WHILE STOPPED MID-RIDE AT A 7-ELEVEN . . .

In the middle of the ride, while everyone else is sitting on the curb guzzling a Big Gulp, spend four minutes fixing your posture. Do three of the exercises described above: sitting torso twist (1 minute); triangle position (1 minute); and wall sit (1 to 2 minutes). This combination will loosen your transverse (twisting) plane and your frontal (side-to-side) plane and reemphasize the sagittal (straight-ahead) plane in a positive way.

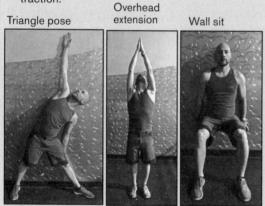

Triangle pose

Overhead extension

Wall sit

Case Study: Phil Curry Goes Straight (His Body, That Is)

He's 6-foot-2, 180 pounds, with a head full of brown hair and "mega-legs" that look like "telephone poles." He's a lifelong athlete, a self-described "kick-ass rider," and a widely recognized merger-and-acquisitions expert who hammers 6,000 miles a year at a relentless 20-mph clip. He can say, without hesitation, that he's able to "power-sprint with elite racers." People are shocked to find out that San Diego investment banker Phil Curry is in his 60s; the grandfather of three hardly believes it himself. He would probably think he was 35 if it weren't for his memories of "The Back."

(continues)

"It started around 1997 or 1998," he said. "And within a year it was bad enough to take me to surgery."

It was a pinched vertebra, an unusual problem for cyclists. The pain went down his right leg from his groin into his right knee. "I couldn't ride without pain," Curry said. "I'd go out on the bike, take a ton of ibuprofen, and pedal until it crippled me up. Finally, after doing a century in 1999, I said this is it. I need help."

Curry sought medical attention from a variety of health-care providers: acupuncturists, physical therapists, sports medicine docs, and chiropractors. He even got epidural shots. "Nothing worked," he said. "Then I ran into a rider who said, 'Go to Symmetry.' Patrick [Mummy] took one look at me and said that I was 'crooked.' I thought, *yeah, sure.*

"But I couldn't argue with the photo."

The photo—the infamous Symmetry Polaroid. Two of them, actually, full-frontal and profile, overlaid with a drafting grid of horizontal and vertical lines. The photos showed Curry's shoulders shifted to the right, his midline off-center, and his hips a mess. Instead of a normal 9-degree forward cant, one tilted 6 degrees forward and the other 2 degrees back. He was, indeed, crooked.

Mummy's Symmetry Pain Relief clinic has made its mark by straightening the crooked. To restore the natural 9-degree cant of Curry's hips, Mummy prescribed a 20-minute sequential routine, which Curry performed before and after each ride. The seven exercises, a personalized combination of yoga and isometrics, included the following:

1. Backdrops: Lie on the floor on your back with your thighs perpendicular to the floor and knees bent at a 90-degree angle, and rest your lower legs on a chair for 5 minutes. This position relaxes the back and prepares it for further exercise.

2. Sit-ups: Remaining in that position, place your hands behind your head and do some sit-ups.

3. Block and strap: Then place a block between your knees and a strap around your ankles and do 50 more crunches, squeezing the knees together and pushing out at the ankles.

4. Strap and block: Do the reverse of No. 3: Place the block between the ankles and the strap around your knees, and do 50 additional crunches, squeezing the ankles together and trying to push out at the knees.

5. Pelvic thrust: With the block between the knees again, thrust your hips upward.

6. Quad stretch: As described in Chapter 1, lie on your side, hold the top of your right foot with your left hand, and gently pull your heel toward your buttocks. Hold for 30 seconds on each side.

7. Wall sits: Standing with your back flat against a wall, slide down to where your thighs are parallel to the ground. You will look like a human chair. Hold for up to two minutes or more.

"I did them religiously, and felt some improvement. My body was straightening out, but I still had pain," Curry said. Turns out that he was too far gone already; a disc was pushing into the nerve and he needed surgery (the cutting away of a fingernail-sized chunk of a vertebra to relieve the nerve). The operation helped somewhat, but he kept up the Symmetry protocol, too; within several months, he was pain-free for the first time in years.

"I've been bulletproof ever since," said Curry. "And as long as I maintain the exercise regimen, I'm confident that there is no chance I'll go under the knife again."

Now, whenever Curry stops to get a Coke at a 7-Eleven, he drinks it while doing a wall sit. "I get the funniest looks from other bikers," he said. "What the hell is wrong with you?" they say. "You think you have an imaginary chair?"

The exercises have paid off in other ways, too. "My wife said I'm an inch taller and I walk straighter," said Curry. "And I've become somewhat of an expert on posture.

"Cycling throws your body off balance. On a road bike, your whole pivot point is your lower back. You develop humongous quads, which get out of balance and overpower your pelvic girdle area. Your hamstrings get tight and pull your spine, so you have to stretch them."

Bottom line: Curry's a Symmetry lifer. "This stuff's not snake oil," he said. "I don't understand acupuncture, but I understand this. I understand the picture of the five-year-old boy, the way we used to be. The exercises Symmetry gave me are making me younger every day."

Jim Ochowicz

THE ORGANIZATION MAN

Friends and former teammates know the former Olympic cyclist and founder of the 7-Eleven and Motorola pro cycling teams simply as Och. It sounds like "ouch" but with a long "o." Longtime followers of bike racing know Jim Ochowicz as the pioneering go-to guy who helped successfully lead the American mission to race across the pond. Back in the 1970s and early 1980s, during the pre-LeMond era, the United States was considered a laughingstock when it came to European racing. Ochowicz, as a racer-turned-sports director, was instrumental in changing that impression and reality. As he told Bike for Life in March 2004 and January 2014, it all happened because he loved cycling and needed to find a way to make a living from it after his racing career was over. His storied résumé includes induction into the US Bicycling Hall of Fame in 1997, president of USA Cycling's board of directors, and men's road coach of the US Olympic bike racing squad in 2004. These days, American racers are a fixture in Europe—much to the chagrin of the French, Germans, Italians, Spanish, and Dutch. Off the bike, Ochowicz was working as a vice president at Thomas Weisel Partners and Merchant Bank in San Francisco. (Note: We have chosen not to edit Ochowicz's 2004 comments on Lance Armstrong and other matters which, with today's knowledge, may appear naïve or amusing. History is history. The cycling world is the way it is today because of

Armstrong's profound influence, good or bad.)

My DAD HAD raced bikes before World War II. I figured that out when I was about 12. He had a box of medals on his dresser. I had a regular 10-speed and started racing around a circular driveway at the cemetery after school with my friends. And I wanted to really try to do it at a much bigger level. So I started riding to bike shops and looking at photos of real racing bikes. I bought a Schwinn Paramount with my paper route money. I started racing in 1966 on the track in Kenosha [Wisconsin] and then Milwaukee. I was 14 and got second in the nationals on the track. Then it was just full gas. I started speed skating in the winter, because I lived in Milwaukee, to stay in shape, so I became a speed skater as well. But my primary focus was on the bike.

I was 20 when I made the US Olympic team in 1972 in team pursuit on the track. And did it again in '76 on the track. Those things were the highlights. At the time no Americans were in Europe racing. A group of us—John Howard, Mike Neel, Dave Chauner—decided to go to Europe and we'd try racing together. And we did pretty well. We did the Milk Race [Tour of Britain] a couple of times and we won some stages. Then Greg LeMond came along. By that time I was transitioning out of the racing part of it; I was getting into sports management. I got married and I had a daughter and couldn't afford to race anymore. So I needed to get into the real world of making a living. And I got a chance to get into sports management by being the manager for the US Speed Skating team in '79 and '80. And of course those were golden years of US speed skating.

Off to Europe with Roll, Hampsten . . . and Armstrong

AFTER THOSE OLYMPICS, my plan was to try to find a sponsor like a European pro cycling team and develop a generation of racers that hopefully we might get to Europe one day and race as a team. And this kinda came on its own. Because when we met up with the Southland people at 7-Eleven, they had just made a commitment to Peter Ueberroth [head of the 1984 Olympic Games organizing committee] to be an Olympic sponsor. They got the sport of cycling and didn't know anything about it. We walked in the door about a week later. At that point, historically, Americans hadn't won a medal in cycling at the Olympic Games since 1904. So these were the 1984 Olympic Games and in L.A., and we felt with the right funding, we could find the right athletes, develop them, and win some medals. And that's what happened.

It was then time to decide what's next. And for me what was next was not gearing up for another Olympic Games, but going over to Europe and seeing what we could do in the pro ranks. So, I talked Southland into backing us financially. We went to Europe, and the very first race we entered, Trofeo Laigueglia, was the kickoff race of the Italian season. Ron Kiefel won. And nobody had ever heard of us before. And he beat people like Francesco Moser and all the world champions.

We did that spring campaign and we got invited to the Giro d'Italia. We didn't have enough riders, so I recruited Andy Hampsten out of his Tour of Texas that spring. We got Bob Roll on. We brought Chris Carmichael in. And we went to Europe and did the Giro. And won two stages. So we were off and running. That set the stage for me to go back in July and meet with Tour de France officials for the first time, convince them to have an American team in the Tour. And so in '86, the first American team raced in the Tour, and in that process we were building another generation of cyclists with a developmental team that we started. And the second generation was started in 1991 when we recruited Lance Armstrong.

Certainly Greg LeMond can take a lot of credit for creating awareness for the sport of cycling. It was televised. We were winning races. People were interested. And for enthusiast cyclists it was a great opportunity to be able to enjoy it from another perspective rather than seeing just Europeans racing. There was an American presence. Lance took it a giant step forward in '99 when he won the Tour. Because he just didn't win the Tour like everyone else won the Tour. He won the Tour having had cancer. And that was a unique story and a miracle, if you want to call it that.

The first year he rode as a pro, he won a stage in the Tour de France. He was [one of] the youngest rider[s] in history to win a stage in the Tour de France. And a month later, he won the World Professional Road Championships. So you're not talking about somebody who wasn't already a very accomplished athlete right from the start. Physiologically, I don't know if anybody is fitter than he is. He's got a great will and determination. He has a winning attitude. He's got a work discipline. All the things you need to be a champion. He was just too young to win the Tour de France in those years and too inexperienced. He still needed to understand what it means to go up the Alpe d'Huez. To understand how big the Tour de France really was and how important it was in an athlete's career to do well there. We focused on the things we could focus on with all of our athletes during that time. Unfortunately, Lance got cancer and we stopped having a team at the same time. And he had a few years with nothing really happening. But all along I believed that he could win the Tour de France. I believed he could win anything he wanted to win. Once he decided he wanted to do it.

The No. 1 thing is, he definitely has the biggest engine. Nobody can push the kind of wattage he can push on the bike and sustain it for as long as he can. We've had some very accomplished athletes in our organization over the years and I've known a lot of very good athletes. But I've never seen anybody like him. So, starting out, that's a huge asset. The second thing is, I've never seen anybody who can train as hard as he can train day after day after day. When he trains with the team, everybody has to take a rest day to stay up with him. He just keeps going all five days. The rest of the guys have to take a day off. He can go and go and go. That is one of the things that makes racing for him not that hard. Until he wants to make it hard. He determines when the race is going to be difficult. And he has done that because he has trained harder than anybody else and is better prepared. Those were some of the things we tried to get him to learn. For example, before we did Tour of Flanders, we'd spend two or three days out there working the Tour of Flanders course. Knowing where the left turns were. The right turns. Uphills. Downhills. Pavement. No pavement. Whatever. And he does the same thing before the Tour de France. Preparation is a big part of being able to compete at that level. And he does it more than anybody else.

Training in Your 40s and 50s

AT ARMSTRONG'S AGE, if you have an injury or illness, you can take time out. I think you can come back up until the age of 32 or so. At 34, it'd be a lot harder to come back. I'm 52 years old. Actually I can ride as many miles as I used to. When you're in your 40s, you can probably do the most training. Your body can really take it. I think you can put in a lot of hours. And you can do it in a bigger gear. If you have the time, you can just do a lot more. The question is consistency. You can't do this for three months and then stop in three months and then come back and do it again for three months and then stop for three months. You need to have consistency. Consistency means you don't have breaks for more than two to three weeks where you're not going to do biking stuff, or some other kind of similar substitute. Like cross-country skiing in the winter or maybe ice skating or running.

I think you can train a lot when you're in your 40s. In your 50s, you can maintain some high level. At least I can. I feel like I can maintain. You're not as strong. No matter what you do, you won't be. But you learn to survive out there by knowing when you can make efforts and when you can't make efforts. I'm not a good climber. But I gotta climb a lot because I live in San Francisco. I ride with people who are better than I am. I don't count miles. I count hours—about 14 hours a week. Which isn't a lot. But it's enough. Because I do more than half of it really fast. Really fast means really fast for me.

I don't get any injuries. Never a bad knee. Never a bad back. I do stretching. Sit-ups, push-ups. Not a lot. A little yoga. If you do 15 minutes a day, that's enough to keep some good flexibility and keep sort of a body balance going.

The older you get, the more you have to consider nutrition. The difference between the nutrition I am looking at and the kind of a nutrition a Tour de France rider is looking at is like day and night. They need to have a very bland strategic diet during and around the Tour, because they need a massive amount of calories and they need to digest that food. And so nutrition to them is a totally different story than to somebody who is just a recreational rider. We can still indulge ourselves with something you may not want on a plate of a Tour de France table. But it is not going to be far off. I am pretty conscientious about what I eat and how I eat it. I follow a low-carb, low-fat diet. I take supplements. Just multivitamins. And try to watch my blood for cholesterol.

You can't deviate too much with diet in professional cycling because of the fact you have to eat so doggone many calories. And it can't be substituted 100 percent of the time with bars and gels and liquids of a sugary nature. We used to race with a bottle of water and a bottle of Coca Cola. That was it. Maybe a sandwich. Or a cookie. You could get cookies then that were wrapped individually. Stick 'em in your pocket so they didn't get all messy. Even today, if you go to the Tour de France there are some riders who just can't eat all that stuff. They can't stand all the sugar content and they get bad stomachs. So there are still people who eat sandwiches or paninis. It's not the fruit. You need some substance to swallow so you think you have a full stomach with food in it, and it can't just be gels and GUs and electrolyte drinks.

Time management is another important aspect of my life. My job is consuming, as most everybody's job is. I've always been pretty good at time management. It's learning how to fit an hour or two hours into a day so that I can maintain a reasonable level of fitness in a sport that I like. So that's not an easy thing to do, particularly if you travel a lot. But I make efforts to accommodate that even in my travels. I bring a bike a lot of times with me. I throw it in a canvas bag. Drag it to the airport and throw it on the plane and put it together and ride if I can. I do that whether I'm going to L.A. or to Zürich, Switzerland. I guess I'm a little more fortunate than the average person because I can keep a couple of bikes around the country. I keep a bike in Austin at Lance's garage—he has a couple of Trek mountain bikes and three or four road bikes. I got a bike in Europe in Eddy Merckx's garage in Belgium. I just go to Eddy's and go for a ride.

The Joy of Wheel-Sucking

I HAVEN'T RACED since 1980. But I like going fast. I find it more fun. I am just competitive. We do races every Tuesday and Thursday down in Palo Alto. Now, they are not official races. But they're races. People meet in Palo Alto. We do a loop. It's an hour-15, an hour and 20 minutes. Everybody goes flat out. Fifty, 60 riders. I'm the oldest dog on the ship, you know? All I got to do is finish and I've accomplished something. I know how to ride a wheel. So I can wheel-suck really good. Survival is probably my forte right now. Because it is fast for me—and hard. But I enjoy it.

We got a guy riding with us right now who just started riding about a year and a half ago. He was a four-minute-miler in college. Went to work, didn't do a lot of athletics. Then got hooked on the bike—and he is a really strong bike rider right now. He is dedicated and can train hard. He's got a big engine. So my advice to him starting out is take it slow. Build a base. He had to work really hard for about six months to build a really reasonable base of miles. Then he started transitioning and developing a little bit more speed, little more style, changing his training program a bit. More from just long slow miles to a little more fast, short-interval training. And today, he's still getting better.

The first thing I'd tell people, don't just get on a bike and go as hard as you can. You've got to learn to discipline yourself a bit. Build a base. And you've got to have someone good—a personal trainer, or someone who knows how to race. Learn about bike handling. And drafting and positioning and riding in an echelon. Do all the things that make riding a bike a lot more enjoyable.

This is true even for recreational riders. I see groups of 5, 10, 15 riders, groups of 40 to 50 riders out on weekends around where I live. And they're all in a big bunch. When you're in a big bunch, you better know something about wheels. What side do you sit on? How close do you get? Those are all just basic skills that every cyclist needs to know. Even at any level, whether you do charity rides or centuries, it's important to know the basics of riding a bike. It's not just how fast you can go. It's how fast you can go, but with a lot more thought put into it.

My middle daughter, 20, trains for speed skating on a bike. She was on the Olympic team in Salt Lake City for speed skating. Then my 15-year-old son just got his first brand-new bike. An Eddy Merckx. And we'll be doing some riding this summer. You know, my father never rode with me. He took me to the bike races. But we never rode a bike together.

Even in this complex world with so many choices, riding a bike is still a lot of fun and interesting. It's an interesting sport for recreation, and because of one's ability to go fast, you have the ability to stay in good fitness and relatively injury-free. It's one of those sports that when somebody does fall upon it or happen upon it in some way, they fall in love with it. That was my case.

Update

AFTER RETURNING PART-TIME to bike-team management in 2010 with BMC, a Swiss bike manufacturer (whose Australian leader, Cadel Evans, won the 2011 Tour de France), Ochowicz went full-time as the team's president and general manager in 2013, retiring from his longtime executive banking job with Thomas Weisel that June. "Everything's changed since 1996" (when his similar job with the Motorola team ended), the 62-year-old said in January 2014, two months after he became a grandfather for the first time. "There was no Internet back then, no real use of cell phones. The bikes today are carbon fiber, not steel and titanium. The teams are bigger, the calendar is much bigger, the season is longer—January through late October, versus February through early October.

"But as for me and my riding, very little has changed," he said. "I still ride 12,000 kilometers (about 7,400 miles) a year, and get up to do the local Tuesday and Thursday morning rides at 6:30 a.m. Consistency is what I'm looking for. So, if I do 1,000 kilometers a month, I'm doing well. It's hard to catch up if you stop riding for too long."

"I don't have the watts I did when I was 20, but I can ride in a group pretty comfortably. I do some body maintenance with stretch bands and yoga, but no weights—there's only so much time in the day. My only problem is weight. I eat out a lot while traveling, so it's hard to keep the good balance I have at home. But besides that, I feel lucky. I still exercise and enjoy it. A lot of my friends the same age are doing the same thing. It's a great space to be in."

9

ACHEY-BREAKY BIKER BONES

How to fight the scary—and until-now unknown—
link between cycling and osteoporosis

In the spring of 2003, while research-ing tandem bikes for one of my Los Angeles Times *sports-gear columns, I called Rob Templin, an old friend who worked as a sales manager at Burley, a leading tandem and recum-bent bicycle maker in Eugene, Oregon. I'd known Templin since 1988, when he was one of the top-seeded competitors in that year's Race Across America (RAAM), which I was handicapping for* California Bicyclist *magazine. A longtime bike racer, Templin never won the agonizing, near-sleepless 3,000-mile race from California to the Atlantic Ocean, but he finished second once and was a finisher four times. He then went on to make a career with Burley, which allowed him to pursue an all-bikes-all-the-time lifestyle. He rode 400 miles per week by commuting to work every day on his bike, taking extra time off in the slow winter months for Southern Hemisphere tours, and representing the company at dozens of cross-state events and endurance rides, such as the 1993 Davis Double Century, which we rode on a tan-dem together. (The guy's an engine with legs; I'd never ridden a 10-hour double before or since.)*

"How's it going?" I asked when he picked up the phone.

"Oh, not too good," he replied. "I've got osteoporosis."

Shock. Silence. Templin was 47, an age when most men don't show any bone loss at all. Most non-cycling men, that is.

Cycling and osteoporosis seem like strange bed-fellows. Superfit humans with powerful hearts and legs like steel rods—oddly coupled with wimpy, brittle skeletons that turn them into bro-ken hips waiting to happen.

Rob Templin surely didn't expect it. Yes, he had always been skinny—bony, really—but lots of hard-core bike people are. He was an aerobic ani-mal, superfit in every way. Or so he thought until he got a call the year before from legendary two-time RAAM winner Pete Penseyres, who was participating in a research study being conducted by a professor at San Diego State University.

Dr. Jeanne Nichols, PhD, a professor of exer-cise and nutrition and a serious cyclist, was con-ducting bone-density studies of veteran bike racers and endurance riders. Ultimately, she ex-amined the bones of 27 Masters racers and en-durance riders, including Penseyres and Templin, who had an average age of 51.2 and had trained an average of 12.2 hours a week for 20 years. Her study, "Low Bone Mineral Density in Highly Trained Male Masters Cyclists," was published in the August 2003 issue of *Osteoporosis International*. And her conclusions, communicated in an article I wrote for the March 2004 issue of *Bicycling* magazine, would stun the bike world: **Anyone who rides a bike as his or her main form of fitness is risking osteoporosis.**

People were shocked. Fit men with thin bones? Wasn't osteoporosis an "old ladies' disease"? After all, four out of five victims are women, whose bone thinning begins at menopause; the "change" causes women's bodies to stop producing estrogen, which helps absorb and store calcium. In 2002, the National Osteoporosis Foundation reported that 44 million Americans over 50 had elevated bone thinning, with full-blown osteoporosis striking 8 million women and 2 million men. In 2004, a Surgeon General's report said that half of all Americans over 50 would soon be at risk for osteoporosis. The disease is blamed for about 1.5 million broken bones a year, including debilitating fractures of the hip and back that leave victims wheelchairbound. Estrogen and other supplements can help prevent bone loss after menopause, although they do not reverse bone loss.

Men are luckier—their bones naturally have a higher bone mineral density (BMD) than women's and usually don't begin to show signs of osteoporosis until 20 years after them.

In Nichols's study of 27 male riders, however, two-thirds showed at least "osteopenia," moderate bone loss. Four of those had severe bone thinning, or osteoporosis. The test group's average hip and spine bone densities were 10 percent lower than those of a control group of similar aged, moderately athletic, non-cycling men.

When I remarked to Nichols that 10 percent didn't seem like a big deal, she was aghast.

"Clinically, 10 percent thinning is significant—not good—almost frightening," she said. "Because, at age 50, average men have *no bone loss at all.*"

The thinning of hip bones and the lower spine early in life is indeed scary, as it accelerates a huge quality-of-life issue by several decades. "Ten percent bone loss today will lead to a much higher than normal fracture risk as they age," explained Nichols. "The debilitating bone fractures that normal men become susceptible to in their 70s and 80s may happen to these superfit guys in the next few years."

In fact, during the time of the study, one participant, 51-year-old bike builder and ex-racer Bill Holland, a personal friend of Nichols, "confirmed" his osteopenia diagnosis with a 15-mph crash that left him with a fractured left hip, broken collar bones, and several cracked ribs. "At that [slow] speed, my riding buddies didn't think anyone's bones could break, but I couldn't get up," he said. That was surprising considering that Holland, 5 foot 10, 147 pounds, was fairly robust, unlike Rob Templin. But riding 150 miles a week took its toll, as 16 minutes in a Dual X-ray Absorptiometry (DXA) bone-scanning machine revealed. Nichols's study measured the densities of the lower spine and hips, the areas at much greater risk (along with the forearms) of orthopedic fracture than other parts of the body. The hip wears away more quickly than other spots because of a high concentration of trabecular bone, the softer inner bone, compared to the tougher, outer cortical bone. The DXA reading would also yield a total body bone density. (The clavicle, probably cyclists' most frequently fractured bone, was not studied. The trauma of falling is most responsible for that, say Nichols and others, with bone thinning playing a minor role, although growing with age.) The experts agreed that one can infer from the hip and spine whether the entire skeleton is thinning.

The results of Rob Templin's DXA scan left him woozier than a sleepless crossing of Kansas at 4 a.m. His lower vertebrae and hip bones were only 75 percent as dense as a normal 47-year-old's, equal to those of a person twice his age. At a time in life when most men's bones are still robust, Templin's skeleton was literally wasting away.

Templin was the worst case of all the 27 test subjects. But not all of his bone thinning could be pinned on cycling, Nichols guessed, partly blaming it on his daily habit of drinking two liters of cola, laden with phosphoric acid that leaches calcium from bones. Cola drinking, one of many risk factors for bone loss, probably explains why DXA scans of other mega-mile riders' bones, though alarming, weren't as bad as Templin's.

Pete "Half-Million Mile" Penseyres, then 58, who had ridden 500,000 lifetime miles in his cycling career, was found to have borderline osteoporosis at his spine and hips. Despite his extreme mileage, his bone thinning was surprising, given his weekly consumption of two gallons of milk and several quarts of ice cream. Dairy products are loaded with calcium, a known bone builder. It was the same story for Don Coleman of San Diego, 42, an amateur racer since his teens, who had borderline osteoporosis in his spine despite his love for milk, cheese, and ice cream.

Among the most surprised of the test group was Dr. Bob Breedlove, 51, who had osteopenia despite a lifelong regimen of weight lifting, another known bone builder. "I was stunned," said Breedlove, an orthopedic surgeon from Des Moines, Iowa, who set a transcontinental tandem record in 1992 and the transcontinental age 50-plus record in 2002. "I thought I'd test normal. I used to run marathons, have no family history of osteoporosis, eat five helpings of dairy a day, and for decades have been lifting three days a week from September through March."

Although the test subjects were surprised by the results, bone researchers were not. While Nichols's study was one of the first to examine bone density in elite male cyclists (most seem to examine women and other sports), the topic has long been in the news, ironically associated with *younger* riders. A 1996 study in *Sports Medicine Digest*, "Rapid Bone Loss in High-Performance Male Athletes," discovered massive bone loss in the vertebrae of four Tour de France racers during the event's three-week time period. In 2000, England's Chris Boardman, the famed Tour rider and World Hour Record holder, retired because of osteoporosis at age 32. Women aren't immune, of course. Pro mountain biker Sally Warner, a University of Washington PhD who published a 2002 study that showed mountain bikers have thicker bone densities than dedicated roadies, was found to have just 83 percent of the spinal bone mass of a normal female her age, then 33.

If you're a little spooked by findings that seem to cut, uh, a little close to the bone, join the club. In Nichols's opinion, bone thinning goes beyond racers and extreme riders. She said average cycling folk are at risk, too.

"Even if you aren't a hard-core racer or RAAM rider, you still are at risk if cycling is your only athletic activity," she said. In other words, it doesn't matter whether your thing is mountain biking, road riding, or Spinning, or whether you do it 20 hours a week or two hours a week. If all you do for fitness is pedal a bike, Nichols believes that you are at risk of wasting the foundation of your body—your skeleton—and turning yourself into a broken hip waiting to happen.

Nichols admitted to me that this conclusion surprised even her. Although she knew from existing research that non-weight-bearing activities like cycling and swimming don't cue the body to strengthen bone the way impact activities such as running do (more on this later), she assumed that hard-core cyclists would certainly have much better bone densities than those found in same-aged non-athletes. "But instead of having similar bone densities, it turns out that the bone health of the cyclists, as a group, was actually worse!" she said.

The bottom line? "A recreational cyclist who rarely does other sports has the bone density of a non-athletic couch potato and is most likely on the road to moderate to severe osteoporosis," Nichols said.

It is important to note that none of the national bone experts I contacted were willing to endorse that conclusion. "This is a good study," said Dr. Felicia Cosman, clinical director of the National Osteoporosis Foundation, after she obtained a copy of it at our request. "But you can't generalize it to all cyclists." Her reason? It wasn't longitudinal [a long-term comparison with several measuring points] and didn't account for heredity, body type, and diet; see "How to Build Better Bones" sidebar, below). And average cyclists don't train 12.2 hours a week for 20 years straight.

Even so, logic seems to indicate some level of risk for tens of thousands of century riders, long-distance tourists, dawn-to-dusk mountain bikers, and four-day-a-week Spin-class junkies. "Big-mile enthusiasts ought to know about this," said Breedlove. "If you're regularly in the saddle for long stretches, it makes sense that some of what happened to us could happen to you."

HOW BONE LOSS HAPPENS— AND HOW TO STOP IT

Cycling's lack of weight-bearing impact and its long hours make it the perfect storm for bone thinning. Add aging and lack of calcium replacement, and osteoporosis is almost a given.

Background: In young adults, 5 to 10 percent of bone is replaced every year. In a process similar to scoring a wall before applying plaster, specialized cells called "osteoclasts" prepare bone for a new layer of calcium by dissolving away surface bone and creating an indentation. Cells called "osteoblasts" then help plaster in a new layer of calcium.

Unfortunately, the process slows, and less of the lost calcium is replaced as you age and reduce your stressful physical activity levels. But the density can be maintained and even thickened by a calcium-rich diet and supplements and two types of physical activity: on-your-feet movement that has impact, G-forces, and vibration, such as running; and any resistance training including weight lifting with free weights, weight machines, or using your own body weight (push-ups, for example).

The rule: Anything that strengthens muscle mass strengthens bone.

It appears that bone responds to stress by building more bone. Repeated jumping and landing, and the pulling and pushing on bones from contracting muscles and tendons, forces bones to adapt to stress, just as muscles do. Additional hormone release and the increased blood flow associated with exercise help to transport vital nutrients to bones.

The results are visible on certain athletes, such as the stronger, denser bones in the dominant arms of tennis players and baseball pitchers and the extra-thick leg, hip, and back bones noted in numerous studies of runners, weight lifters, and volleyball players.

Impact and resistance build bone for people of all ages. One Oregon State University study had kids jump off 2-foot-tall boxes 100 times, three times per week, for seven months. The result was 5.6 percent higher bone mass in those kids than in a control group who did only stretching and nonimpact exercise. "That translates to a 30 percent decrease in the risk of a hip fracture at adulthood," said study director Christine Snow.

A study of triathletes aged 40-plus found that the bone-building potential of running apparently is powerful enough to counteract the bone-losing potential of cycling and swimming. A survey by the Veteran Affairs Medical Center of San Diego of triathletes who competed in the 1999 Hawaii Ironman found that female triathletes who trained intensively had just as much spine and upper thighbone strength as their male triathlete counterparts. The same bone-building triggers exist in animals, too. Sheep placed on a vibrating platform for 20 minutes for five days a week increased their hipbone densities by one-third.

For pure cyclists, however, the news ain't so good. Sports physiologists have surmised for years that cycling's seated, off-the-ground position, which eliminates weight bearing and impact on the legs, does not trigger the body's bone-building mechanism much or at all. Cycling is not alone in this regard; bone thinning is also associated with low- or no-gravity activities such as swimming, or, to a radical degree, space flight. (You'd have to ride intensely for 100 years to equal the bone damage incurred on a two-month space orbit, according to Nichols.) Injured athletes also suffer bone loss from inactivity.

The Calcium Sweat-Loss Theory

Despite cycling's lack of running-style, weight-bearing impact, I wasn't convinced that the bone-loss story ended here. Riding your bike up a hill puts plenty of stress on muscles and tendons, and by extension, bones. Even Nichols admitted that logic dictated that the "heavy tension on the pedals while standing and climbing, especially, probably builds some bone."

After calling bone experts around the country for comments on Nichols's findings, one remark nagged at me for months. Dr. Eric Orwoll, director of the Oregon Health and Science University in Portland and one of the nation's foremost authorities on male osteoporosis, called Nichols's study "provocative." But he was certain that under-nutrition, not cycling, was the culprit.

"You can speculate all you want about cycling and osteoporosis," said Orwoll, "but get enough calcium and vitamin D and you're okay."

That's logical—just get enough calcium. But as I was thinking about Orwoll's statement several weeks later, a lightbulb went off: Getting enough calcium is not easy for cyclists.

The recommended daily calcium requirement for an average adult, according to the National Institutes of Health and several other government organizations, ranges from 1,000 to 1,200 milligrams (mg). But wouldn't this be too low if you were partaking in activities that burned up a lot of calcium? Even if you steered clear of eating

disorders, adult lactose intolerance, or overconsumption of soft drinks (all of which lead to bone thinning), could a cyclist's calcium stores still get hammered by the sport's unique capability for seemingly endless hours of hard training?

Orwoll, clearly not a cyclist (I could tell because he referred to them as "cyclers"), was probably not aware that cyclists can ride all day long. I know from decades of putting in 12-hour days in the saddle during tours and endurance events that we cyclists lose tons of minerals through calorie burn and sweat—salt, potassium, you name it. After all, that's what Gatorade is all about. So what about calcium? Could it be that all that riding was chewing up all the calcium those old bike racers took in—and more?

For years, Gatorade included no calcium among its ingredients (although the newer Gatorade Endurance formula does have a small amount). Calls to RAAM contacts revealed no calcium in the most-used ultra-endurance drinks. I had to go all the way back to a RAAM rider from the 1980s to find an energy drink with calcium in it: GookinAid Hydralite, now used in the tennis and rehab markets. GookinAid was concocted in 1968 by a top US marathoner after he left "green puddles" in his wake (i.e., he puked) during an unsuccessful afternoon at that year's US Olympic Trials.

"Turns out that you sweat out a lot of calcium," said Bill "The Bagman" Gookin. Dissatisfied with his Gatorade experience, Gookin, a biochemist, gained local notoriety by taping plastic sandwich bags to his back, chest, and armpits to gather sweat samples for analysis. "It was no surprise that sweat is composed of water, potassium, sodium, magnesium, calcium, amino acids, vitamin C, and other noxious substances. All these need to be replaced," said Gookin, who went on to ride the Race Across America with GookinAid in 1985, crossing the country in 11 days.

How much calcium comes out in sweat? Dr. Christine Snow, the Oregon State University

Bone Research Lab director, told me that an average-sized man engaged in intense training loses 200 mg of calcium in sweat per hour. But she said not to worry. "The NIH recommendation of 1,200 mg of calcium per day has enough padding to handle one hour of exercise," she said.

But then we did some math. Given that cyclists can easily ride four, five, six, even ten hours per day, a seven-hour century ride could sweat out 1,400 mg of calcium—more than a day's recommended intake. At 12.2 hours of weekly training, the participants in Nichols's study lost 2,440 mg of calcium—two full days' worth a week, year after year. No wonder their bones were disappearing.

With typical energy drinks containing little, if any, calcium, century riders would have to down an extra dozen servings of milk or yogurt per week on top of an already healthy diet. Otherwise the calcium they sweat out could come from only one place: their bones.

Like other bone experts I interviewed, Nichols seemed surprised and amused when I called her to share my theory that sweat loss could be a major factor in a cyclist's bone thinning. She told me that her three-person medical-journal peer review board, in addition to other bone experts interviewed for this story, hadn't considered sweat loss a factor. But confronted with the above math, and being a serious Masters cyclist herself, Nichols admitted it couldn't be ignored.

"Losing calcium through sweat is a plausible explanation, but not the whole explanation," she said.

As it turns out, there are precedents for calcium sweat loss, which does not discriminate by age or sport. Robert Heaney, PhD, a nationally known calcium researcher and professor at Nebraska's Creighton University, liked my sweat-loss theory. He told me about a 1996 study, "Changes in Bone Mineral Content in Male Athletes" (*JAMA*), that found sweat-loss-induced bone thinning among basketball players at the University

of Memphis by Robert Klesges, PhD. DXA scans over the six-month season showed significant thinning. To find out why, Klesges's team wrung out the players' sweaty jerseys after practice. "Our analysis showed huge expenditures of sodium [salt], which we expected," said Klesges, "and surprising amounts of calcium, which we didn't!" Fortunately, what comes out can be put back in. During the 1996 season, Klesges supplemented each player's daily diet with up to 2,000 mg of calcium, stirring low-cost calcium lactate into their energy drinks. Lo and behold, "Bone loss was virtually eliminated that season," he says. Memphis players drank extra calcium the next five years, with the same results.

Klesges's findings exposed a common shortfall in the American diet: too little calcium. "Most people don't even come close to the US-RDA of 1,200 mg," he said, "but that amount is still not enough for an athlete exercising over an hour each day."

And it's even worse for a cyclist. "At least the basketball players minimized the calcium loss with weight-bearing vibration and a limited season length," said Heany. "Cyclists don't have that." Add decreased sex hormones (which helps thin bones) in endurance athletes (1998 *Journal of Orthopedic Surgeons* report, "Exercise-Induced Loss of Bone Density in Athletes"), that many cyclists are thin (and thin-boned) to start with, and that long hours in the saddle can leave little opportunity or desire for bone-building activities such as weight lifting, basketball, jumping rope, or running. "Face it, it is an axiom in bike racing that 'If you're not riding, you're resting,'" said Nichols. "Fact: Most cyclists hate running."

That comment reminded me of the time I asked Greg LeMond, who was just back from doing the TV commentary on the bike leg of the Hawaii Ironman, if he would ever consider doing a triathlon. "No way," he said. "I find running painful." Maybe not as painful as a broken hip when you're 70, though.

The Logical Fix—and the Mixed Results

Bone loss is difficult to reverse but it can be done with dedicated weight training, cross-training, and calcium supplementation programs (especially when the calcium and vitamin D is taken 30 minutes before your ride—see "Bone-Up Plan" sidebar). How has it worked out for some of the people profiled in this chapter? Dr. Bob Breedlove, who tragically died after a collision with an errant driver on a lonely highway during the Race Across America in 2006, was a good example of the difficulty of rebuilding bones. He religiously followed many of the bone-building recommendations listed below. He added more weight lifting to his program and more calcium to his diet (to 2,000 mg a day) while training for his 2002 transcontinental ride and the 2003 Paris-Brest-Paris. But he got disappointing news at his DXA scan in November 2003. Since Nichols's initial test two years earlier, Breedlove's hip-bone density was down 3.7 percent, although his lower spine was up 1.5 percent.

"My radiologist told me he's seen couch potatoes with stronger bones," Breedlove told me. "Of course, their cardio system ain't worth stink. So pick your poison." But he didn't give up the fight. After his second test, he increased his daily calcium intake closer to the 3,000 mg ceiling that Christine Snow deems safe, began lifting weights all year round instead of only during the off-season, substituted running for cycling some days, and in 2004, began taking Fosamax, a bone-building drug.

Rob Templin, the grandmotherly boned ex-RAAM rider with osteoporosis told me in late 2013 that he mountain bikes more, goes hiking and running, eliminated his case-a-week addiction to cola, and for the past 10 years has taken the bone-builder Fosamax, calcium, and vitamin D supplements. Also, every day for the past six years, he's used testosterone gel to raise his low T levels, which supposedly helps enhance bone density. He knows he should lift weights (which he hates) and eat more yogurt. He travels the world with his company, Second Summer bike tours, and says he's successfully turned cycling into a "lifestyle" rather than an obsession—even though he still rides 300 miles a week, down from 400.

And his bones? Ten years after Templin got his diagnosis, they are as thin and porous as ever.

But he considers that a resounding success. "I'm maintaining," he said. "I haven't gotten worse. So in a way I'm actually gaining in that I'm not declining with age, like everyone else."

Bill Holland, the bike builder with osteopenia, had more success. He still rides a lot but now downs 1,200 mg of calcium a day and rotates thrice-weekly 4-mile runs and weight-lifting sessions. The results are upbeat; since his first bone scan in 2001, he's reversed his bone loss and seen 1 to 2 percent annual increases in density. "Someday, if I live long enough," says Holland, "my bones might even be back to average."

THE PLAN: HOW TO BONE-UP

Don't wait until you break your hip. Bone thinning appears to be endemic to cycling. The more you do, the more you are at risk. So, what to do?

Get more calcium into your diet and more balance into your athletic life. Make cycling your main thing, but not your only thing. Add weight lifting, running, hiking, and impact exercises. Eat more dairy, cut smoking, and reduce soda consumption. Take some powerful new bone drugs, to possibly build back some of the bone you've lost. These actions will you're your skeleton strong, still let you ride a lot, and give you better all-around fitness. The details:

(continues)

THE PLAN: HOW TO BONE-UP *(continued)*

1. Take calcium supplements: Get at least 1,200 mg of calcium per day. The National Osteoporosis Foundation (NOF) recommends 1,000 mg daily for those under age 50 and 1,200 mg for those 51 and up. According to the National Institutes of Health, less than half of men get 1,000 mg. Vitamin D intake, says the NOF, should be 400–800 IU for both men and women under age 50 and 800–1,000 for those above age 50. Good supplementary sources of calcium include calcium tablets, Calcitonin (a non-estrogen hormone), Tums, low-fat yogurt, and raloxifene (an oral tablet that mimics estrogen in the bone but not in breasts or uterus). Help your body absorb the calcium by taking 400 to 800 IU of vitamin D per day. Mega-milers should increase their calcium load by 200 mg for every training hour beyond an hour per day. A study presented at the 2013 meeting of the Endocrine Society found that cyclists who took 500 to 1,000 mg of calcium and 400 to 2,000 IUs of vitamin D 30 minutes before and one hour after a 35K time trial had less bone density decrease than those who did not. The Before group loss less than the After group.

Note: Some research has shown that too much calcium may actually increase the risk of prostate cancer, kidney stones, and heart disease, but the vitamin D in dairy products (see below) can offset that.

2. Add calcium-rich foods: Got milk? You'll build bone—and lose weight, too. Add more milk (any type) and other dairy products, such as yogurt or Swiss and cheddar cheese, as well as calcium-fortified orange juice, salmon with bones, and other high-calcium foods during your regular diet and post-ride refueling. Each serving contains 200 to 230 mg of calcium.

Incidentally, studies show that increased dairy consumption may have another benefit: weight loss. Eating an extra three servings of yogurt a day caused men in a 2003 University of Tennessee study to lose 61 percent more body fat and 81 percent more stomach fat over 12 weeks than men who didn't eat yogurt. Why?

"Calcium helps the body burn more fat and limits the amount of new fat your body can make," said Michael Zemel, PhD, the study's author. Other studies have backed the finding: Teens in Hawaii with the highest calcium intakes were thinner and leaner than those getting less calcium, and a test comparing groups of mice yielded similar results.

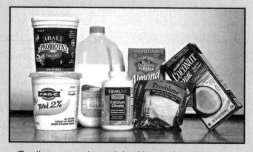

Cyclists, at serious risk of bone-thinning, need to load up on calcium-rich foods and supplements.

3. Add more protein: Several studies show that consumption of relatively high amounts of protein (higher than the RDA) can actually improve bone status. Older studies showed that additional protein significantly improves recovery from hip fractures. This makes sense for two reasons. Throughout history, humans have adapted to higher rather than lower protein intake. And bones, being made up of about 50 percent protein and living tissue always rebuilding itself, require a significant amount of replacement protein from the diet.

On the flip side, those with the lowest daily protein intake in a Tufts University study of 600 men and women also had the weakest bones, especially in the hips, thighs, and spine. In a University of California study, researchers found that for every 15 grams of protein you add to your diet each day, your bones become exponentially stronger.

4. Add more magnesium: Magnesium may help to keep the skeletal system healthy by preventing calcium and potassium from seeping out of bones. "Magnesium is most abundant in unprocessed, whole foods—the very foods that men

(continues)

THE PLAN: HOW TO BONE-UP *(continued)*

don't get enough of anymore," said Katherine Tucker, PhD, a Tufts University epidemiologist and professor of food science quoted in *Men's Health* magazine. Her recommendation: Protect your bones by adding one serving of spinach, yogurt, brown rice, bananas, or almonds to your daily diet.

5. Lift heavy, all-body weights: Heavy weights, used in two or three sessions per week, put maximum stress on muscles, and, by extension, bones, cueing the body's bone-strengthening mechanism. "Heavy weight shocks the muscles like running does, signaling the bones to grow," said Dr. Warren Scott, former director of sports medicine at Kaiser Permanente Hospital in Santa Clara, California, and head of the medical care unit at the Hawaii Ironman Triathlon. When muscles contract and pull, they produce electric currents in the bone tissue. Maximize the effect by lifting heavy—enough so that you "max out" (i.e., reach failure or lose form) at 6 to 10 reps per set for three sets. Lighter weights (sets of 11 to 20 reps) build bone at a slower rate, but still help. Do at least one set for each major muscle group (chest, back, shoulders, arms, and legs); two or three sets would be even more beneficial.

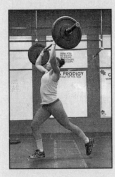

Weight lifting's load flexes the bones, which stimulates growth.

6. Do push-ups at home: Can't get to the gym? Try exercises that use body weight or a resistance band. Conventional floor push-ups and handstand push-ups against the wall, for example, can help strengthen your shoulders, chest muscles, and triceps.

7. Do back-strengthening exercises: Protect the lower vertebrae, which become particularly weak in cycling due to lack of movement, by working the oft-neglected spinae erector (lower-back) muscles. At the gym, do back extensions every time you finish doing sit-ups; the two exercises are complementary.

8. Run, jump, and do other impact activities: Jogging, uphill and downhill hiking (especially with a heavy backpack), skipping rope, doing jumping jacks, climbing stairs, dancing, or simply jumping up and down for 10 to 20 minutes several times a week helps jump-start bone growth with weight-bearing vibration.

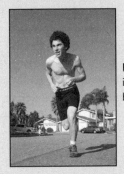

Running's G-force impact also stimulates bone growth.

Weight-bearing exercise on the major muscle groups releases hormones that trigger bone cells to multiply as much as 2 percent a year. (Note: Swimming won't build upper-body bones, since it isn't weight bearing.)

The impact must be significant. Cycling vibrations aren't enough. A Johns Hopkins study, published in the November 2002 issue of the *Journal of Internal Medicine*, found that light-intensity activities like walking did not strengthen bones. A Hebrew University study found that running was the only exercise that strained the shinbones enough to strengthen them.

Must you run a 10K to build bone? Length of time is being debated. Some studies say just a minute of impact is enough, but to be safe, do 20 or 30 minutes, Snow said. An OSU study found that bone density increased in postmenopausal women who jumped up and down 50 times a day

(continues)

THE PLAN: HOW TO BONE-UP (continued)

three times a week and did squats and lunges while wearing vests weighted with 1 to 10 pounds. Another study ("Good, Good, Good . . . Good Vibrations," *The Lancet*, December 2001) placed sheep on a vibrating platform for 20 minutes each day for five days a week over a year; results showed a 32 percent increase in the hipbone density of the sheep.

9. Stand up on the bike: Standing on the pedals loads all your weight on the legs. Many cyclists never get off the seat, especially since the advent of aerobars. Add more standing, especially during climbing, which puts very high torque on your muscles and bones.

10. Mountain-bike more: Sally Warner's PhD study, "Bone Mineral Density of Competitive Male Mountain and Road Cyclists," found significantly higher bone density in mountain bikers than in road cyclists, particularly in the upper body, probably owing to the occasional hiking, the jarring ride, and the high-torque climbing of mountain biking.

11. Cut back on smoking, excessive alcohol, and soda: All of the aforementioned are known bone thinners. One study found that the more cigarettes smoked, the more bone was lost. Soft drinks and even sparkling water are loaded with phosphorus, known to leach calcium from bone. Alcohol is toxic to bones, and alcohol abuse is associated with accidental injury, nutritional deficiency, and hypogonadism. One study found that long-term hard drinkers lost almost 70 percent more bone than nondrinkers. Recommendation: Swig less than 60 grams per day (less than two cans of beer or 2 ounces of hard liquor).

12. Know your risk factors for osteoporosis: If you're skinny, Caucasian, Asian, have a family history of osteoporosis, were trained to excess as a youth (e.g., female gymnasts), or have taken steroids, you have a higher propensity for osteoporosis.

13. Get a bone scan: Know where you stand, skeleton-wise. Insurance companies won't pay for the DXA bone-density scan ($200–$250)

until men are 65 and women are 50—unless you appear to slump when you see your doctor, complain of aches, and mention that your wife or friends say you look shorter, which could indicate premature "kyphosis," a grandmotherly forward slump.

14. Get some summer sun: Your skin cranks up production of vitamin D and banks it for later in the year during the summer, so give yourself 10 to 15 minutes in the sun before putting on sunscreen, or take a short walk outdoors during lunchtime three times a week with your sleeves rolled up. According to Dr. Michael Holick, a professor at the Boston University School of Medicine and author of *The UV Advantage*, chronic lack of sun exposure due to covering up and sunscreen can lead to a vitamin D deficiency that can increase the risk of bone thinning, muscle pain, multiple sclerosis, and colon and prostate cancers.

15. Try powerful bone-building drugs:

1. Fosamax, manufactured by Merck and approved in 1995, reverses some of the effects of osteoporosis by slowing bone-destroying cells, and thus allowing more time for bone-building cells to catch up. A study published in the *New England Journal of Medicine* (*NEJM*) in early 2004 found that the bone built by the slower turnover was as solid as normal bone. A later *NEJM* study in 2004 found that Fosamax keeps strengthening bones for at least a decade, dispelling fears that it might eventually boomerang and start making hips and spines brittle and prone to breaking.

2. Forteo (Lilly), a faster-acting drug, was approved by the US Food and Drug Administration (FDA) in 2003. It is an injectable form of human parathyroid hormone (PTH). Side effects include growth pains similar to those experienced by fast-growing teenagers.

3. Strontium ranelate, shelved for 50 years, is a "new" drug that was found to increase bone density in postmenopausal women, according to a study in the January 2004 edition of the *New England Journal of Medicine*. Mixed with water, it is a powder composed of the mineral strontium

(continues)

(discovered in lead mines a century ago) and ranelic acid. While Dr. Felicia Cosman of the National Osteoporosis Foundation warned that it is no better than any other bone drug, strontium ranelate is noteworthy because of its easy absorption and lack of side effects, except for diarrhea, experienced by 6 percent of patients in the study. In other words, it can be taken for years without concern, a big plus considering that other bone therapies have some downsides. Fosamax, a biphosphate, can cause stomach cancer. Estrogen, which keeps bones healthy, has been linked to a slight increase in strokes and blood clots and can have side effects such as vaginal bleeding, mood disturbances, and breast tenderness. Raloxifene is generally free of serious side effects, but it can cause hot flashes, leg cramps, and deep-vein thrombosis, a blood-clotting disorder.

Forteo can cause nausea and cramps and is also linked to cancer in mice.

16. Take folate, B vitamins, or a multivitamin tablet: The aforementioned drugs work by reducing levels of homocysteine, an amino acid that, at high levels, can double the risk of osteoporosis-related fractures (and also raise the risk of heart attacks, strokes, and Alzheimer's disease). A standard multivitamin, taken once a day, does the trick, according to Dr. Douglas P. Kiel, senior author of the Framingham study (published in the May 13, 2004, issue of the *New England Journal of Medicine*) and director of medical research at the Hebrew Rehabilitation Center for Aged Research and Training Institute in Boston. Foods naturally rich in B vitamins and calcium—including dairy products, broccoli and other greens, leafy vegetables, carrots, avocados, cantaloupes, apricots, almonds, and peanuts—can also reduce the risk of broken bones.

INTERVIEW
Eddie B
THE WORKAHOLIC POLE WHO CHANGED AMERICAN CYCLING

"We had a complex about the Europeans, with their three lungs, four hearts, and five legs," said three-time Tour de France winner Greg LeMond. "Eddie B helped us get over that."

With that introduction, Edward "Eddie B" Borysewicz (Bor-say-vich) stood up to a rousing ovation at the Endurance Sports Awards dinner in San Diego in February 2004. On stage he was greeted by LeMond and all eight members of the 1984 US Olympic team, whom he had coached to a record nine medals, including four golds. They had come to honor Eddie and to participate in a cycling fantasy camp that raised money for the reconstruction of Eddie's home, which was destroyed in a massive San Diego fire several months earlier. For the moment, Eddie was living in an 8- by 10-foot pool house.

"He was the John Wayne, the catalyst," said 1980s star Alexi Grewal.

"He took us young cowboys, and made us real cowboys," said LeMond.

In the 1970s, the US national cycling team program was in shambles and the sport was underdeveloped. Then, in 1976, Eddie B defected to the United States from his native Poland and resuscitated the team with his common sense and Eastern bloc training methods.

In Poland, Eddie had won two national junior championships and two national championships,

and he had been awarded the highest sports award in Poland: the "Special Champion in Sport." Damaged by aggressive treatment of a misdiagnosis of tuberculosis, he began preparing for a coaching career in his 20s, earning a master's degree in physical education, physical therapy, and coaching. He went on to coach a leading Polish trade team and 30 national and world champions, including bronze and silver medalists at the 1976 Olympic Games. Soon thereafter, he defected to the United States and became coach of the US national team for the US Cycling Federation [now USA Cycling]. During 12 years of coaching, his American riders won 30 world championships, 9 Olympic medals, and 15 Pan-American medals. In 1988 he left the USCF and with investment banker Tom Weisel created the Subaru-Montgomery team, which later became Montgomery-Bell and then the US Postal Service team.

Throughout his coaching years, Eddie B developed and coached some of America's greatest cycling stars, including LeMond, Lance Armstrong, Olympic medalist Steve Hegg, and six-time world champion Rebecca Twigg. Since 1996, Eddie has been running training camps in Ramona, California; his clients have included many national and world Masters medalists. Speaking with a thick Polish accent and ungrammatical English, Eddie B was interviewed originally in March 2004 and again in

February 2014. Variously described as "blunt-spoken," "really tough," and even "cold" by his adoring riders, the intense Polish immigrant put performance first and America squarely on the world's cycling map, where it has been ever since.

FROM YOUNG AGE, I read everything. I read the Italian CONI blue cycling book [*Cycling*, a manual put out by the Central Sports School in Rome in 1972 and sometimes called the "blue book" of cycling]. Later I read papers from the Polish Sports Institute and from the Soviet Sports Institute. So maybe my fate to coach.

I was born in Poland in 1939, on the Nemen River on land that now in Belarus. Before World War II, Stalin take eastern part of Polish country. In fourteenth century Poland was the biggest country in Europe, did you know it?

Cycling was a big sport in my country when I grew up. I was good at cycling almost all my life—but was a better runner. I run very well, 400 meters excellent. At age 17 I run 51 seconds with no training. I have natural stride.

The coach even take me to national team. Then he give me a racing bike for fun, to help run training, because he knew I was crazy about cycling. So, I start to compete in bike races. First year I race in 30 events. I was double junior champion in 1958 at age 19.

My progress stop when I go into military. I supposed to be privileged in sport, to go to Sport Battalions like other athletes, and continue training, [but] wasn't allowed to do athletics for one year because my father was anticommunist. They didn't do me any favors. They made it hard for me. Did not to do any training at all for cycling.

My club and my federation really fight for me. After one year, I move to a regular division, where was a little sport program. But when I there just for a few months, everything canceled because of Cuba problem [Cuban Missile Crisis]. East bloc forces went on alert. We have to send bicycles home and are regular soldiers again.

Nothing about the military helped my cycling. I did a lot of cross-training on my own. Everything I can to keep in shape. It was like being in prison; I do what I have to do.

Fate Intervenes

AT 21, ONE season after getting out of military, I was already on national team again. I start winning races. Everything incredible. Then my cycling career was change by a doctor decision.

In an exam, doctors discover I have a little point under my left collarbone they think is indication of contact with TB. The doctor thinks this is a new thing, because nobody sees before. I spent four months in the hospital. This guy screwed up my career.

I probably had TB when I was little boy during the Second World War and my body just took care of it. But it left a little scar, like scar tissue. Like a little bean you can't see on the X-ray when my arm hang down, but is visible when I lift my shoulder high.

So here I am, winning races and making national team, one of the strongest guys, achieving all my dreams. Then I go into the hospital for four months, and in two weeks I might have killed myself. I was very depressed. So I don't talk to anybody. Even right now hard to talk of this, because it touched my heart.

Half season after hospital, I am back to national team. I am good again. But I know I am not going to be as I was. Because after 100K when I was on the break, I used to get better and better. Now, after hospital, I have pains with my liver.

So, at 22, I know my future. I love cycling so much, but I'm not stupid. I know my best thing is over. So I went to Academy Physical Education and I change my goal, because I know I am not going to be world champion. But I am going to develop world champions.

I rode very well for three years more as member national team. I did well at nationals, and I compete with our national team in different countries. I wasn't a good climber, like when I was junior. I was different guy after the hospital; I pick up like 25 pounds and only lost 15 or 10. So I become heavy guy, muscle guy. In team time trial I was excellent. Also in crit and classic races that did not have hilly stages. I didn't make selection for some stage races with one-third mountain stages. I did pretty good on the road—a few times top 20.

I was two-time national champion of the track and national champion of the road, but I not make any progress. So I study hard.

I kept riding until I was 29 only because I love cycling—and the life. I was amateur by license, but of course I really a professional. I rode bike for very good money, for a communist country. So I had very good life and I do what I like to do: pursue my physical education studies. I graduate Academy Physical Education. Next, I graduate special after physical therapy and coaching school. I spent 22 years in school. Results always "A."

Coaching Career
WHEN I WAS 29 to 30 years old, I plan to race two, three years more. One Sunday, I won a classic race. On Monday, I am called by secretary from office of chief of sport this region, and told please come to see. When I come, he told me name of some person who is president/CEO of different club. "That is your new boss," he said. "Excuse me if I don't understand it," I say. "Please just do," he said. And that is it. He tell me I have to work. So I have to quit being a bike racer.

He told me I now head coach of different club.

I not afraid at all. I was coach even in my last years of competitive cycling.

My nickname as bike rider was Professor. Two reasons: One, I only guy with master's degree. Two, I always thinking. My friends ask many times for advice, even when I still a bike rider. I always analyze.

My generation was exactly similar like in United States. No professional coaches, only ex-bike riders, with no education. That eventually changed in Poland; now you can be only coach if you have get a master's degree in PE [physical education], two years after graduating coaching school. Besides studying, I listen old guys. I try to learning from everybody and I read every book. Anything that can help me. That was my second education. By this experience, learning a lot, learning hard way.

A good coach is combination of things learned in school and developed on your own. You have to always think, "I am . . . teacher." I know cycling because I race hard and many years and successful. School is important too. Both things together and not other things. You must really be dedicate. You must love. You must be passion. Okay? Impossible different.

It takes much time, this passion. During our divorce my ex-wife said, "We weren't married for 21 years because he was on the road 255 days a year."

Now always I lecture. I tell people, "Don't be crazy and be imbalance with work and family." Because family is very important and I miss this. I have two nice, smart kids and I have good relations with my ex. But I was a divorced single guy at age 55.

Coaching Philosophy
COACHING PHILOSOPHY FOR me is: you must be educated. You must have cycling [experience]. Not necessary best in country or best in the world. But you must have professional experience. That help. Bigger that help. Many times superstars cannot be coaches. I don't know superstars can be coaches. Because these guys have no education and think what is good for them must be good for everybody. So for me cycling experience, practical experience very important. Education very important. And next self-education. You must know how to use this university stuff in practice.

My own experiences as a cyclist taught me a couple simple truths: Hard work is equal important as rest. You must work very hard. And you must rest well. You have to relearn how much is too much.

People absolutely don't rest enough. Rest is ignored. It is key.

And so is analyz[ing]. I check my pulse all the time after two years racing. There were no heart rate monitors then. I was only guy checking pulse in two positions, horizontal and vertical [lying down and standing]. Both are important. Vertical can be horizontal same. For example 42 and 42. But usually vertical was, 55 for example, always higher.

I taught myself to take pulse. I always talk to doctors. I gauged my fitness by my pulse. In my time on the national team we have always a blood pressure check, a pulse check, weight check, urine check. Nurses did it; it was expensive, took much time, very complicated. So many different things can be checked. For me, pulse is simple and very good. That's enough for me. We can't do everything.

The pulse is a simple, accurate gauge. On day before race [Saturday], pulse should be low, perfect. On Sunday in morning, will be higher from adrenaline. After race on Sunday your pulse is [naturally] high; when was hard race, my pulse must be up. Monday pulse always is higher. Tuesday it is still higher than normal, but going down. Wednesday almost perfect. My philosophy is day after race is easy recovery ride. Second day after race [Tuesday] is a test to see how you feel. Do light warm-up, then speed work—jumps or sprints. If feel weak on the second sprint, do not [do] any more sprints that day. If feel good, do more. Depends on my feeling.

The coaches did not tell me to do this. They had us doing a regular workout the day after a race. I was one of first to say we need a recovery day after hard workout.

And I was first guy in Poland to have a longer crank arm. We all used 170 mm steel crank arm.

It was primitive; we used hammer to change them. On visits to France, I discovered aluminum crank arm. Every year, when I'd go there, I'd always collect money beforehand from riders and go to bike shops to see latest stuff. One time when I said I wanted aluminum crank arms, shop owner say, "Which price?" I was surprised. This was first time I heard of different prices and sizes. I picked up a 170 and told him that this size was normal for us. So he recommend me a 172 and a half. I say, what else do you have? He say 170, 172½, and 175.

"Give me 175," I said.

"No, no," he said. "This going to be *grande problema*."

I was always the thinking guy. Longer crank arms will give me advantage in climbing. So I stuck to 175. We argued. I took the 175s and a bottom bracket home on Friday, put them on, then go to the big classic race on Sunday: 240K, 250 starters.

After 50K, only 14 guys were left. It was the crosswinds—in Poland, there is a lot of crosswind, "devil wind," we say. But I outsmarted devil, I thought. After 50K, I passed everybody. Oh, so smart! My crank arms—wonderful! They work! At 50K, I'm not usually trying to win. I usually take over after 100K. But now I jump after 50. And it is not long before I have a cramp. And I lose.

I said, My God! Uh oh! I was one of seven guys to finish the race. I always finish first, but now I was the seventh. I rode cramped all the way. The hardest race in my life. I knew the problem was not the crank arm. The problem was the big change. The Frenchman in the shop was right. Change crank arms for 2½ mm. But not for five. It was a very good lesson I learn. Something I pass on to my students.

Coming to America

WHEN I WENT to United States, I never believe I am going to be coach.

I did not come here for coaching. I quit cycling just six, seven months before. I get divorced because of cycling. I was workaholic. That's my problem. I work from 7 [a.m.] to 11 [p.m.]. You know in Poland, I was full-time professor in University of Poland. I teach PE and physical therapy, was a full-time coach, and head coach of club. I was national coach for juniors. And I was tour guide for some times. I was incredibly busy. And I threw out my first marriage by being workaholic. So in 1976, I say no more cycling in my life!

At that time, already I develop world champions. Olympic medalists. I was most successful coach in Poland by results. So I say, "Good-bye sport!" Unfortunately, I have this sport in my blood. After break of 10 months, I met [USCF board director] Mike Fraysse and I see what they got in US. He offers job and I back to coaching again.

Main difference in the way I coach: I am not a guy who tell you how many repetitions you have to do. I explain how you have to train and how hard you have to train. So you make decision of one more repetition or not. Because you are the captain of your body, not me. And always I explain what's going on. I always honest with my client.

Client must come to my place. I never ever coach anybody by Internet I never see. People offer me more money. I say: Sorry, thank you, good-bye. I have to see this body. And I have to set up position on the bike. I have to talk about life, training, recovering, nutrition, discipline, and on and on. Okay? And for me is very important self-discipline. Not discipline. I never ever check riders 10 o'clock is in room?

If you ride for me, I need to know about him. I have to see him on the bike. I need to see his VO_2. I have to see his blood. Next we can start program. And I push him to the max. Because only [when you] push hard and recovery well you can produce. Always I am monitoring his training.

When you racing once a week, I always explain to riders, four different training days.

Monday is recovery ride, Tuesday is testing day—sprints—so I can see how my recovery is going. It is going to give me information about what kind intervals I'm going to do next day. Wednesday is super-hard training—intervals, maximum, harder than race! That's maximum. My intervals, my philosophy is different than other people. Some people for me don't know what they are talking about. Must know what is different between sprints and intervals. Absolutely big difference. Thursday is endurance. Friday is recovery day. Saturday is a warm-up day. And you ready. Sunday is race day.

Recovery ride means you riding when you want it, with who you want it, how you want it, and where you want it. Everything what you want it. Important is even with who you riding. Where you riding. In other words, I say you riding bike with good rpm, with gears you not feeling you pushing pedals. You listen the bird. And looking like grass growing. Or ride on the beach and see nice jogging women. Look at the scenery, Okay? Heh heh. For how long recovery ride depends on who you are. Everyone is riding differently. Professional rider is two hours. An amateur, about hour. And that is individual. When he don't like to ride after 30 minutes, he feel bad, psychology bad, go home. Try afternoon maybe for another half hour. That's fine, too.

The second day [after the race or hard training effort] is "testing day"—you are testing yourself with speed work. Testing day means testing your performance. Testing who you are. How you recover. It's a two-hour workout. In this plan, many coaches follow me. After all, I am in this country 20 years. Before I come to this country, I learn only one thing about American sport cycling: LSD—long slow distance. More you are riding, the better you are.

For touring, LSD yes. For recreation, LSD fine. But not for competition. Speed work, intervals, endurance, and recovery—is necessary for Americans to be good. You must have a balance.

Americans were not doing speed work before me. Nothing was organized. It was really wild in cycling.

Here's how to do a test: warm up for 15 to 30 minutes, depends on who you are. Then maximum strength about 50 seconds—where you pushing body to the max. Your heart to the max. Blood pressure to the max. Maximum acceleration and hold. And always your legs feel like table legs. Before you do again, allow full recovery. Your pulse going the same level as when you start ride bike.

Sprints and intervals are different thing. My God! Sprints are 15 seconds. Intervals different—there is five different kinds of intervals. Is different for crit, is different for time trial, is different for hill climbing. Different for road race. And only big difference is time, is speed and recoveries. Because with sprint, recovery is maximum. Speed is not important. In interval, speed is important. Because you must simulate race.

My philosophy is two days after a race and two days before a race I always [use the] same training principles. How many days I have between races [and the two-day cushion on each side of them] is how many days I really train. I have one day I combine intervals with endurance. When I don't have more than four days [to train], that is recovery stuff.

I dunno what US cyclists did before me. But my program become very detailed. For two years, I work with Ed Burke [University of Colorado professor and prolific cycling health writer], who die unfortunately last fall. Every Friday, we fly to different place around the country and do clinics for 100 to 150 people. And I give always 40 pages information about cycling. My ex-wife say why I don't give one page to marriage?

His Stars and His Health

MY PROGRAM WORK for everybody to get better. First you need the right position on the bike. Next, knowledge to make you better. But not anyone can be champion. Need genetics.

LeMond was 16 when I met him. He had incredible body and personality; I immediately say "this guy can be world champion." One of the best I've work with. The natural athletic body. Without it, cannot be a world champion. I gave him the structure. Now only ones like LeMond I meet are older. Vic Copeland, doctor from San Diego, we work together I dunno how many years, 10, 15. Was just marathon or triathlon racer when we met, not so great. In two, three years with me, began winning. Now, he is not beatable. Not touchable. He is better than younger guys. Mr. Thom Weisel, [former] CEO and owner Montgomery Securities [he sold it—ed.], is another incredible athletic body. Too bad we cross each other not when he was 16, like LeMond. He was already 45. After one year he won national champion. He win five times national champion. He becoming world champion in Masters category. He or Vic could have been another Greg LeMond.

I love cycling and always will, but only ride three or four times a year. I swim every day, but it not like going out for a two-hour ride. That makes you feel so good and sleep so deep. Had two bikes on the porch of my home in San Diego that burned down in the fire [of 2003]. Too busy. But after the fire, LeMond sent me his stationary bike. I put it between the pool and the sliding door, so I am forced to ride it.

I'm 65 now, alone. Twelve years divorced. My grandfather lived till 90 and had all his teeth. The swimming keep me with 50 heart rate, 110/70 blood pressure, and 140 cholesterol.

American people eat too much. I eat six times a day fruit and vegetables. My biggest meal is lunch, like in France. Noon to 2 o'clock. They got it right. When you eat too late and go to bed, that's how you store fat.

I worked so hard. I wanted to make better team to win Tour de France. Now I coach six hours a week in the velodrome and three hours on the road on Sunday. Otherwise, I worked on my house farm—three horses, 50 chickens, cats, dogs. I dream of riding three times a week. I always said I'd ride tomorrow, but tomorrow never came. When my home is rebuilt, I will ride again.

Update

EDDIE B, AGE 75 when we talked in February 2014, had an eventful decade after his original *Bike for Life* interview. Still on crutches while recuperating from a two-year period that included two hip-replacement surgeries and five back surgeries, the latter the result of twice being hit by cars while riding, he spoke of many successes. His popular 1985 book, *Bicycle Road Racing*, was republished; his home was rebuilt with the help of donations of $120,000 raised through bike-industry fundraisers; and in 2006 he was recruited by Poland to coach the Polish national team in preparation for the 2008 Beijing Olympics (he advised the team through 2011). "Poland won its first medal in the worlds in the points race in the velodrome while I was there," he said proudly. "My system always gets good results." He coached a crew of California athletes at the 2011 USA Cycling Masters Track National Championships, and after 16 years of being single, he got married again in 2012. He continues to coach part-time at the velodrome, rides often, and trains cyclists of all abilities in San Diego County (eddiebcycling.com).

10

ROLL MODELS

There's nothing stopping you from riding at 60, 70, 80, or 90, or with a broken body, or even with just one arm, as Gerd Rosenblatt, Alejandro Oporta Reyes, Bill Walton, Russell Allen, Heart Akerson, and Don Wildman prove.

John McEnroe just couldn't stop talking about the Wild Man. I was in the tennis great's dressing room at the Craig Ferguson Show at CBS Television City in Los Angeles one day in 2009 interviewing him about his mountain-biking prowess for Bicycling magazine—but he didn't want to talk about himself. Mac always kept coming back to his Malibu neighbor, a local legend he rides with. "He's 76!—Can you believe it?" he raved. "And he's the orneriest, funniest, toughest old bastard I've ever seen in my life. . . . He pumps weights for two hours before we ride. He stand-up paddleboards for two hours afterward. And then we start riding the whole way up this massive, steep climb for a solid hour—and he doesn't drink any water. He doesn't even bring any!"

"His name is Don Wildman. He used to own the Bally fitness chain. You ought to be writing about him."

Well, I did. After my L.A. Times article came out, the emails poured in. People were turned on by Wildman, inspired by him, and embarrassed by their own laziness, their surrender to age and sloth. The theme was clear: If this old guy could work out five hours a day at his age, what in the heck is my excuse?

Role models are those who lead us by example, break barriers, push on when the going gets hard, and show us what's possible. They let nothing stand in the way of their goals, no matter their years or their physical challenges. Since Bike for Life is all about "riding to 100 and beyond," meet the "Roll Models," cyclists who keep on pedaling despite it all: 80ish UC Berkeley professor turned double-century Hall of Famer Gerd Rosenblatt; the amazing one-armed rider of La Ruta, Costa Rica's Alejandro Oporta Reyes; maybe the tallest (and most injured) bike-loving man in the world, retired NBA basketball superstar Bill Walton; my friend Russell Allen, who was the longest living member of the 1932 Olympic cycling team; the toughest, most colorful 60-plus gringo at the world's toughest mountain bike race, Heart Akerson; and, of course, the Wild Man himself, Malibu's irrepressible Don Wildman.

ROLL MODEL #1
GERD ROSENBLATT:
IT'S NEVER TOO LATE TO START

This wheel-sucking, hill-climbing professor did his first double century at age 70—then did 37 more.

The finish line of the Furnace Creek 508 is a surreal scene. Riders emerge from the darkness after 30 or 36 or 40 hours of riding 508 grueling miles north from Santa Clarita to Death Valley and back south to *the I-15, utterly wasted and relieved and grateful to have survived. Relatively fresh four-man teams coming in while it's still light often stay to celebrate the arrival of two-man teams and soloists, each progressively looking more beaten-up. In 2004, fresh and showered after a 30-hour finish with my four-man team of 40-somethings on Team Sasquatch, I was hanging out at the finish line about midnight when 71-year-old Gerd Rosenblatt, a UC Berkeley professor, came in after 36 hours, half of a two-man team with his 69-year-old partner Ron Way. 71? I was amazed—but Gerd was actually just getting started. Three years later, he and a female partner would set a mixed-team two-person record of 33:18. That was pretty impressive for a guy who didn't even do his first century until age 67, or his first double until 70.*

In the next seven years, Rosenblatt racked up 38 double-centuries—including six at age 76 in 2009— and was inducted into the California Triple Crown Hall of Fame. Slight of frame (5-foot-4 and 117 pounds) and a longtime tennis player and walker before he took up cycling, Rosenblatt always finished in the top 50 percent overall in his events, sometimes in the top 10 percent. Unfortunately, at 78 (in 2011), Rosenblatt's beloved double-century days abruptly ended with a broken pelvis—he'd been a victim of the osteoporosis that threatens all hard-core cyclists (see Chapter 9). But he's still doing centuries—on a three-wheel recumbent—and vows to do it until the very end.

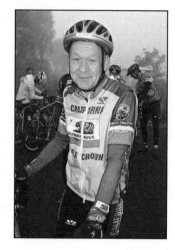

Meet California endurance legend Gerd Rosenblatt.

"Nobody older than me has ever beaten me," jokes Rosenblatt, a professor emeritus at Berkeley who taught at Penn State and worked at Los Alamos before coming west, studying high-temperature materials chemistry (how materials behave at high heat) and Raman spectroscopy (a technique using lasers that identifies molecules through their vibration and rotation). He uses that line often, because it's fun and it's true. Due to a late start, age 70, he has always been the "oldest guy" at each of his 38 double-century rides.

Rosenblatt doesn't ponder what "might have been" if he'd started cycling decades earlier. He just feels lucky that he rides at all. "It wouldn't have even happened if it wasn't for the fact that I just wanted to be able to do road rides with my wife," he said.

His wife, Susan, whom the widower Rosenblatt married in 1990 at age 57, was an enthusiast cyclist used to taking one- and two-week bike-tour vacations. But her husband, who was busy teaching classes, running his research lab, and raising his teenage son (an older daughter was long gone), didn't ride with her more than a couple of times a year on his old Peugeot 10-speed. "She'd race her bike up and down the Berkeley Hills, where we live," he said, "and I'd walk my bike up the half-mile, 14 percent incline on Centennial Drive from the office to home."

The walking changed to pedaling in April 1993, when he discovered gears. The Rosenblatts bought a pair of REI mountain bikes to go with their new vacation cabin in the Sierra foothills. "And I liked it!" he said. "I really enjoyed mountain biking—all those gears! If you believe in physics, cycling is easy: Just gear down. You can climb anything." Soon, when his son and Sue bought him a Specialized Stumpjumper dual-suspension mountain bike, he was doing just that—including conquering Centennial Drive on his sixtieth birthday later that year.

That was the start of something big. (A YouTube video, entitled "Super Gerd Rosenblatt," filmed 14 years later, shows the 74-year-old climbing 25-percent-grade Marin Avenue in the Berkeley Hills.) In 1993, Rosenblatt started racing in the 60-plus age group, taking a fourth and a sixth at the Sea Otter Classic cross-country events over the next few years. In 2000, preparing for a six-day bike tour that included a 100-mile day, Gerd and Sue did their first century ride at AdventureCORPS' Death Valley Century. They followed that with the weeklong Tour of Colorado, where he finished in the top third of the field and discovered the art of drafting.

"I found that I'm a good wheel-sucker," he recalls. "Drafting helps a lot in these long rides—especially in the wind. Especially at my size behind a big guy. You can go 17 mph drafting against the wind but only 12 mph alone."

In 2003, when he was 69, riding in the lead pack at the Wildflower Century, Rosenblatt noticed some people wearing jerseys imprinted with the words "California Triple Crown." So he inquired about what it meant.

"Wow!" I said. "Three double-centuries in a year! I needed to do that. On the drive home, Sue and I discussed it. There was a double century in Bishop in three weeks, a couple days before my seventieth birthday."

Battered by headwinds, far and away the oldest rider in the field, Rosenblatt was tired and sore when he finished. "But I finished mid-pack," he said. "And everyone was so nice—that's what got me hooked."

Having done a lot of sailboard racing in San Francisco Bay, Rosenblatt was used to amped-up competitors cussing and screaming at one another. "But at the doubles, it feels like everybody's on the same team helping each other," he said. "You draft. You wait at the rest stops when it gets dark and ride in together. You get a personal challenge and camaraderie that helps you push yourself."

So Rosenblatt kept pushing. During the next seven years, he collected five of the cherished Triple Crown jerseys, ultimately accumulating

38 double-centuries by 2010. He did 19 different doubles. "I did each of the hardest rides on Chuck Bramwell's list—the Terrible Two, Devil Mountain, Mulholland, you name it," he said. But after 2010, there were no more.

Because at age 77 came the accident: a 1 mile-per-hour fall in his driveway that shattered the professor's pelvis in a dozen places and left him immobile for 10 weeks.

The fractures occurred because Rosenblatt had severe osteoporosis, a major risk factor of endurance cycling, which was first discovered by researcher Jeanne Nichols in 2003. Rosenblatt, informed of her findings, reasoned that the bone loss came from his long hours of sweating while riding. (Lack of impact, another cycling-related bone-thinner, probably affected him less due to his history of playing tennis and walking.)

Today, Rosenblatt takes vitamin D and calcium every day and gets two infusions of Fosamax every year. He added upper-body barbell exercises to his lifelong morning calisthenics routine of jumping jacks, sit-ups, and running in place. And he's back on wheels—but not a bike.

A trike.

"I got conflicting advice from the physicians," he explained. "Some said, 'Get back on the bike,' but an endocrinologist said, 'If you fall and break your hip again, you will die.' So I switched to a recumbent trike in January 2011—a $3,000 Catrike 700.

"It's risk management. The statistics show that you crash once every three years on a bike while cycling at a reasonable speed riding 6,000 to 10,000 miles per year."

The trike has slowed Rosenblatt's speed by about 25 percent, and changed him from a very fast climber to the slowest climber in the group. He notes other downsides to the trike: You need two different-sized spare tubes, it doesn't fold well, so no more European travel, no more mountain biking. But that hasn't stopped him. He still does centuries. He's even done Lon Haldeman's 18-day PAC Tour on Route 66 from

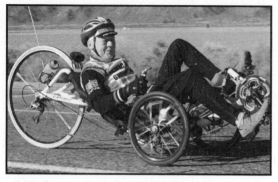

Rosenblatt's osteoporosis led him to a trike.

Santa Monica to Texas three times on three wheels, versus twice on two wheels.

"The trike hasn't diminished my love for cycling. It's actually fun, like being in a human-powered go-kart," he said.

"I love cycling and hiking because they defer the toils of time. They let you do the same things you could do when you were younger. If you stay active, it doesn't feel much different. And that's the key to being happy."

ROLL MODEL #2:
ALEJANDRO OPORTA REYES:
DON'T LET A DISABILITY STOP YOU

**Meet La Ruta's amazing one-armed rider—
and his one-leg fork.**

Blood, broken bones, carnage. The legendary descent down the back side of the Irazu volcano at the La Ruta de los Conquistadores stage race is always dangerous—rainy, freezing, and out-of-your-mind j-j-j-jarring, a 20-mile, 4,000-foot drop down a road made entirely of mud-slathered rocks. For those without good technical bike-handling skills, it takes forever. Even with skills, you work so hard to stay upright and balanced through the bumpy minefield that your body feels rattled and drained to the core—as if you'd been blasting your arms, shoulders, and back in the weight room all day and then been caught in an endless earthquake.

That's why, in 2011, after working my way through the most treacherous part of this crazy descent, then stopping to catch a breath and shake out my

braking-fatigued hands, I did a double take. A tiny, jacketless rider appeared out of the mist with his right jersey sleeve blowing in the wind. He was holding his handlebar with only one hand. Amazingly, this man, who I found out later was on his way to completing his fifth La Ruta, did not have a right arm.

I was dumbfounded. How in the world does a one-armed man balance, shift gears, and brake on flat ground, much less survive one of the most epic downhills in the mountain bike world?

In 2003, construction worker Alejandro Oporta Reyes, then 39, had his arm crushed so badly in a traffic accident that doctors amputated it all the way to the shoulder. That might be traumatic for most people, but Oporta stayed remarkably calm in the days and decade afterward. Because the way he figures it, he gained a lot more than he lost.

"First, I thanked God that I was alive," he said, through an interpreter. "Then I decided to keep doing what I had always done: Challenge myself."

Unmarried and childless, the 5-foot-4 Oporta had once worked as a cowboy and often did bull riding for fun at "Turno" rodeo parties with his

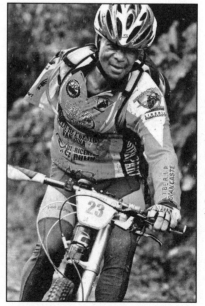

Alejandro Oporta Reyes has done the world's hardest mountain bike race—with one arm—five times.

friends. Now, with one arm, he found that he could easily keep playing soccer. And when his friends Victor and Alberto Meches wanted to ride the two-day, 180-kilometer (112-mile) Lake Arenal bike race a few months after his accident, the one-armed man did not hesitate. He grabbed his old Trek 4300 sitting in the garage. It had been modified so that the front and rear brakes could be actuated from the left grip.

"All the other racers were wondering how I was going to shift gears. It wasn't easy; you have to do it like this," he pantomimed, darting his hand two feet across an imaginary handlebar to an invisible right-hand gear shifter. "It's a challenge, but I'd gotten good at moving my hand fast while riding that bike to the market every day."

Riding in the beginner class at the Arenal race, Oporta was surprised to find that he was fast. Limiting his gear-shifting when he could, he did not crash, and finished in the top third of the pack. He yearned to do more.

A couple years later, atop the same Trek, Oporta did *way* more: the Guanaride, a 450-kilometer (280-mile), five-day stage race in the northern coastal provinces of Guanacaste and Puntarenas. It featured climbs, descents, long flat plains, and river crossings through beaches, rainforest, and the famous "Dry Forest."

When Oporta finished without incident, he naturally set his sights on Cost Rica's ultimate challenge: the granddaddy of mountain bike stage races, the world's most feared off-road event, La Ruta de los Conquistadores.

He trained for two years for the 2006 La Ruta. "I gave it my best shot, but I did not finish any of the three days," he said, without shame. "The stages were too long, too steep, too grueling, too technical. I had to walk too much. But that just made me more determined to come back stronger."

In 2008, Oporta rejoiced when he finished the longer, more grueling *four-day* La Ruta. And then, unexpectedly, the one-armed man retired the old Trek for something that would take him to a new level, a machine custom-matched to his riding style, his sensibility, and his body: a one-legged bike.

Guardian Angels

"He did this amazing thing—and his bike is a piece of junk. We have to do something."

It was 2007. Brecht Heuchan, a Tallahassee, Florida, lobbyist and mountain biker, then 37, had just finished reading an article in *Dirt Rag* magazine authored by writer-photographer Manuel Maqueda. It was about Oporta.

"I was so touched," said Heuchan. "Alejandro had an impact on me—on everyone. What drew me to him was less about his bike-riding skill—which is amazing—but the effect that he has on other people. The way he's content in his own life, the way he talks, like the way he thanked his sponsors, 'Banco Nacional and God Almighty.' He's a special person, a legend in Costa Rica, but he's mild mannered, not beating his chest, kind of shy."

"I dream of having a lighter bike someday," said Oporta in the article. "Maybe a Cannondale, because I am, too, a lefty"—a reference to Cannondale's signature one-legged suspension fork.

Heuchan was galvanized. "Long story short, it got put on my heart to do something," he said. "So I called my lobbyist buddies, all mountain bikers and good-hearted people, and said, 'Wouldn't it be cool if we could help this man out?'"

His friend Mike Harrell offered to lead the financing effort. Then Heuchan made his pitch to Todd May, owner of the Higher Ground bike shop, a Cannondale dealership that sits at the highest point in Florida, 222 feet above sea level.

"I told Cannondale the story," said May, "and we all pitched in and built him this kinda cool custom bike."

The team first called La Ruta founder Roman Urbina to get Oporta's dimensions. Within a couple weeks, the factory sent a beautiful black

2008 Cannondale Rush Carbon Team dual-suspension bike with a 110-mm Lefty fork, 100-mm Fox PR3 in the rear, Mavic Crossmax SLR wheelset, Hope superlite disc brakes, Shimano XTR drivetrain, and Cannondale Hollowgram Si crankset, all weighing in at 10.2 kilograms. Retail price: $6,899. It was Cannondale's top-of-the line marathon bike, specifically designed for events such as La Ruta.

Reviewers, including the BikeRadar website, had called this model "quite possibly the best single-pivot cross-country/marathon bike ever," its 4.3 inches of suspension travel said to be perfect for all-day riding and its featherweight 22.5 pounds perfect for long, sustained climbing. Most important, of course, was the Lefty fork, a perfect complement to Oporta's left arm.

May's first step was trying to figure out how to move all the controls to the left side of the Rush's carbon-fiber handlebar. That was not a major problem for a man who runs a high-end bike shop with a reputation for building special-needs machines for amputees.

"It was trial and error," May said. "We cobbled together various brake and shift levers, turned 'em upside down and backward, shortened the bar, and got it tested in 15 or 20 hours."

"Then," said Harrell, "with it all built and paid for [between $3,500 and $4,000, based on dealer wholesale costs and labor], we put it in a box with a helmet and a Higher Ground jersey, crossed our fingers, and sent it off."

The fingers were crossed because the guardian angels didn't know if the bike, meant to be a surprise to Oporta, would get through customs in time for the 2008 race—or would get stolen, since no one knew when to expect it. In fact, when Heuchan saw Oporta at the start of La Ruta on Day 1, he was riding his old Trek. Customs still had the bike, requiring $700 in taxes to release it to La Ruta personnel. It took several weeks to authorize the expense.

The customized bike finally cleared Costa Rican customs the morning of La Ruta's last day—then was rushed to the Caribbean port of Limón, where the race ends at a giant beach party.

The Cannondale was presented to a surprised and overjoyed Oporta at the finish line. He picked it up with his only hand and rejoiced the way any hard-core rider would: "It's so light!" It was more than 10 pounds lighter than his 15-kilo Trek.

Heuchan would have loved to have seen the presentation. "By the time I finished, they'd already called Alejandro up on stage and given him the bike," he said. "He finished ahead of me. At least I got a picture of him and me. He had no idea who I was. Finally, after a while, I mentioned how we put it all together for him and gave him my email. He was beyond grateful."

Poetry in Motion

Heuchan's only La Ruta was the "single hardest thing I've ever done," he said, adding that his two Ironman triathlon finishes "didn't come close." Of all the things that stand out about the 2008 La Ruta for him, nothing topped the descent off the Irazu volcano.

But not his own descent.

At several points, Heuchan stood absolutely transfixed as he watched Oporta make his way down the rock-strewn mountain road. "I was astounded by his technical skills," he said. "Trashed bodies were being carted off the mountain bleeding and broken—and they all had two arms. And he comes out without a scratch!"

Oporta must get off the bike to handle the roughest stuff, and, of course, cannot stand out of the saddle. "While climbing," said Heuchan, "he looks like a sewing machine—precise up-and-down leg movements, with the upper body super-still and quiet. Descending, his balance is exact and perfect to watch. Dismounting, he's so smooth getting on and off the bike that it resembles getting out of a chair. It's poetry in motion.

"If he had his second arm, could he be more efficient? It doesn't look like it."

Beyond form, Heuchan was struck by how Oporta seemed to embody the concept of *pura* vida—"Pure Life," the national slogan of Costa Rica, which alludes to an intrinsic enjoyment of the moment. "One thing you can't miss is how happy he looks riding a bike. Other people are out there suffering—and you can see it in their faces and on their bodies, with heads and shoulders drooping and everything looking bad as they labor. But he holds his proud form, and radiates a pure joy.

"When you see people like that, you can't not be inspired. You think, 'Here I am, able-bodied and wasted. I want some of his energy'—because he's giving off tons of it."

When you ask Oporta about the loss of his right arm, he evinces no sign of regret or self-pity. "Psychologically, I wasn't really affected," he said. "I just thought of it as another one of the normal troubles you run into in life, and you have to move on." In fact, given all that happened, he's hard-pressed to find a downside.

Oporta certainly doesn't blame his missing arm for the crashes that left him with a broken leg in 2009 and a broken jaw in 2010, the latter causing him to miss La Ruta that year. After all, if he still had his right arm, he might not even be a cyclist. He would not be inspiring people wherever he rides. And he certainly would not own his beloved, one-of-a-kind, one-legged, one-handled Cannondale Rush, on which he has finished another four Guanarides and three La Rutas.

Living off a small government disability pension, Oporta said he has only one simple goal in mind for the future: "Keep on riding."

As he does, he'll keep touching people like Heuchan. "He's just out there doing his thing," he said, "and making the world a better place by doing it."

ROLL MODEL #3
BILL WALTON: CYCLING'S BIGGEST FAN

With a love of cycling and a broken body, the 6-foot-11 NBA Hall of Famer sees his 72.4 cm custom road bike as his wheelchair, his gym, and his church.

On the afternoon of April 17, 2010, hanging out at the finish-line area of the Mt. Laguna Classic, a challenging century ride that climbs the highest point in San Diego County three times for a total elevation gain of 10,200 feet, I see a very tall rider on a gigantic custom bike come in. He's exceedingly happy, grinning from ear to ear, his massive white teeth beaming like a searchlight. He'd completed the first two loops—77 miles with 7,700 feet of elevation gain—on flat pedals while wearing massive, bootlike basketball shoes. Now, done for the day, overjoyed with his accomplishment, he happily poses with normal-sized folk who instantly recognize him. I got my photo-op, too, and then, a few days later, interviewed one of America's all-time greatest athletes, 6-foot-11 NBA Hall of Famer Bill Walton, then age 58. Walton won two NBA titles—one each with the Portland Trail Blazers and Boston Celtics—and earned two NCAA titles at UCLA. He was named NBA Most Valuable Player once and College Player of the Year three times. As big as Bill is, his personality is bigger, making him a natural in front of the camera, as his two-decade run as an ABC and ESPN commentator on NBA and college telecasts attests. All the while, he's been an enthusiastic supporter and participant in Southern California bike events. He told me about his lifelong passion for the sport, how it helped keep him out of the doghouse with his college coach John Wooden, the relentless injuries that brought him to the point of despair, and the joy of cycling that brought him back.

Q: Bill, why were you so happy at Mt. Laguna the other day?

This was my comeback ride after my back surgery, and I didn't know if I could ride something like that again. Cycling's a huge part of my life; I ride everywhere, every day if I can. I've been doing all-day rides since I went to UCLA—doing centuries before we called 'em centuries. I did the Rosarito-Ensenada and Tecate-Ensenada rides in Baja for years, and the Death Valley Century every year starting in 2005, until the operation in 2009.

Q: During your NBA career, did you manage to get in any riding during the season?

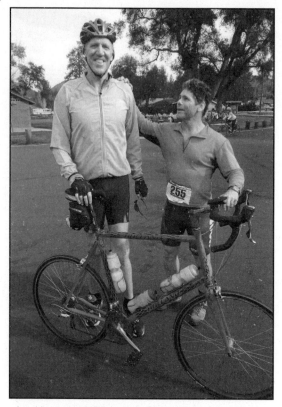

Looking up to NBA legend Bill Walton, at the 2010 Mt. Laguna Classic in San Diego County.

I rode wherever I played—Portland, San Diego, and in Cambridge, with the Boston Celtics. With the Trail Blazers, when weather permitted, I'd ride my bike to the games; I just lived a couple miles from the Coliseum. Funny story: When we won the NBA championship in 1977, I rode down to the parade. The starting point was jammed like the parking lot at a Grateful Dead concert [he's a huge fan, with a Dead skull painted on his headtube], and I immediately got separated from my bike. It was just gone. After the parade was over, I announced over the PA system, "Will the guy who has my bike please bring it back, so I can get home?" And I got it back.

Q: In 1985, you cowrote a book on bikes, Bill Walton's Total Book of Bicycling—*still on Amazon .com. When did the love affair with cycling start?*

When I could walk. As kids in San Diego, we'd buy bikes for $5 at police auctions, fix 'em up and ride 'em all over town. At UCLA, my bike got me to class fast, without being noticed. I joined group rides on the Westside and at the Encino Velodrome, even rode with [three-time Olympian] John Howard, one of my heroes. One summer at Sonoma State, I'd ride every day in Napa, Marin, and Sonoma after classes for 8 hours— from 1 to 9 p.m. I love the freedom, the motion, the gliding, the adventure, the environmentalism—there's an endless list of positive reasons why I ride my bike. And it's my time to be with myself.

Q: What do you mean?

My greatest inspirations and creativity come in the weight room, where I am regularly, or on my bike, where I wish I was all the time. In that space of freedom and imagination, you have the time and ability to organize your dreams beyond the tight boundaries of your normal life. When I come back from my rides, my wife, Lori, always has to remind me, "Bill, don't forget: I wasn't part of that 6-hour conversation that you just had with yourself."

Q: Was finding a bike to fit you a problem?

When I got my first 10-speed, I always had an extra-tall seatpost. It'd be like a foot above the handlebars. I finally got a custom frame in the early '80s, and now have a beautiful bike from [custom builder] Bill Holland.

Q: At UCLA, didn't your bike once help keep you out of the doghouse with your coach, the legendary John Wooden?

I fought Coach Wooden on every issue, every subject: dress code, hair length, facial hair, social issues, economics, Vietnam. He had a rule that hair could not touch the ears and you had to be clean-shaven every day. So when I showed up for the first day of practice my senior year with one day of invisible beard and hair just touching my ears, he said I couldn't practice. Of course, I argued. He said, "Bill, you may be the two-time college player of the year and an academic

All-American, and I deeply admire your principles. But we will miss you." Fortunately, I always rode everywhere and kept my bike right in the locker room. I rode as fast as I could down to Westwood, jumped in a barber's chair, grabbed a plastic razor, and raced back up on my bike right into Pauley Pavilion. I parked it on the side of the court, then stood at the end of the line, hoping that he wouldn't notice that I was late.

Q: *You're the only NBA Hall of Famer who missed more games due to injuries than you actually played. When you packed up after Mt. Laguna, I noticed the handicapped sign on your van.*

I have three bone fusions—both ankles and my spine, which has a titanium rod in it. So I have limited motion, but at least the fusions have enabled me to get back in the game of life. There are three athletic things I can do: I'm in the weight room, I'm in the pool, and I'm on my bike as much as I can. I'm not unique in that those are really the sports at the end of the line for everybody. But they are also sports of choice. These days, my bike acts as my wheelchair, my gym, my church, all in one. I live to ride, and ride to live. Always, my first question to the doctor is: Will I still be able to ride my bike?

ROLL MODEL #4
RUSSELL ALLEN: HOW TO RIDE TO 99
Take a look back at the well-lived life of America's oldest Olympic cyclist and a long-forgotten pro-cycling world.

When I first met 1932 Olympic cyclist Russell Allen in September 2005, he was going non-stop. Two or three times a week, he rode his bike on the beach bike path. Other days, he'd hit the card clubs in Gardena for a couple hours of Texas Hold 'Em, stop at the gym for an hour of weights and a Spin class, then rush home to cook dinner for his daughter Susan, with whom he lived in the Topanga Canyon section of Los Angeles. Not bad for 92.

When Audrey Adler, his Spin instructor at the Spectrum Gym in Santa Monica, told Allen that John Sinibaldi, one of his teammates on the '32 US team,

was still alive in Florida, he whipped out his checkbook and said, "When do we go?" The three of us flew east in mid-December. Allen and Sinibaldi had been 19 when they'd last seen one another 73 years before, but it was like no time had passed when they met. They were inseparable throughout the "Ride with the Legend" weekend organized by Sinibaldi's son, which drew 500 people from 14 states.

With Sinibaldi's death just three weeks later, Allen became America's longest living Olympic cyclist. A professional six-day racer in the 1930s, he'd married at 28, had three kids, then didn't ride again until he retired at 62, making up for lost time with regular 60-mile group rides into his early 80s. He led large groups of kids to venues at the 1984 Olympic Games, at 91 set a Guinness World Record by becoming the oldest person to bungee jump off the famed Queenstown, New Zealand, bridge that started the sport, and still had serious power in his legs at 93, when we rode a tandem together at the 2006 LA Marathon bike ride. Classy and handsome until the end, Allen led a remarkably rich life, with every goal seemingly accomplished except one: riding to 100, which he missed by one birthday.

How did he account for his remarkably fit and healthy longevity? "Even when I stopped riding for years, I never stopped working out," said Allen.

Born in 1913, Allen was the middle child of three raised in Huntington Park, near East Los Angeles, by a single mother. His father, an alcoholic, shot himself. Allen got his first racing bike at 13 and was soon riding with the prestigious Krebbs Cycle Club of Long Beach. A prodigious sprinter, "Legs," as he was nicknamed, won a spot on the US Olympic cycling team and raced the four-man pursuit event on a wooden track built inside the Rose Bowl.

"We lost the first race against Italy, the eventual winners, and that was it for us," he said. "But we had lots of fun going to all the events. I met the great Finnish track runner Paavo Nurmi [who won nine gold medals in three Olympic Games in the 1920s]. I shook hands

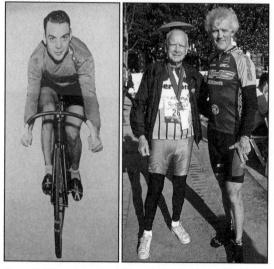

Russell Allen was age 19 when he competed in the 1932 Olympics.

Allen, 93, and John Howard at the 2006 LA Marathon bike ride.

knew a lot of girls. We had a ball there. Then we went on to New York."

Soon, Allen was racing twice a week at the outdoor track in Nutley, New Jersey, winning enough to move into a New Jersey boarding-house that charged $10 a week. The goal was to do the six-day races (which involved two-man tag-team riding non-stop) in Madison Square Garden. "Sometimes I made money at Nutley, sometimes not," said Allen. "There were a lotta good riders back there, and getting into the six-day races in the Garden was tough. I trained 100 miles a day on the road to be ready." Within a month, Allen was competing in the Garden.

The six-day races started with 15 teams of two riders, half of them from Europe—usually French and Germans, said Allen. Teammates alternated for six straight days. "The field often declared a truce for a couple hours in the early morning and you'd ride on the flat with handlebars up as your partner slept; nobody could gain in that time," he recalled. "You had little covered bunks around the track where you could get three, four hours of sleep from 2 or 3 in the morning to 2 in the afternoon, when the crowd started coming. Starting at 5, we'd have dinner."

Two or three thousand fans would show up. Admission was only 25 cents, box seats a dollar. The show featured motor-paced team races.

"I never won a six-day race," said Allen, "but came close with different partners; my first, Dave Lans of New York, crashed on the third day. So I teamed up with his old teammate."

Drugs were already part of cycling, he recalled, "although back then we didn't give a thought to what our trainers were giving us. On the last day of a six-day race, last two or three hours, they usually had some sort of pep-me-up drink—and you'd drink it. Stimulants, cocaine, we had no idea what was in there. But it was something."

As always, the money made it worth it. "The minimum pay was $125 a day—a fortune in the

with Jim Thorpe and Johnny Weissmuller, and the great Hawaiian swimmer-surfer Duke Kahanamoku. Met quite a few celebrities, too. Later on, in a six-day race in Hollywood, I met Clark Gable."

After the Olympics, a wild decade of professional racing all over the globe ensued for Allen. In 1933, after a winter season of six-day races at Gilmore Stadium in Hollywood, just in back of the Farmers Market (still an L.A. landmark today), he headed for the big time. "We knew where the money was—in New York and New Jersey," he said. Allen's pattern for the next five years became heading east in the summer, then to South America in the winter.

"A lot of teams from the East had come west to the 1933 winter races in L.A. and San Francisco, and I made friends with a French rider named Felix La Fonette," Allen recalled. "He had a car. He said, 'Russell, you come back to New York with me. My mom and dad have a place at 59th and Broadway, with a spare bedroom. Won't cost anything to live with us.' So we drove all the way on Route 66. In Cleveland, he

Depression," Allen said. "But you had to pay your trainer and your own meals, so you'd end up keeping $600 out of $750 [for the six days]. Some of the Europeans got $200 to $300 a day. The organizers up you [raise your rate] every time you ride.

"It was a lot of money, especially considering that you could take a girl to dinner and the movies for a buck, but it goes fast," he said. "Sometimes I flew between L.A. and New York. Sometimes I took the sleeper train. It was the good life."

Of course, that included women.

"I had lots of girls; we had 'em just like any athletes," said Allen. He noted that cycling wasn't as popular as baseball back then, but neither was basketball or football. Even so, baseball players weren't making that much—Mickey Mantle was making $5,000 to $6,000 a year at first.

Living *la dolce vita*, Allen didn't have any regrets over not being able to go to the 1936 Olympics in Berlin. "I was a professional. I got a letter at home from [then–US Olympic committee chairman] Avery Brundage; boy, he was tough. You sneeze, and he'd throw you off the team. There was a woman backstroker who was caught taking a drink of champagne on the ship to Germany, and they threw her off.

"I was actually on board the ship the day of the night that the US athletes sailed for Germany. I knew a lot of 'em, wished 'em luck, and went back to my place in New Jersey."

Allen kept the life going—New York in the summer and South America in the winter—until late '38, when war broke out in Europe. "When Hitler started gobbling up all those nations, the Europeans couldn't come over here anymore. That was the end of my cycling. Some riders continued for a few years—but I didn't."

In 1941, at age 28, relatively late for that era, Allen married a neighborhood girl who had gone to grammar school with him, wooing her on a tandem he bought when he was making a lot of money. "Rose was the only girlfriend I had—and I had plenty—who never saw me race in New York, San Francisco, anywhere. But she was a good rider. We went everywhere."

When Allen volunteered for the navy in 1943, he found that his cycling background kept him out of harm's way. Assigned to the Tooney School of Athletics in Bainbridge, Maryland, as an athletics instructor, he led marching and exercise drills. He was then shipped to Coral Gables, Florida, to teach swimming and survival skills to naval gunners. "We'd show them how to take your long-sleeve dungaree shirt, tie a knot in the bottom, wet it, and scoop air, so it's just like water wings. You're safe for hours. When it's dry, you wet it and scoop it up again."

Over the next 30 years, Allen worked for a time as a Chevrolet and Cadillac sales manager before eventually becoming a full-time professional gambler, a fact he successfully hid from his family—"although we did wonder why he always had a quick supply of $100 bills on him," said his daughter Susan. He played golf at Los Coyotes Country Club near his Buena Park home, and never rode at all—although he used an exercise bike and lifted weights two or three days a week at a health club.

At his wife's urging, he saddled up again after he retired at 62. "Rose still worked, and I had the time," Allen said. "I joined a club and ramped up the miles. In my 80s, we'd ride down the San Gabriel River to Seal Beach and as far down as Laguna and back." He qualified for the Masters nationals year after year until his late 80s, when he gave up competition for good.

A widower at age 87 after 59 years of marriage, Allen could still crank it up to 20 mph on the bike path at 92, when I met him in 2005. He credited his lifelong gambling and exercise addictions, plus a good diet, for keeping his mind and body sharp.

"I've never really been sick—just a two-day cold every few years—and a lot of that is because

I've eaten well all my life," he said. "My mom used to make salads for the market, and she threw away the frying pan; we always baked or broiled, and had tons of vegetables, pickles, you name it. I kept those habits. Oh, I ate fast food. But as a rule, I took care of myself." A single evening cocktail was his only vice (not counting the gambling).

Although Allen's card playing constantly exposed him to secondhand smoke, with no apparent ill effects (he's a non-smoker), he figured the gambling was a big plus for longevity.

"It's important to stay in circulation, to get away from the TV, and, as you get older, to pal around with younger people," he said. "My wife and I always became friends with our children's friends—and stayed close with our kids."

Besides his safe assignment in World War II, Allen derived many benefits from his Olympic connection over the years. In 1984, he carried the Olympic flame for a mile in the torch relay in Los Angeles, rode on a float at Disneyland, and received passes to every event at the Games. He was delighted to visit Sinibaldi in 2005, meet fellow Olympic cyclist John Howard in 2006, and be the guest presenter of the 2006 Competitor Cyclist of the Year award to soon-to-be-deposed Tour de France winner Floyd Landis, in 2007.

In his last decade, Allen lived with all three of his kids—at their invitation—and visited them often. He went bungee jumping once a year with his youngest daughter, who lives in New Zealand; at 91 set a record as the world's oldest bungee jumper; and at 92 spent three weeks traveling around the Middle East with one of his daughter's friends from college. Right after his ninety-ninth birthday in 2013, just as he was about to fly to New Zealand to see his daughter and reclaim the title of world's oldest bungee jumper, he died.

"The smartest health decision you can make is to educate your kids," Allen often said, noting proudly that all three of his, as well as his wife, graduated from UCLA. "They'll return the favor down the road."

ROLL MODEL #5:
HEART AKERSON: FINISH OR DIE

Failure is no option for the shirtless, longhaired La Ruta legend, who completed 14 consecutive editions of the world's toughest mountain bike race.

"My god! A homeless guy with hair down to his ass and no clothes on a mountain bike! All I could think was, 'Is he racing or going to work or escaping from an insane asylum?'"
—Rich White, Big Bear, California, at La Ruta de los Conquistadores, 2005

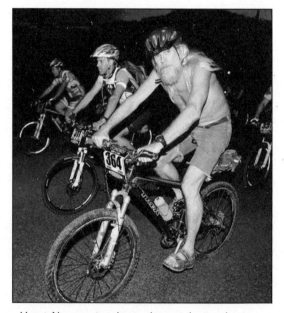

Heart Akerson, toughest gringo at the toughest mountain bike stage race.

Appearances notwithstanding, Heart Akerson is not homeless or insane. Just the opposite. A 63-year-old (in 2013) father of 9 and grandfather of 12, with a foot-long Father Time beard, white hair past his shoulders, cut-off jeans, and no shirt, he's a wealthy businessman and trained physicist. He invents medical products and runs an alternative energy company he said will revolutionize electric power, all from a sprawling Costa Rican oceanfront estate where engineers and programmers come to work and family members have been known to walk around naked.

And athletically, Heart's a warrior.

It was 1998 when Heart first lined up at the start of La Ruta de los Conquistadores, a three-day, 200-mile crossing of Costa Rica from the Pacific to the Atlantic by mountain bike that is so hard that 50 percent of all competitors, most of them around half his age, don't finish. The ordeal involves slogging through a sweltering jungle rainforest under the blazing equatorial sun, through endless lakes of thigh-deep mud, over dilapidated half-mile-long railroad bridges, and up a storm-lashed 10,000-foot volcano drenched in hypothermic freezing rain.

In this event of mind-boggling difficulty and unpredictability, Heart established an enviable record that no other American has surpassed: He completed the race for 14 consecutive years, finishing every stage of every race he started, usually in the middle of the pack.

Heart's La Ruta streak ended in 2012 after Day 1—but not because he missed a time cutoff. As strong as ever, he withdrew in protest from the race when his son Rom, a pro rider who finished third that day, was disqualified for illegally accepting a water bottle from a spectator on the course. Heart vowed never to do La Ruta again unless the race organization gave him and his family an apology.

In his seventh decade, Heart Akerson arguably remains the toughest gringo to ride what may be the world's toughest mountain bike race. And he has always done it in no shirt, cut-off jeans, and sandals.

🚲

"I thought he was a hermit, a crazy person. He reminded me of the Governor, a recurring character in Carl Hiasson's books, who was once the governor of Florida but now lives in the Everglades swamps, subsisting on snakes and roadkill." —Peter Dollard, Kennebunkport, Maine, at La Ruta, 2011

Heart was not the countercultural love child of reefer-smoking beatniks. Just the opposite. Born in Maine, the offspring of a homemaker and a Honeywell computer salesman, and raised in country-club estates all over the United States, he was a brilliant student and a classically trained pianist. Throughout junior high and high school, he wanted to be a nuclear physicist after reading about the Manhattan Project, but that changed when he was at the Virginia Polytechnic Institute in the turbulent era of Vietnam. With protests all around, it was "a very active time to think," he said. By his 1972 graduation with a bachelor's degree in theoretical physics, Heart had hair down his back and played keyboard, drums, and guitar for Andromeda, a hard-core rock band that sang against nukes. "It was heavy metal—even through that genre didn't officially exist yet," said Heart. "Me and the engineers and computer science guys in the group interpreted it as literally being against heavy metals that were destroying the earth: uranium and plutonium."

Surviving on his savings from music gigs and his Mr. Fixit mechanical skills, Heart traveled for a year in India and the Himalayas after college, sailed a boat around South America, then breezed through the PhD program at the Institute of Theoretical Science at the University of Oregon. Yet even with corporate America beckoning, he moved south to a primitive hippie commune near Ashland, Oregon, where he wore a buckskin loincloth, grew his own crops, and cooked over an open fire for three years. After fathering two daughters with a commune resident named Honey, he built a 41-foot, ocean-worthy trimaran and led his family and several others on an open-ended sailing adventure up and down the coast to South America.

One radical shift after another had taken Heart worlds away from his conservative upbringing. "The shift is what makes life interesting," he said. "The black and white instead of the gray, the waves instead of the calm."

Three more children were born in the next few years as the Akersons sailed the Pacific and returned during part of the year to Seattle, where Heart made good money selling solar panels. Dissatisfied with the transverters that convert solar energy to usable electric power, he founded a company to do it better called Heart Interface.

During numerous sailing trips down south over the succeeding years, he and Honey fell in love with a pristine ocean bluff on Tambor Bay at the end of Costa Rica's Nacoya peninsula. When he sold his company, he and Honey bought 240 acres of land there, determined to nurture their growing brood in a natural state unencumbered by clothing and societal expectations.

"When I saw him, I thought, 'Here's some expatriate who's been living in the jungle for 20 years like one of those Japanese soldiers in the Philippines still fighting World War II. And he's going to do a race that I trained six months for?'" —Robert Forster, Santa Monica, California, at La Ruta, 1998

Although Heart hadn't participated in any athletics since his days on the high-school football team, he had ridden a bike 20 miles a day to and from his grad-school classes. That's why he was not intimidated when a close friend challenged him to do the 1988 Ironman Canada, a day's drive from Seattle.

"It damn near killed me," said Heart. "I froze because I had no wetsuit for the swim. I rode a Huffy that was way too small for my body. The announcer thought it was a joke—me running in cutoffs, barefoot. But I did it the way I was comfortable."

Heart had started going barefoot back in college and taught classes shoeless at the University of Oregon. "I learned long ago that taking your shoes off in a temple was a sign of respect," he said. "As I traveled, I began to have a hard time determining boundaries. As far as I can tell now, the whole world is a temple."

Being shoeless (and shirtless and shaveless) for years toughened more than Heart's soles. "It actually puts pressure on you to be good," he said. "You can't relax; you gotta get it together. People see someone like me and look for weaknesses, something to criticize. But they'll tolerate you if you have a great idea or perform an impressive sporting feat." Like technology that'll halve their electric bill—or the ability to finish an Ironman. Heart ultimately did four straight Ironman Canadas, taking an hour off his time each year.

Heart thrived on being different. "It's like the [Johnny Cash] song, 'A Boy Named Sue,'" he said. "At first the boy cursed his dad for naming him Sue, then after a while he liked it; it made him tough."

After Heart moved to Costa Rica, it was only a matter of time before he heard about the toughest event in the neighborhood: La Ruta.

Ironically, riding a bike—and walking through airport customs—was one of the rare times that Heart actually wore shoes. Being a high-tech aficionado, he was drawn to the sleek, carbon-fiber frame of the radical (for 1994) Trek-Y22 dual-suspension mountain bike when he decided to buy bikes for his kids. When his fellow American-expatriate neighbor and buddy Nat Grew, a wealthy cattle rancher and marathon runner in his 60s, told Heart about La Ruta in 1998, Heart upgraded his components, bought a pair of Shimano SPD clipless-pedal sandals, and started training.

"I saw Heart for the first time on the breakfast of the second day, the climb up the Irazu volcano. 'Is there something wrong with him?' I thought. This is not for real. He had no shirt. I had two layers and a rain jacket. That year it was freezing. Eventually, halfway through the day, he put on a plastic trash bag. I talked to him later. Very nice guy. He has thick skin,

like a turtle. It has to be, to take that punishment. Back in the day, I was naïve, I didn't really know what hard-core was. Now I do. Heart's one of my heroes." —David Gomez, Miami, Florida, at La Ruta, 2000

People normally train for months, sometimes half a year, for La Ruta. For his first race in 1998, and all those that have followed, Heart trained only once a week.

"Hey, I'm extremely busy," he said. "But all my family is very fit just from our normal lifestyle, from walking around our huge piece of property. We can drop what we're doing and run and swim until we fall asleep. We always ate wholesome organic food prepared from scratch. My wife coordinates the biggest weekly organic produce market in the country. My kids grew up running naked in a natural paradise—hey, my two-year-old granddaughter just ran by! So to prepare for my first La Ruta, I did the Pre-Ruta (an abbreviated version of the event the month before) to know what I was getting into. Then I did a hard 60-miler once a week."

The race wasn't a piece of cake. Heart crashed four or five times on Day 1 and was plenty tired. But quitting or slowing down was simply not an option. At age 48, he finished mid-pack.

"I take it for real," said Heart. "For me, it's finish or die."

Over the years, through endless rain and mud, hailstorms, 95-degree heat, and 100 percent humidity, Heart's 14-for-14 La Ruta streak largely proceeded free of drama. The only exception was the 2003 race.

"I don't have time to get sick—but I did get sick that year on Day 1," he said. He found himself throwing up all night, with acute diarrhea and a heavy fever.

"My wife said, 'You're not going out tomorrow for Day 2.' But I knew I had no choice. After all, I put out all this heavy rhetoric—'Finish or die'—so it's time to walk the talk. To flush the sickness out of me, I drank water all night—no food. I arrived at the start line completely empty, like I'd been fasting.

Heart lined up beside his sons Rom Kanga, Orion Orca, and Nyo Stream Falcon, who've all been doing La Ruta for years. (These sons and his other children, including Teal Oceans, Forest Bear, Zan Wolf, Silke Grasshopper, Eden Spring, and Shade Bamboo, were all born doctor-free at home in natural childbirth and named after "walking through the world with them on the first day of their lives," said Heart.) Rom, 18 in 2003, became a top Red Bull–sponsored rider who would go on to finish as high as second in La Ruta 2011. Youngest child Nyo Stream finished twenty-fifth at age 17 in the 2006 edition. When the gun sounded on Day 2 in 2003, the brothers left their father in the mist. Heart was hurting.

"It was the hardest thing I ever did—climbing 8,000 feet up Irazu on just water, not even a piece of papaya or banana, not even an electrolyte drink," said Heart. "They tried to stop me on the last two stations because I was already past the cutoff time, but I just rode right through. And I made it to the Day 2 finish line in Turrialba before the cutoff."

"We just call him 'The Hippie.' We consider him a local. He always finishes everything he starts. He just did the Chirripo [trail-running] Race with four of his five sons, was the only one barefoot for 21K up Costa Rica's tallest mountain, 15,000 feet, all rocks. We don't understand him. He makes a lot of money. So why doesn't he shave his beard? Why does he walk into our office barefooted? Why does he look like that?" —Luis Diego, La Ruta race manager, 2006

Talent and willpower have helped Heart Akerson shape his life in his own way on his own terms. Now he is gearing up for his most formidable challenge of all.

"We have a serious problem in the world now," said Heart. "It's on the verge of becoming dysfunctional—and we're running out of time. Environmental catastrophe and the vast infrastructure differences between the developed and undeveloped worlds are creating economic and political pressures that are already exploding. We need clean energy for everyone—now." After years of focusing on medical products, like a beeping intubation tube that can prevent fatal operating-room mistakes, Heart returned to the renewable energy businesses with the Heart Transverter, which builds on his previous concept of seamlessly patching solar, geothermal, fuel-cell, and wind power into the existing energy grid at no expense.

Can one man and one idea make a difference?

"You know the whole spiritual path that a lot of people work for—the all-one-god, all-one-consciousness, the spirit, fate or Jesus or whatever they want, right?" said Heart. "That's one direction to go. To me, quite a long time ago, I went the other direction—I marvel at the feeling that we are individuals. Then I use individuality or ego or whatever you want to call it as one of many tools to get things done."

Like La Ruta 14 straight times—and bigger challenges to come.

ROLL MODEL #6:
DON WILDMAN: GET YOUNGER FRIENDS

That's the key to super-fitness for this Malibu legend, weight trainer, big-wave surfer, and cyclist extraordinaire, who's faster than ever at 80.

We're 45 minutes up a forbidding Malibu dirt road that climbs 2,200 feet in 4 miles, and the Wild Man is ahead. Way ahead. Out-of-sight ahead. And my excuses begin: "I'm a mountain biker, but I've never ridden right after a grueling, two-hour, all-body weight-room workout before." "It's so hot—90 degrees and rising—that I'm literally blinded in my own sweat." "I'm bonking because I haven't eaten a thing in over three hours."

But, of course, the Wild Man hasn't eaten, either. He lifted the same weights I did, probably more. And, amazingly, he hasn't swallowed one sip of water all morning; he didn't even pack a water bottle on his bike. So at the top, when he greets me with his typical upbeat attitude—"Wow, I'm really getting strong; that's the first time I ever rode this in my middle chainring"—I look at the leathery brown face, the slightly stooped shoulders, the washboard abs and bulging biceps, and face reality: A 76-year-old man just kicked my butt.

And then: I better train harder.

Malibu resident Don Wildman, possibly one of the fittest septuagenarians on the planet, has always had that galvanizing effect on people. The founder of the company that became Bally's Total Fitness, the giant health-club chain, Wildman not only made a career out of telling people to get fit, he fit the part himself, packing his life with daily workouts and an endless parade of grand physical challenges—world-class sailing races against Ted Turner, 90 holes of golf in a day, nine Hawaii Ironman triathlons.

The activities didn't retire when he did in 1994. On one vacation, he paddled the length of the Hawaiian Islands. Every Monday, Wednesday, and Friday, he leads "The Circuit," a grueling two-hour weight workout at his gargantuan home gym that has become legendary in Malibu. He rides seven days a week and paddles three.

"I don't rest," he said.

A month after I rode with him, Wildman was racing across the country for 3,000 miles on a road bike as part of "Team Surfing USA," a four-man team competing in the 2009 Race Across America from Oceanside, California, to Annapolis, Maryland. Team Surfing, which paddled 115 miles from Malibu to the start and planned to paddle to the Statue of Liberty after the finish, used the event to raise money and awareness for several causes, including ALS (amyotrophic lateral sclerosis, or Lou Gehrig's disease; see Augies

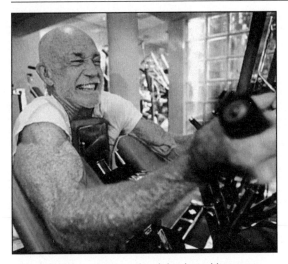

The Wild Man, convinced weights keep him young, pumps up to three days a week.

Quest.org), autism (BeautifulSon.org), and cystic fibrosis (http://sca.cff.org/pipeline2009).

This was Wildman's second RAAM, having done the race at age 60 on a 1994 team that finished second with a time of 5 days, 21 hours, and 24 minutes. In 2009, the father of three grown sons was old enough to be the dad of two of his RAAM teammates—Tim Commerford, 41, the bassist for the rock group Rage Against the Machine, and 45-year-old Laird Hamilton, the famed big-wave surfer. And he could have been a grandfather of the third, Jason Winn, 27, owner of Bonk Breaker energy bars. Their difference: a mere 49 years. (Note: Team Surfing led the 2009 RAAM into West Virginia, until it was knocked out when Jason was hit by a car.)

Back in Malibu, Wildman, Winn, and I coasted down Winding Way. In my early 50s at the time, I'd wondered if I could hang with the Wild Man after hearing those raves about him from McEnroe. With that question clearly answered, we braked at his stunning, tropical-themed, five-acre cliff-side estate and stashed our cycling gear in one of his four bike-and-Porsche-crammed garages. Then we hopped into a souped-up golf cart and took his winding

private road to his one-room beach house on the shore of Malibu's Paradise Cove. Next on the agenda: an hour of stand-up paddleboarding.

Before we wrapped up the nearly five-hour workout—a normal day for Wildman—he jumped up to a bar and reeled off 12 full-hang pull-ups, his lats flaring out like a cobra. I eked out 11; between gasps, I said, "I'll get you on these next time, Don."

"Yeah, but you better do those overhanded," he said. "You know those underhand ones are a lot easier." Of course, he's right. I need to train harder.

Some people keep very fit into their 40s and 50s. Wildman is heading full-speed into his 80s.

The Wildman Luck

Nearly six decades ago, a rail-thin, 6-foot-2 17-year-old from Burbank High muffed the kick-off in the last football game of the season. "I kicked the ball about 15 yards—then ran over and dove on it. Coach yelled out, 'Great on-side kick, Wildman.'

"A teammate looked at me and said, 'Don, you're the only guy who can fall on an outhouse and come up smelling like a rose.' They called it The Wildman Luck."

As the troublemaking, street-fighting, evolution-believing son of Pentecostal preacher Al Wildman, an acolyte of famed evangelist Aimee Semple McPherson, Don always managed to make the best of a bad situation—even when he was shipped out to the Korean War before graduation to "get me on the right track."

His first day in Korea, Wildman found himself a medic in a wiped-out convoy surrounded by dozens of dead American boys and thousands of Red Chinese soldiers pouring south across the border.

"I high-tailed it across a frozen river, certain I was going to die," he said. "I wanted to shoot myself in the foot, break my hand, anything to go home. Then I met other survivors: If they could take it, I could, too.

"When I got home, I had a reference point for the rest of my life. Nothing was as bad as Korea. If it wasn't life or death, I could deal with it."

Back in L.A. in 1953, Wildman worked construction, sold insurance, got married, and, to put some bulk on his skinny frame, began working out at a Vic Tanny gym in Burbank. He ended up running the gym for 10 years, battling the stereotypes that claimed fitness was dangerous for women, and that men with muscles were dumb—even as he built up his own.

"I tried to lead by example," he said. "Unlike these MBAs who never worked out, I had to look the part. When I started out, it was a selling business—and I was a muscle-head who totally believed he was a better salesman. I guess because my father was a minister, I naturally ended up doing the same thing: changing lives."

Wildman began preaching the fitness gospel to a much larger audience when Tanny went bankrupt in 1962. "It was the Wildman luck again—I was in the right place at the right time," he said. Creditors contacted him about taking over eight clubs in Chicago. Soon he was buying big and small chains in other cities, always careful to maintain their separate identities to avoid the system-wide scandals that plagued the fitness business. Driving traffic with ads featuring celebrities like Raquel Welch, he rode the fitness and racquetball wave to ownership of 17 nationwide chains under the umbrella of his Health and Tennis Corporation. By 1993, when he retired from running Bally's, the successor company that had bought him out a decade before, there were 400 clubs, making it the biggest health-club company in the country.

All the while, Wildman kept working out. His time crunch, and the advent of multi-station weight machines in the '60s and '70s, led him to clear messy barbells off the floor and experiment with what became known as "circuit training," the rapid movement from one exercise to another.

"I think I invented circuit training because I had to—I didn't have the time to rest. You work one muscle group, then the opposing group—and you're done in half the time." Circuit training was a huge hit—especially with women, who flooded into his clubs. Training at 6 a.m. every day, Wildman built up to 237 pounds at age 37, leaving him time to pursue his big hobby, sailboat racing.

In 1982, the morning after Wildman and his crew of 20 became the first to win all three of the Chicago Yacht Club's famous Mackinac races in one season, a *Fortune* magazine writer asked him what was next. Drunk on champagne, Wildman remembered something about a new sport he'd recently seen on TV, and blurted, "I might do that Ironman."

"That ended up in the article," he said. "Now, I had to do it. So I started running."

The Ironman Decade

In October 1982, Wildman flew to the Big Island of Hawaii with a bike, running shoes, swim goggles, and a small transistor radio. Instead of carrying a cassette player and tapes, he had rented a local radio station for the day to play his own music—the Rolling Stones, AC/DC, the Cure, The Beatles, and Talking Heads.

He finished in one minute over 12 hours, second in the 50-plus age group to Canadian Les MacDonald, who would be his rival for the next decade. Running 100 training miles a week and cycling three or four times that, Wildman leaned-out to 175 pounds. He scored his personal Ironman record of 11:23 at age 60 and finally beat MacDonald, the president of the International Triathlon Federation.

"I did the Ironman until my knees were wrecked," he said. "A surgeon told me no more running—'You've got bone on bone.' But I don't blame it all on the running; the bump skiing and the golf every morning—all that torque—helped, too."

But Wildman didn't slow down. After his last Ironman in '93, documented in an NBC profile, he moved on to his newest loves: snowboarding, windsurfing, and cycling, both road racing and mountain biking.

His Advice: Weights, Races, and Younger Friends

Today, Wildman said that his cycling is stronger than ever. "My bike speed is similar to my Ironman days—and there's a reason for that," he said. "Strength helps cardio. In the last decade, I started to try to keep my strength up. As you get older, the fall-off in strength is greater than the decline in VO$_2$ max—unless you fight it."

Wildman took his old circuit-training routines and ramped them up into what he calls "The Circuit," his now legendary two-hour blasting sessions. One wing of his estate, stocked with a couple dozen machines, free-weights, and inflatable exercise balls, looks like a condensed version of a Bally's gym.

Everything gets used.

Wildman usually doesn't work out alone. Joining us were his Team Surf teammates Commerford and Winn. Hamilton is also a frequent workout partner, along with McEnroe, 50, and Detroit Red Wings star Chris Chelios, 47, when they're in town. A pattern emerges: None of them is within a quarter-century of him.

Wildman eats healthy, takes lots of supplements, fills his radiant, *Architectural Digest*–worthy home with happy photos and paintings, and is always up for fun. The night before, he and his friends piled into a limo and went to a Lakers playoff game. But a key element to his fitness strategy clearly is finding younger friends.

"Old guys don't train anymore, so all my buddies are real young," he said. "They're more fun. They push you and you push them, and you forget how old you are."

Young friends also teach him new games. "When Laird met me in 1996, he saw that I was an aggressive snowboarder—and thought I'd make a good tow surfer," said Wildman, who often joins Hamilton on surfing and paddle-

boarding adventures in Hawaii and other big-wave hot spots.

Conversely, he got Hamilton hooked on mountain biking, an obsession since he moved to Malibu in 1983.

Of course, acting like a man 50 years younger carries some risks. In 2006, Wildman tore his rotator cuff while snowboarding in Argentina. Heliboarding six months later, he drove his left femur through the end of his tibia, shattering the latter. ("I couldn't walk on it for 12 weeks, but I could cycle with the other leg," he said.) In the winter of 2009, he broke his left femur at a right angle when his mountain bike slipped on black ice in Utah. Ten days later, he was doing chin-ups; two months later, snowboarding.

When he was surfing in Hawaii with Hamilton in September 2008, a barrel slammed Wildman into his board, puncturing his lung and breaking a rib. A month later, he won three golds and four silvers in cycling events at the World Senior Games, which he has competed in since 2004.

"Seeing high-level people your age once in a while is important," he said. "It tells you that you're normal."

If all goes as planned, there will be many more accidents and Senior Games to come, because The Wildman Luck is genetic, too. His dad lived to 88, his mom to 94. He's had no medical problems, other than an overactive thyroid 30 years ago. He rarely gets sick.

Wildman likes being a role model, but finds it ironic that he usually inspires younger people, not his chronological peers.

"When I met the Wild Man, I was in my late 30s and already starting to think slowing down was natural," said Commerford, as an excited Wildman personally serves us raspberry yogurts at his downtown Malibu yogurt shop, his latest passion. "Then we rode together, and the same thing that happened to you happened to me: I thought, 'What's my excuse? I gotta train more!'"

"People my own age say, 'It's too late for me,'" said Wildman, "but all kinds of studies show that even nursing home populations can improve with exercise. And you get the reward for it: the endorphins. So pick something that you really like doing—cycling, trampolining—and just do it.

"As a kid, you go out and play. As an adult, you want the same fun, the same excitement," he said. "So when people say to me, 'When are you going to grow up?' I always say the same thing back: 'I hope I never do.'"

I followed up with the Wild Man in October 2013. Eighty now and still sounding as buoyant as a 30-year-old, he was on his way to the Senior Games in Utah, where he again won a number of medals. Always looking forward to new adventures, he was putting together another Race Across America relay team for 2014. He was also excited about marketing his new invention: a giant motorized skateboard for golfers.

Despite two knee replacements three months earlier, Wildman said he could still leg-press 635 pounds and do 22 full-hang pull-ups. He had fallen in love with his 35-year-old nurse, a mountain biker who, he raved, was a "10."

"You look and feel 20 years younger if you lift weights and associate with younger people," he reiterated when asked for the keys to athletic longevity and success. "About 400 athletes show up at the Senior Games, and all of them except me and a Navy Seal have scrawny upper bodies. You can't let yourself get fragile.

"Because growing older is not for sissies."

INTERVIEW
Marla Streb
A PhD IN THE DOWNHILL SCIENCES

It's difficult to imagine a greater bundle of contradictions than champion downhiller Marla Streb, who prefers to take the least direct line—unlike descending—through life. Growing up in Baltimore, Maryland, she trained as a classical pianist, supported herself through college as a cocktail waitress, did her postgraduate work as a research chemist studying oysters and mussels, then discovered the joys of mountain biking in her late 20s, after doing the bike-relay leg in a local triathlon. She moved out west to La Jolla, California, in her VW microbus named "Indifference," picked up a job in a medical lab testing HIV strains in monkeys, and filled her free time exploring San Diego's sprawling network of canyons, gullies, and hills on her mountain bike.

Streb soon graduated to racing cross-country and accelerated up the amateur ranks. She looked forward to a potentially lucrative career as a pro rider, until reality in the form of a VO$_2$-max lab test suggested that genetics can't be fooled. Her coach recommended that because she could never be the fastest cross-country woman biker—her lung capacity for precious oxygen molecules was not high enough—she should rethink her role in the sport. You can't argue with data; Marla knew that from years working in the labs. So she took up downhill racing. And she became increasingly more proficient at taming gravity despite a litany of injuries. In fact,

she became celebrated for her starring role in an off-beat television commercial for VO$_2$-max energy bars in which she barreled into a tree on a downhill run. "That commercial paid for my house," Marla told Bike for Life, before she won the national championship at age 37. Her autobiography, The Life Story of a Downhill Gravity Goddess, *opens with this passage: "I used to be a normal woman with a promising career as a research scientist, but a mountain biking bug bit me, and I changed." She was interviewed in March 2004 and again in January 2014.*

I'VE ALWAYS HAD an awkward approach to everything I do, especially forming sentences. For some reason, I abhor predictability. I've broken up with boyfriends because of it. Conforming makes me uncomfortable and weak. That's why I was initially so reluctant to wear sponsors' logos all over my body and look like a "team member." I felt like a sell-out. And in that respect I'm now the Gravity Goddess of Sell-out. But if it can further what I love to do and help with this great act of nonconformity, then I have to concede.

Unlike many women, I am reluctant to get married or commit to a relationship. I often refuse to drive in a car. I'll go to great lengths to get somewhere—hitchhiking, difficult train schedules, dangerous bike routes, et cetera—just for the principle. I'll put my life in jeopardy to get there "my way."

Babies frighten me. I sought out the most broke life-partner, Mark, I could find. Guys with money turn me off. Mark doesn't have a bank account or a dime to his name—perfect! I don't smoke pot. Although I own three houses and a 50-foot sailboat, I still sleep in my VW bus or the cold floor of my garage. I prefer to sleep outside alone than stay in a comfortable house with friends.

Of course, biking is beneficial to relationships, because it's a stress reliever. I'll go out for a long, painful one after a difficult day, and I come home relaxed. It is a problem though if a couple tries to ride together and they have different riding philosophies. My boyfriend and I will fight bitterly, so we don't go on "rides" together anymore. Just happy, slow commuting after I've already trained that day.

My pride or insecurity is my motivation. I go out on a massive cross-country ride with no food or water and get dreadfully lost and bonk terribly, eventually finding my way back home in the dark. Then I feel much better. If I am ever feeling apathetic, which can happen after 11 years of racing, I don't try to force an aggressive feeling. I just enjoy the moment of being able/paid to ride my bike in the woods on a weekday at a beautiful mountain resort. Then something always kicks in when that start beep goes off and the throttle always opens. Usually a more relaxed downhiller is a faster one. But some people perform better if they think of their competition as the enemy. They think of something that pisses them off. It always worked for [wildman downhiller] Shaun Palmer.

Breaking Ground—and Bones

I HAVE HAD my share of injuries. I've broken my right collarbone five or six times. I broke this mostly during training, a couple times getting hit by cars (one lady gave me her car, a Daihatsu,

for my compensation). This was during my steep learning curve. I finally had a piece of it removed, so now it's collapsible. A collapsible shoulder can be a huge benefit, so I try to fall on that side when I tuck and roll. It literally folds inward on impact. But even if your collarbones are intact, I recommend tucking and bringing your arms into your body and rolling to the side. You want to get as small as possible.

I broke my ankle during the World Cup qualifiers in South Africa. Two hours later I had my mechanic duct-tape my foot to the pedal and I went on to place third in the race.

I broke my arm during practice for a Mammoth Mountain NORBA. This injury was responsible for a 70 percent salary cut the next year.

I've broken several fingers—in training mostly, but no big deal. I usually just race right through these—as with all the other injuries, I suppose—and tape my fingers together.

I had a torn thumb ligament, but this happened in high school. The lack of a ligament caused my hand to slip off the bars occasionally. So I voluntarily had my thumb joint fused together so it "hooks" on to the handlebar.

I haven't found any pain more intense than the pain of a scratched cornea. I did this at an IMAX movie shoot, where I poked my eye putting on a street motorcycle racing jacket (from the Velcro of the arm). I crumbled over and couldn't walk for seven hours, my eye spasming while I lost control of all my other bodily functions.

In a qualifier, I crashed and my leg hyperextended behind my head, tearing my hamstring. I continued down the course and crashed and tore it almost completely. This was my second most painful injury ever.

At an X Games winter competition, I impacted an icy jump with my hip at about 50 mph. The bruise lasted for two years, and now I have a small, gelatinous, melon-shaped protrusion on my butt. Looks like a nasty saddlebag.

I broke my leg with torn PCL [posterior cruciate ligament] from riding motocross. This was my most expensive injury. I've had it operated on three times now, and the cadaver graft with complicated bolt system's really holding up!

And I have a shattered ego, which happens frequently in racing and training.

As I get older, the only noticeable change has been a slowdown with recovery from several hard training days strung together. I still have to maintain a higher fitness level than my competition (from what I've read), and this seems to cancel out the slower recovery. Often at the end of the day, my 21-year-old teammate is more beat that I am! Perhaps because I tend to be very mellow, my high-strung younger counterparts get worn out equally.

For the last few years, I've tried to incorporate protein in every meal, even snacks. Seems to starve the craves. I used to eat zero animal flesh, but I got too skinny and kept breaking bones. Now I'm much healthier with vitamins and daily salads. Although I still have a problem with sweets, coffee, and multiple Red Bull vodkas. But that makes me happy and that's what life is about!

In the off-season, my weekly training is two to three dirt-bike sessions, one BMX/downhill workout, two cross-country rides, lots of road (usually commuting, of which I am a big advocate), gym two to three times, running on the sand dunes two to three times. In season, it's one big cross-country ride, one easy run, four days downhill or mountain cross-training/racing.

The most important thing that mountain biking taught me is that if I can climb a mountain, I can do anything. Mountain biking taught me that I am strong, tough, and brave. That I am never too old. That I like to get dirty and play like a child. It's taught me that guys like women who can beat them at something. That there's a lot more beauty in the world than what you can see from the sidewalk or the driver's-side window.

Update

WHEN *BIKE FOR Life* reconnected with Marla in January 2014, it became clear that life after cycling could include a lot more cycling.

Retired from racing since 2009, the mother of two girls (born in 2006 and 2008) reported that she was riding every day ("unless the temperature drops below 20 degrees—which happens in Baltimore"), running and skateboarding for cross-training, and working out at the gym. She was planning to return to competitive racing this year at age 48. But instead of the downhill, she's aiming for "Enduro" races, a popular discipline introduced in the past decade that combines downhilling and climbing in lengthy time trials.

"A good thing about gravity racers is that we don't lose our skills," Streb said, "So Enduro is perfect for old downhillers like Brian Lopes and Steve Peat, who both do it. It's the best of both worlds for me since I was known as the fittest downhiller. Actually, I had to be, because my downhill skills weren't that good."

The skills were still pretty good as her career wound down. She won her second Single Speed World Championship in 2005 (the first came in 1999), and took third in the US national championships' downhill and super-downhill in 2006, just a few months after giving birth to her first daughter. After that, as Streb phased out of racing, she moved back to her Baltimore home town from her base in Costa Rica and took a desk job as the general manager of the Luna team in 2009. But it only lasted a year and a half.

"I found out that I wasn't an office person who could do a regular eight-hour-a-day job," she says. "It's like a lot of ex-pro riders. In our racing careers, we do one thing—work out where we want and when we want, and only need to show up at the starting line on time. But cycling still was my career, even though I wasn't competing."

Streb and her husband, Mark Fitzgerald, founded Streb Trail Systems, which designs hiking/biking trails in the United States and Latin America. She teaches bike safety and bike commuter advocacy for Bike Maryland, and she teaches mountain bike riding skills in her own clinics. Motherhood led her to create "Bike, Baby & Beyond," a seminar delivered at bicycle festivals touting the fitness advantages of cycling throughout pregnancy, including the day before delivery. Her best advice (quoted in the *Monterey Herald* on April 21, 2012): "Take the seat and the seat post off the bikes during the first trimester and do all of your rides out of the saddle. Without a seat on your bike, you can get back on your bike postpartum in just a few days, if you like."

She was riding within a week after both births, she says. In lieu of preschool, she took her kids for daily rides on a cargo bike outfitted with a huge basket filled with toys and books.

"I wear a lot of hats—and everything I'm doing, I love doing," Streb says. "I'm getting people on bikes. I'm working with athletes. I'll be competing again. I'm 90 percent car-free. Luna still sponsors me and I ride Orbea bikes. How could it get any better?"

Well, there was one more thing: A few months later, in Crested Butte, Colorado, she was inducted into the Mountain Bike Hall of Fame.

11

BIG-TIME MOTIVATION

Nine case studies show that fun, challenging, team, family, and philanthropic events can provide a key human connection and a lifetime of motivation.

On April 21, 2013, I rode with my 17-year-old son Joey, my 16-year-old nephew Jake, and 150,000 other people from downtown L.A. to Venice Beach and back. It was another CicLAvia, Los Angeles's grand three-times-a-year experiment in closing down huge swaths of asphalt just for human-powered vehicles. Since it began in 2010, I haven't missed a CicLAvia, an idea copied from bikes-only Sundays in Bogotá, Colombia, as well as in Mexico City, and pushed by L.A.'s mayor from 2005 to 2013, Antonio Villaraigosa. And I've seen more of this city at 2 to 8 miles per hour than in half a century by car. At various CicLAvias, I've seen the African American Firefighter Museum on South Central, mariachis playing on Soto Street in East Los Angeles, bogus green cards being peddled at MacArthur Park, and dragon-embossed gates in Chinatown. I've pedaled around the Frank Gehry–designed Walt Disney Concert Hall and down the steps at the beautiful Civic Center Plaza downtown. Best of all, I've seen teeming masses of humanity on bikes—thousands of all ages and races on all kinds of bikes, everything from beach cruisers and Kmart mountain bikes to $10,000 Italian dream machines—and even a 12-foot-long dinner table on wheels pedaled by 10 diners at 4 mph, and a 20-foot-high bike that perched its acrobatic (insane?) rider at traffic-signal height. And I've adjusted the

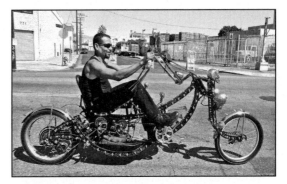

CicLAvia: You won't see this at a bike race.

too-low seat heights of dozens of scrunched-up people who clearly hadn't been on a bike in decades.

At the June 2012 CicLAvia, I saw mountain bike star Tinker Juarez pedaling at 5 mph as he shepherded his wife and young son through the bike-clogged streets of Hollywood. Later that year in the fall ride, Joey and I posed for a picture with Mayor Villaraigosa himself when we joined his retinue as they cruised south through downtown—which led to an interview in his office for a Los Angeles Times story about how a broken elbow he suffered from a bike crash led him to implement many recent bike-friendly measures in the city.

Down at Venice Beach, Joey and Jake and I posed with the Watts-based Real Rydaz bike club and their crazy chrome- and mirror-studded contraptions (the best one is pictured here). We shared a $12, two-pound bacon-laced Fatburger. We marveled at a giant mural of Michael Jackson painted on an abandoned building on the way back to downtown. With the crowds, the kooky photo-ops, and all the conversations, we were thoroughly wasted by the time we arrived back at our car at 5 p.m.—35 miles and eight hours after we started. That may not sound like much to a hard-core rider, but it was the most the boys had ever ridden solo. And at least a dozen people, noncyclists in normal life, personally told me that the distance had motivated them to train for the event.

Yes, you can stay pretty motivated with hard-core stuff like multiday stage races, double centuries, Masters racing, gran fondos, and cross-country tours. I do a lot of these rides many times a year, and I'll never stop, because they fire you up, get you excited about staying fit and eating right, and take you to beautiful places, both geographically and psychologically. But you shouldn't skip fun events like CicLAvia, which epitomize what I think is the most beautiful motivational aspect of cycling: that you can do it with your family, your friends, your BFFs, and strangers ranging from the Real Rydaz to disabled vets on adaptive bikes. In the early 1990s, my extended family used to do an annual 40-mile post–Thanksgiving Day ride; we still talk about it 20 years later. My brother-in-law told me he misses it because it motivated him to stay in shape. My wife and I did our honeymoon on a 600-mile tandem ride from Nice, France, to Rome, Italy; in the rough times, just talking about it would lighten the mood and get her thinking about getting in shape again.

Every year since 2000, my friend Rich and I and a dozen of our friends do an epic mid-June birthday ride—an all-day century road ride or a dawn-to-dusk mountain bike adventure to celebrate our almost-identical birthdates that month. Sometimes it's the only time we've ridden together for months. But it sure motivates us to train hard in May—as I hope it will for at least the next 50 birthdays.

We're human, not robots. To ride to 100 and beyond, you're going to need some compelling motivation. The nine case studies in this chapter, with their promise of fun, adventure, ego-gratification, and hard challenge, provide powerful inducements to stay excited about the sport and do the underlying hard work—the weights, the stretching, the diet, the training. As important, they should fire your creativity. Think of them as catalysts to create your own crazy events, to get out of your comfort zone, to squeeze more cycling into your life. Some of the examples, like decades-long riding streaks and turning blasé business trips into epic bike trips, are solo affairs. But others, like a father-and-son cross-country tandem tour, weeklong buddy trips at the world's toughest mountain bike stage races, and 500-mile fund-raising rides for charity, have a lot in common with CicLAvia, that kooky 4-mph party of 150,000 Angelinos: They are priceless, shared experiences that'll keep you motivated to ride your bike.

MOTIVATION CASE STUDY #1: CLIMB YOUR BRAINS OUT

Go to the Big Island of Hawaii for the world's steepest, tallest sea-to-summit ascent.

I was a little scared. Fourteen or fifteen thousand feet of climbing is a lot in one day. So I sought spiritual guidance from Pastor Ka'apu, the white-haired holy man.

"Bring a ho'okupu—a small gift of significance—to acknowledge that the spirit of the sacred mountain allowed you to transcend," he said, clasping my shoulder after giving a traditional Hawaiian prayer at my hotel. "And good luck."

At sunrise the next day, 6:54 a.m., I dipped my front tire in the Pacific Ocean and grabbed a small seashell. My plan: Deposit it later that day at the top of the sacred mountain, Mauna Kea, Hawaii's highest mountain and the steepest and highest sea-to-summit hill climb in the world: 13,796 feet in about 46 miles.

The payoff at the top promised to be spectacular: winter snowdrifts 30 feet high (Mauna Kea

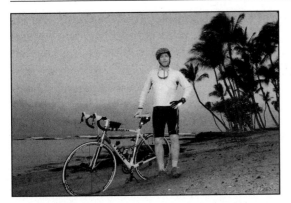

The world's highest, shortest sea-to-summit rise, up 13,796-foot Mauna Kea, began on the beach at 6:54 a.m.

means "White Mountain" in Hawaiian) and the world's clearest views of the stars, which is why 13 national observatories from 11 nations are located up there, their white and metallic domes making it look like a surreal neighborhood of giant igloos. The peak's isolation in the middle of the vast Pacific Ocean and lack of light pollution not only make it an astronomer's dream, but sacred ground to native Hawaiians, tourists hunting for a Kodak-moment sunset, and spiritual groups seeking nexus points of the universe. In 1994, I'd driven up to the top of Mauna Kea with my wife. I vowed to climb it someday by bike.

That day arrived in February 2011 with a business trip to the Big Island to interview some pro triathletes training on the nearby Hawaii Ironman course. Although the Mauna Kea climb has long stretches exceeding a 17 percent grade, 40 percent less oxygen in the air at the end than at the beginning, several miles of gravel-dirt road near the top, and no access to food or water before or after the Visitor's Center at 9,200 feet, I wasn't worried. Several times over the years, I'd biked Maui's well-known 36-mile, 10,003-foot climb up Mt. Haleakala, the world's steepest continuous all-paved sea-to-summit road, in about five hours. Although not particularly fast (the record is half that, 2:32:51, set by Canadian pro racer Ryder Hesjedal in 2009), I naturally assumed it'd be a simple matter of knocking off

4,000 more feet of elevation in another two or two-and-a-half hours, max. Having read on the Internet of a man who did Mauna Kea in six hours, I told my crew and a photographer, "I'll be done in eight hours—by 3 p.m." That would give us plenty of time to make it back downhill to catch my flight home at 10:30 that night.

It was a fool's math.

I didn't realize that while the shortest climb up Mauna Kea is 46 miles from the east coast city of Hilo, it's 13 miles longer, with an extra 1,000 feet of climbing and descending, on a route from my hotel on the Kohala coast, on the Big Island's west side. The extra distance would take its toll.

I left the coast after 10 miles and began the climb. The lush tropical scenery faded into grassland and then rocky scrubland by the time I reached the Saddle Road, the sole cross-island route between Mauna Kea and its smaller southern sister, Mauna Loa, an active volcano just 120 feet shorter. I stood on the pedals, because the Saddle is nasty-steep for 90 minutes before it flattens in the island's wind-blasted, slow-to-a-crawl midsection, which travels through US military weapons training grounds complete with sounds of distant explosions and screaming jet engines. I reached the turnoff to Summit Road, the last road to the top, about 12:30 p.m.—more than five hours after I started. I'd ridden 46 miles and climbed 7,500 feet—and was at least 90 minutes behind schedule.

I thought I could make up time on the final push to the top, but that proved delusional, because it was about to get a lot worse: Reaching the observatories, 14 miles up Summit Road, required another 7,500 feet of climbing. I didn't fully appreciate the task until mile 4, when the grade went to 17 percent.

At 17 percent, you push one pedal at a time as if it bears the weight of the world. At 17 percent, you can barely ride faster than you can walk. As the elevation went to 7,000 and then 8,000 feet, I walked half of it. When I reached the Visitor's Center at just over 9,000 feet, it was 2 p.m.

Waiting there was my crew, a group from my trip sponsor, Trek Bicycle. I couldn't have done this without them. Trek had loaned me my bike, and the crew had brought me something to eat and drink a few hours earlier.

Unfortunately, they also brought me bad news: The road ahead was even worse, including miles of gravel and dirt, and they had to leave me because of a meeting. They wouldn't be able to ferry me down the mountain to the hotel after I reached the top. That meant I would be in serious risk of missing my flight. They suggested I bail.

I shook my head. I'd done way too much work to turn back now. I'd just hitch a ride home at the top. I was going to finish this. It was just another 8 miles. Another 8 miles with 4,592 feet of climbing. Starting at around 9,000 feet high.

The first 4.6 miles of the final stretch was unpaved—"to discourage tourists and bicyclists," joked a ranger at the Visitor's Center. "It's only paved after that to stop dust that could clog the telescopes." He was right—it was discouraging. Mostly walking, occasionally riding in solid spots, I finished the first mile in 23 minutes. At home, with sea-level oxygen, I can happily *walk* a mile in 15 minutes. But in the dirt, with 20 to 40 percent less oxygen in the air, a mile seemed to take forever. My lungs began audibly heaving for breath. Step-by-agonizing-step, I slowed into 30- and 40-minute miles. As I was occasionally passed in a cloud of dust by vans ferrying tourists to the top to see the famous Mauna Kea sunset, my relentless optimism began to break down.

"I am an idiot," I began to mutter at around 12,000 feet.

It was now late afternoon. The sun drooped and the temperatures fell. I could see the paved switchbacks to the top just ahead, but they seemed to grow no closer. I grew despondent. I put on my vest against the looming chill and wallowed in utter dejection and self-damnation; I was going to miss the sunset, miss a ride home, and miss my 10:30 flight home.

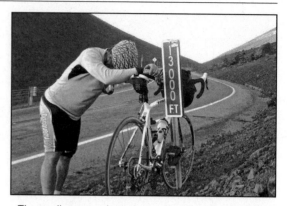

Three miles to go: beat, but not beaten, by miles of dirt road, thinning air, and lack of food at 13,000 feet at 5:42 p.m.

Finally, when I had 3 miles to go, the road turned back to blacktop—but it was too steep to ride. At 5:42 p.m., walking, I reached the road sign marking 13,000 feet and hung my head in abject hopelessness. The remaining 1.5 miles and 796 feet of elevation seemed impossible.

Finally, as the sun started to flirt with the horizon, the grade moderated. With a desperate burst of energy, I pedaled the last couple of switchbacks through mile 8 at 6:18 p.m., and came upon the surreal neighborhood of round white and metallic observatory domes, the horizontal rays of a dying sun glinting off them like blinding welding-torch flames. Parked on the ledge were half a dozen red tourist vans. Almost 12 hours after I'd started, I'd made it just in time to see the sunset!

Lightheaded, dehydrated, I dismounted and began to stumble over to the viewpoint. Then I noticed a handful of young Japanese adults in bright orange parkas running at me with a weird, wild-eyed hysteria. They were screaming something over and over. It took a second to understand it through their accents, but they were saying, "Heeero! Heeero! You a heeero!"

Yes, after walking most of the last 11 of the slowest, most challenging miles of my life, I'd become their *hero*! From their vans, they'd all seen me trudging along the dirt road. A dozen of them now swarmed around me, shaking my hand and

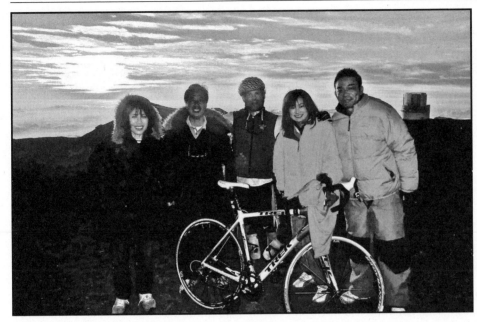

After Roy reached the top at 6:23 p.m., Japanese tourists called him a "Heeero!"

posing for pictures with their wasted, 55-year-old American "heeero" and his borrowed bicycle.

Feeling almost drunk, giddy from the lack of air and food, I started laughing uncontrollably. As my reward for riding 15,000 feet from sunrise to sunset, it seemed like I'd just won some sort of prize on a kooky Japanese reality TV show. How could I ask for a better ending than this?

Actually, it does get better. Quickly, I started to freeze. After being turned down for a hitch-hike by all the tour-bus drivers ("Legally, no can do," they said), I spotted a white four-door Ford truck and knocked on the window. It was the friendly Australian couple, Ruth and Andre Fletcher of Melbourne, who'd stopped halfway through the dirt road and given me some desperately needed water. I hopped in the back seat. We finished watching the sunset fade from orange to red to purple to black. And for the next two hours, the Fletchers drove me back to my hotel on the Kohala coast. I made it to my flight with five minutes to spare.

When I was flying back to L.A. that night, I realized two things: There weren't any 30-foot drifts of snow up there (it had been a warm February; it was almost all melted), and I'd forgotten to leave my ho'okupu—the seashell from the beach—at the top of Mauna Kea, as Pastor Ka'apu had advised me. So first chance I get to visit the Big Island again, I vowed to go back up there and do it right.

Only next time, I'll probably do it by car.

MOTIVATION CASE STUDY #2: START A WOMEN'S MOUNTAIN BIKE CLUB

L.A.'s 500-strong GGR says girls bond better without boys.

In 2005, 41-year-old Wendy Engelberg needed something new in her life. Stressed out by an ugly, dragged-out divorce, bored by her job as an auto-parts store manager, she had no kids or compelling hobbies to distract her. So on October 31 of that year, she showed up, a little scared, at Malibu Creek State Park for an event called Fat Tire Fest that she discovered on the Internet.

"I always wanted to try mountain biking," she said. "I was fit from aerobics class, so I thought I could do it. I was a little scared." This would be her first ride on the new $450 bike she'd bought. In fact, she hadn't ridden a bike since childhood.

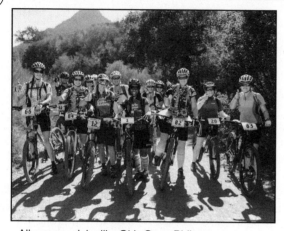

All-women clubs like Girlz Gone Riding are booming because females empower one another, they say.

"After two hours, I hated it," she said. "Mountain biking is hard. I fell again and again. But it was therapeutic. It immersed me in a whole new world of learning and challenge and fun that took my mind off the divorce. By the end of the day, I was hooked."

Eight years later, Engelberg had six bikes in her garage. She had become a hard-core endurance rider who was spending every weekend at a bike race or cycling adventure.

And although her picture does not appear in any magazines, some say she has emerged as one of the most influential people in the country in getting women in their 30s, 40s, and 50s out on the trails through the women's-only club she founded: Girlz Gone Riding.

Started in 2011, GGR grew to nearly 500 members by December 2013, making it one of the largest women's mountain bike clubs in the country. The numbers get attention. Some of the world's largest bike companies get in line to sponsor its events. And in the tradition of women's-only running races and triathlons, which have been magnets for introducing hundreds of thousands of women to endurance sports in the past decade, some say that GGR is inspiring thousands of women to get out on the trails in a way that co-ed bike clubs simply can't.

"There are no men there," said Mark Langton, who runs a weekly skills clinic that many Girlz have attended. He is the president of CORBA (Concerned Off Road Bicyclists Association), the organization that sponsored the event in Malibu Creek. "Women empower other women when they ride together. They love to get out and exercise—but they don't like doing it with men. They get turned off when there's too much testosterone floating around."

The Problem with Men

Men ride too fast and don't wait. Men are impatient. Men aren't supportive or nurturing.

They're too competitive. No matter what level she rode at, Engelberg heard the same complaints. She heard them while riding the Santa Monica Mountain fire roads three or four days a week with women she met at Fat Tire Fest. When she moved up to technical single-track trails, bought a fancy $3,100 dual-suspension bike, and began taking road trips to mountain bike meccas, from Sedona, Arizona, to Whistler, British Columbia, with the 700-member-strong North Ranch Mountain Bikers, the biggest (and mainly male) club in the West, she still heard the same thing: It's no fun riding with men.

Endless races, road trips, and new friends followed. There were downhill races at Tehachapi and Los Olivos; adventures with friends in Mammoth, Kernville, and Bend, Oregon. "I was happy again," she said. "The divorce was done. Now, everything revolved around mountain biking."

With no need or desire to go home, she kept pushing further, doing all-day 25-, 30-, 40-mile rides. But when one of her friends suggested the Rwanda 50 Ride in Orange County, that seemed like too much. "Come on—we're already riding more miles than that, anyway," her friend replied.

Naturally, Engelberg went out and bought her fourth bike, a long-distance-oriented Specialized Epic 29er. When the girls began cross-training on the road, she added a road bike, her fifth.

In January 2011, Engelberg went to a happy hour with several women mountain bikers. Again, they began ranting about how they disliked riding with their boyfriends.

"We realized it wasn't really the guys' fault," she said. "Men and women have fundamentally different approaches to life and sports. Guys are hard-wired to be competitive. Girls are there for the experience, to talk, to support each other, to stop and wait for one another. They enjoy riding at a slower pace where they can talk and share."

That's when the big idea hit: a club just for women. After some serious drinking and brainstorming, they settled on the name Girlz Gone Riding, and immediately planned their first event at Malibu Creek State Park for the following month. It included three levels of guided rides, guest speakers, coaching clinics, and gear donated from local bike shops for raffles.

"We expected 20 or 30 girls to show up," Engelberg said. "So we were shocked when we got over 100!"

The women's ages ranged from 30-somethings through 60-somethings, with the majority over 40. Most had the same story: They liked to ride, just not with their impatient husbands and boyfriends. "When a second event in October 2011 drew over 100 women, we knew we were on to something," Engelberg said.

Strength in Numbers

GGR's growing membership includes a handful of male bike-shop managers and CORBA board members. Most of the Girlz are from their late 30s to late 50s, with the club's toughest riders being two 76-year-old triathletes. "They kick our butts," said Engelberg with admiration.

Club activities include quarterly rides, "Wenches on Wrenches" workshops at Pasadena Cyclery and Newbery Park Bike Shop, day trips to Mt. Pinos, a three-day September trip in conjunction with the Kernville Fat Tire Festival, and the annual Rocktober Gala at Malibu

Creek State Park, which usually draws 150 Girlz. The club inspired a racing offshoot, the SoCal Endurance Ladies team, which soon had 49 members, making it one of the biggest women's teams in the country, according to Engelberg, who's on it. Two of them did the Leadville 100 in 2013.

GGR's big membership numbers get attention. "We have an enormous presence in L.A. now," she said. The club gained a sponsorship from Liv/Giant, the female division of Giant Bicycles. World champion endurance rider Rebecca Rusch conducted an online clinic for the club, and famed downhiller Leigh Donovan came in for a hands-on Downhill 101 session.

Besides the fact that there are no dues, Engelberg thinks the best benefit of the club is the girlzgoneriding.com website and GGR Facebook page. "It's very active, with people hooking up for rides every day, selling parts, going to races," she said. "Whenever and wherever you want to ride, you have people to do it with."

And the best thing about all the club's connections, activities, stars, and industry contacts, she said, is that "women are sticking with it. We keep gaining members and not losing any. Women are continuing to mountain bike instead of getting discouraged and leaving. The difference is that we aren't cliquey. We wait for them. Nobody gets dropped."

That is partly due to the collaborative female nature and partly because of the way the rides are designed. Every GGR ride is broken up into Beginner, Intermediate, and Advanced groups, and then subdivided into fast, medium, and slow. Each group has a ride leader up front, a sweeper in the rear, and a floater, who goes back and forth to help out wherever needed.

"This way, it's not intimidating," said Engelberg. She guessed that "probably more than half of our members would not be riding regularly if not for the GGR. The bottom line is simple. Whether it's riding or shopping, we would rather do it with women."

BIKES IN HER IMAGE
KNOCKED DOWN, SUPERSTAR JULI FURTADO CAME BACK WITH HER OWN WOMEN'S BIKE LINE

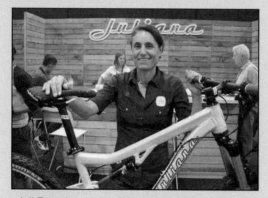

Juli Furtado with her Juliana brand bikes.

Juli Furtado was on top of the world. After exploding on the cycling scene with a victory at the first World Mountain Bike Championships in 1990 (at Durango, Colorado), and winning 23 major races in a row in 1994, the future Mountain Bike Hall of Famer took it to a new level in 1996, winning both the NORBA nationals and her third World Cup title. She was 29, the best in the world, with a long career still ahead.

Then it all fell apart. After a poor showing at the Atlanta Olympics, in 1997 she was diagnosed with lupus, a chronic, incurable inflammatory disease that occurs when your immune system attacks your own tissues and organs. It attacked her skin and joints, causing severe fatigue. Some days, she could not function at all. And just like that, her career was over.

Furtado had seen a career in sports disappear before. In the late 1980s, at age 15, a series of debilitating knee injuries knocked her off the US National ski team and into cycling. But what to do now? Her career as an athlete was done.

"It was really hard. After my skiing experience, one of my goals was to go out on my own terms, to retire when I wanted and how I wanted. I hadn't begun to think of what's next."

Lost and seeking change, she moved from Colorado to Santa Cruz, California. "I don't know why . . . it was different," she said. "I went through a period where I thought 'Oh, I don't need to accomplish any more. I've had this accelerated life.'" That didn't last long. She worked as a radio announcer for news-hour drive time, went to Africa on safari, and rode her cruiser bike a lot. And she had an idea for a women's-specific bike.

"I just knew there was a market, because . . . women are different," she said. "Women want different experiences from biking, from shopping, from bikes that look and feel different. When I raced, I changed the saddle, the grips, the handlebar—everything was custom. These things matter. So I wondered: Why don't we make bikes for women that already have this?"

Furtado incorporated a company that made bars, grips, and stems. She called it Juliana. In 1999, she licensed the name to Santa Cruz Bicycles, which then made the Julianas, one of the first women's-specific mountain bikes. "Men use their names—Fisher, Lemond, Eddy Merckx. Why not women?" she said.

"The bike did real well," said Furtado. "Santa Cruz goes through a lot of models, but they never dropped the Juliana. It always sustained an avid following." In 2003, she began working part-time at the company in marketing.

By 2011, noting that the big companies all started making women's bikes, Furtado proposed turning Juliana into an entire line.

At the 2013 Interbike, Santa Cruz debuted the five-model Juliana brand of hard-tail and dual-suspension mountain bikes with aluminum and carbon frames in three wheel sizes.

The line is "doing great," said Furtado a year later. And so is she, despite the lupus. "For the average 46-year-old mother of a five-year-old boy, I have a pretty active life," she said. "I ride when I can and don't when I can't." In a typical week, she'll do two days of trail running, two days of mountain biking, a road ride, and tennis. Increasingly involved with events, she helped open a high-school bike league in Arizona. In a sign of the times, girls are often half the riders.

"Everyone said, 'There's no market for this,'" said Furtado. "Today, you're missing out if you don't have dedicated bikes for women."

MOTIVATION CASE STUDY #3:
DO A TEAM EVENT

Find out why the camaraderie of 24-hour racing goes way beyond your team.

"Did you charge your lights? Are you sure you charged your lights?" Rich screamed.

"Yes, yes, yes," I assured him. "Don't worry. Brand-new. Used once. Recharged for hours back home. Done deal."

And so began the most memorable lap of 24-hour racing in my life. Which might seem kind of strange, given that it was a lap I didn't ride.

While I retreated back to the campfire, reached in the cooler for another beer, and dangled another hot dog over the flaming logs, Rich rode off into the night. With my lights. Under my name.

You see, I was supposed to be riding in the 1996 24-Hours of Moab, not him. But the day before the event, as the members of Team Mountain Dogs, our bike club, casually pre-rode the 10-mile loop, I bit the dust. Hard.

Distracted by a "Hey!" yelled by a photographer off to the left, I buried my front wheel in a rut and face-planted. I have no memory of falling or of the impact. When I awoke, my friends said I'd been unconscious for three minutes. After another two minutes, I began to remember my own name. By the time I was able to recall the name of my 1-year-old son Joey, a four-wheel-drive ambulance had arrived to take me to a Moab hospital.

That night, the sight of my face actually compelled a child at the local McDonald's to clutch his daddy's leg in fear. On race day, with six stitches in my lip, a throbbing sensation in my cheekbone, and an oozing crust congealing over the right side of my mug from mouth to eye to ear like a gory *Phantom of the Opera* mask, I decided it was best to let Rich take my place.

Not that anyone seemed to mind. Mountain Dog founder Rich "The Reverend" White, known for his passionate pontificating about all things mountain biking, is a superb rider, way faster than me. Although he hadn't planned to race—he was chronically short of cash and didn't want to pay $100 for his share of the entry fee and expenses—he had a confirmed seat on the 12-hour road trip from L.A. because we all wanted to channel his energy. In fact, I was here in Utah because of Rich. Four years earlier, after we'd met when I tried to sell my first book to the bike shop he managed, he'd taught me how to mountain bike, introduced me to the beauty of the mountains. I was almost honored to will my lights to him.

Still, I was bummed—this would have been my first 24-hour race. Now, it was a lost weekend.

The Revelation

In the hours before the race, I pondered the gruesome shell hardening over my face and watched with envy as the Mountain Dogs scurried about, worrying over this and that. I had no purpose; I was worthless. But as I moped around the 1,000-strong tent city, something strange happened.

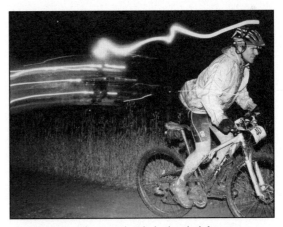

In 24-hour racing, you battle in the dark for your teammates.

A camaraderie. A getting-away-for-an-adventure-with-my-friends vibe. A "where-ya-from-dude-and-what-the-hell-happened-to-your-face?" neighborliness. It was infectious. And suddenly, riding or not, this event was giving me something I needed, something I craved, something I didn't experience much in everyday life: the feeling of being part of a team on a great quest.

I'm no psychologist, and I know that lots of women do these events too, but it seems that 24-hour races tap into a primal compulsion that men can understand best: the need to get together, take on a challenge, get sweaty, get bloody, and, most of all, get tales to tell. Tales for next week's ride. Tales for the next family barbecue. Tales for 50 years from now, when we're using wheelchairs instead of bikes, pacemakers instead of HRMs, and diapers instead of Lycra shorts.

If I'd known then that I'd do half a dozen 24-hour events after this, including a solo, I wouldn't have been surprised. If you'd have told anyone at Moab that by 2005 there would be dozens of 24-hour races across North America, 20,000 participants, NORBA-sanctioned team and solo championships, and a solo world title race with hundreds of age-group participants, they might have said "of course." After all, we'd been practically crying for something like this for years.

Yes, I was out of the race as a rider. But a team needs more than that. There would be chains to lube, dozing riders to wake, beers to chill, hot dogs to roast, and stories to record for posterity. And who better to do that than me, a former wedding videographer?

The Guardian Angel

It's midnight, about the time I figured Rich ought to be finishing his lap, and the start-finish zone is electric. Too early to sleep, too dark to ride without fear, hundreds of spectators and competitors clogging the finishing chute in a frenzy of sound and sweat. In the middle of it all is yours truly, a regular Geraldo Rivera, asking the hard questions on videotape. "What's it like to share the same bike shorts for 24 hours?" I grill two clothes-swapping members of Team Largeass.

Soon it's 12:10, 12:15, and I pan over to Craig, our Mountain Dog teammate awaiting the baton. Where's Rich? He shoulda been here by now! Did he crash? Is he hurt?

Finally, at 12:20, Rich comes flying into the pits, drenched in sweat and quivering with excitement. He hands the baton to Craig. And he tells me something that makes me cringe: "It was the lights."

My lights—the ones I assured him were potent enough to beckon a supertanker to harbor. They burned out around 11:30, halfway through the most treacherous part of the 10-mile loop. I remember his words as if they were my own: "Suddenly, I find myself blind, invisible, freezing, and terrified in the wet, moonless night. One false step in my slippery clipless shoes could put me into the path of mountain bikers flying downhill at 30 mph—or plunge me 50 feet into jagged rocks below. So I inch along in baby steps. At this rate, it'll be hours before I get back."

I feel like hell. I let a teammate down. I start to apologize. Then Rich stops me. "Roy, don't worry about it," he said. "Because of those lights, this turned into one of the greatest rides of my life."

Huh?

"After about 20 minutes in the middle of nowhere," he explains, "a featureless biker screeches to a halt, his handlebar-mounted lights blazing like the eyes of a snarling animal. 'Get on my wheel, now!' he barks.

"And for the next 30 minutes I hang on for dear life, tethered to the halogen beams of a human seeing-eye dog who screams at me to stay with him, to speed up, to turn right or left or stand up, to ride with more exhilaration and terror and pure speed than I've ever ridden in my life.

"Who he was, I don't know. But he was an animal. A guardian-angel animal!"

The second he says that, I notice a muscular, dark-haired biker from L.A. whom I've interviewed several times before. It's Johnny G, renowned fitness guru and inventor of Spinning, the ultra-popular health-club stationary cycling program. He'd brought a team to Moab—Team Spinning, of course. He'd just finished a lap in 1 hour, 5 minutes—which was quite fast, especially at night. I remark how impressed I am with his time.

"I might have gone even faster," he notes in his distinctive South African accent, "if I didn't have to stop to tow a guy in."

I'll never forget seeing Rich grab Johnny's hand and shake it, especially since the moment is immortalized on videotape. "Thank you, thank you, thank you," he babbles to his rescuer. He becomes almost reverential when he looks at the posted standings, which show Team Spinning in the top five.

"Wow, you're a contender," Rich said. "And you stopped to help me. Unbelievable."

Johnny G, always the motivator, shrugged off the thanks. "Above everything, these 24-hour events are all about teamwork," he said, his tone modulated like an Indian wise man. "Even if it's not your team."

Wow. Teamwork—even if it's not your team. I bask in his words, so true, so poignant, so perfectly capturing the beauty of this remarkable 24-hour bonding experience. Then I put the camcorder down. Johnny's eyes instantly narrow, then dilate.

"My god, Roy," he said, "What in the hell happened to your face?"

MOTIVATION CASE STUDY #4: THE FAMILY TANDEM TRIP

Father and son learn to work together pedaling from Portland to Yellowstone.

"Buddy, you gotta help me here. My body's wearing out. I'm totally fatigued, beat up, wasted. I can't recover. Everything hurts. Honestly, you gotta push harder."

Surprisingly, my son Joey, a 15-year-old non-stop talking machine, listened to my plea and didn't say a word. Halfway through our 850-mile tandem tour from Portland, Oregon, to Yellowstone National Park in August 2010, he did not respond with his usual lame "I *am* trying, Dad!" or his smart-alecky "In your face!" For the first time in his life, he kept quiet—so I had no idea what he was thinking. Was he reflecting? Was he psyching up? Was he mad that he even agreed to do this epic tandem trip with me in the first place?

After all, not only was Portland-to-Yellowstone Joey's first bike trip, it was completely alien to his way of life. Although he'd attended a once-a-week karate class for years, like most of his peers he was way better at surfing the net than throwing a football, shooting a basketball, or riding a bike. My overprotective wife had lobbied relentlessly against the trip, arguing that the kid couldn't handle 11 days in the saddle—until I politely reminded her that she was totally unathletic yet somehow handled an 8-day, 600-mile tandem ride from Nice to Rome on our honeymoon in 1994. Since Joey was a byproduct of that ride, popping out nine months later, I saw a father-son trip on the same bike, our 1993 Santana Sovereign, as completing the circle—sort of a genetic symmetry.

There was also an urgency to doing the trip in the summer of 2010: The next year Joe would turn 16, get his driver's license, and never want to hang out with his parents again.

I tried to make sure Joey was ready physically and mentally for what I called "The Last Chance Tandem Trip." I dragged him along on every gear purchase—new shifters, Aerospoke wheels, stoker seat, racks and panniers, tent, sleeping bags. To build up physically, we did eight progressively longer tandem rides starting in May, topping out with a century from Irvine to Oceanside and back the week before the trip. To keep motivation high for the big ride, it had an epic payoff—Yellowstone Park. And so it would start off as easy and fun as possible, I chose a route that

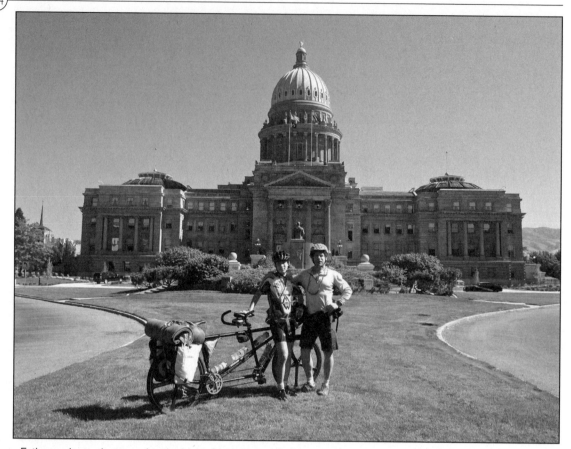

Father and son pit-stopped at the Idaho State Capitol Building in Boise.

headed east through the speedy, spectacular, and sightseeing-laden Columbia River Gorge.

The Columbia River, which serves as most of the border between Washington and Oregon, is the only low-elevation gap through the Cascade Mountains. That's why, combined with the Snake River to the southeast, it was the route that Lewis and Clark and the pioneers of the Oregon Trail took to the Pacific Ocean. A greenish splendor loaded with waterfalls—77 of them on the Oregon side alone—the Columbia River Gorge not only would start the trip off with lots of cool Kodak moments, like 620-foot-high Multnomah Falls, the second-highest year-round falls in the United States, but help power us along like an extra engine. That's because of the wind.

The steep Columbia Gorge walls, combined with the atmospheric differential between the cool, moist, dense maritime air west of the Cascades and the dry, hot, less-dense air to the east, create a wind-tunnel effect that has made it a world-famous mecca for windsurfers and kiteboarders. In the summer, that relentless 35-mph wind—up to 50 mph when Pacific storms hit—blows west to east up the Columbia. I envisioned us easing into the trip and loosening up our muscles while being whipped east on those gorgeous tailwinds for 200 miles, like passengers on a bullet train.

But that was not to be.

The Hellish Triple H

When we rolled out of the Portland airport on State Route 30, the Oregon Scenic Byway, we were slammed into what we would soon call "H-cubed." Heat, headwinds, and hills. Very quickly, it was clear that the pleasure cruise I promised was a pipedream.

An extreme mid-August heat wave in Oregon transformed the easy easterlies into hellacious headwinds and broiled us alive; temperatures hit 100 degrees every day and went as high as 106. A couple days later, when we pulled into the small, Columbia River town of Arlington at 6:40 p.m., the temperature was exactly 100 degrees. Staying hydrated was a real problem. Normally, I don't touch soft drinks; but now, pushing our two-wheel Winnebago 7 or 8 mph against the wind, I was draining two water bottles and guzzling a 44-ounce, quickie-mart root beer every hour.

Another big miscalculation was unrealistic expectations. Old cyclists like me are comfortable with the strange cycling concept of "suffering"—taking it to the edge and keeping it there for a long time. But that is not normal behavior for untrained folk. Did I actually think that a teenager who had never pushed very hard athletically could hammer for more than a few scattered seconds at a time?

"Dad, you sweat like a pig," Joey would say.

Yes, I'd think to myself, it's not easy fighting headwinds in 100-degree heat while lugging a tent, sleeping bags, a bunch of gear, and an extra 130 pounds of inactive human flesh. "Please push a little more, buddy," I'd reply. I repeated that request so frequently, often using less than polite tones, that I quickly began to irritate both of us.

That doesn't mean Joey wasn't working harder than he'd ever worked. He was getting quite dehydrated, too. Since H-cubed did not let up, we both needed an extra-long time off the bike during our breaks to recuperate, rehydrate, and refuel. Every stop was necessary—and often memorable.

In Cascade Locks, we saw the renowned Bridge of the Gods over the Columbia and ate half-pound hamburgers at the iconic CharBurger. In Arlington, we slept on a boat dock on the Columbia River. We ate at Bozo Burger on Boardman, and

the Dairy Queen in Pendleton. We learned about Lewis and Clark and the Oregon Trail in museums in Oregon and Idaho, and even rode our bikes on the covered-wagon wheel tracks. We swam in two of America's biggest and most historic rivers, the Columbia and the Snake.

Of course, we also met the weirdest characters and heard the craziest life stories at restaurants and rest stops, which gave us hours of conversation later on the bike. A truck driver from Riverside, California, begged us to let him ferry us over the mountains. A blond, Irish-looking half-Indian man told us how his darker siblings called him "limey," while he called them "savages." At a Motel 6, a friendly Nazi fellow with chest and arms covered in giant tattoos of swastikas graciously helped me maneuver my bike out of a doorway; we wondered how helpful he'd have been if he'd known we were Jewish.

On a bike trip, even the crummiest moments become valuable lessons, such as the time Joe reminded me, after our sixth front flat tire in five days, that I hadn't been following my own basic rule of repair: Run your fingers across the inside of the tire before you put a new tube in. That's how we discovered a couple of embedded, tiny, virtually invisible wires, courtesy of the shredded chunks of steel-belted tires littering the shoulder of I-84.

That shoulder was our home for 10 days starting in The Dalles, 90 miles east of Portland, where the green of the forests was replaced by brown, treeless high desert. On that 8-foot-wide strip of heat and wind, our only shade came from an occasional overpass.

As early as Day 2, I could feel my body breaking down. After a week of H-cubed, including an abrupt 4,000-foot climb into the thickly forested Blue Mountains of eastern Oregon that just about killed us, I was seriously worried that I was becoming a candidate for rhabdomyolysis. That's the condition in which the body, unable to get in enough nutrients and recovery to support its activity level, starts eating its own muscle.

The Magic Moment

After we made the climb, alternately walking, running, and riding, I-84 was a joy. The weather was beautiful and a bit cooler through the Blue Mountains as the interstate angled southeast to Boise, Idaho. That would normally have called for a celebration, as we had finished the first half of the trip and now would be riding in the Snake River Plain, a relatively flat depression that follows the curve of the mighty river for 400 miles from the Oregon border to the Yellowstone foothills. But instead of getting stronger as the days went on, I was getting weaker. Ten miles east of the Idaho state capitol building, on a cloudless, sweaty, 90-degree day, my thighs were crying—and our schedule increasingly hopeless.

The plan was to meet my wife, who was flying into Salt Lake City and renting a van, at the gates of Yellowstone. At 65 miles a day, however, we weren't going to come close. The headwinds had eased, but we were still riding so slowly over the gently rolling countryside that we couldn't build up enough wind to cool off my face, which felt like a radiator about to blow.

Joey is a happy, smiley kid who had been remarkably upbeat the whole trip, even as I got increasingly on his case asking him to pedal harder. He'd just say, "In your face, Dad!" and push for 10 or 15 seconds. But now, with my strength evaporating and desperation setting in, I tried two new tactics: begging and embarrassment.

"Buddy, I'm breaking down. My muscles have no more power. We're supposed to be a team, not a horse and his rider. You're going to have to make a more consistent effort to help. I can't go any harder, so our speed is actually controlled by *you*. You told your friends that you were riding to Yellowstone. Well, whether we make it or not on our own power is entirely in your hands."

And that's when Joey, who normally never lets a comment go by without a 10-minute response, became strangely silent. He didn't say much as we made a one-hour pit stop at a combination Burger King, convenience store, and gas station, each of us sucking down a 44-ouncer and three bacon burgers. But about 30 seconds after we hit the road again, he uttered three words that I will never forget: "Let's get moving."

And just like that, for the first time in a week without any prompting by me, Joey stood out of the saddle and pushed hard. "Stand up with me," he commanded. "Let's do 5 of these markers"—referring to the 4-foot-tall metal posts on the side of the road spaced about 50 yards apart.

We hammered those markers so fast that I was stunned. It turns out that several factors had coalesced at once: We'd crossed the county line and were now riding on a shoulder of perfectly smooth concrete. And the headwinds had disappeared.

Thirty seconds later, Joey stood again. "Six markers," he said.

Soon, we were up to 8, then 11, then 16 markers, shoving it in higher gears and taking shorter rest periods each time. We weren't just riding—we were interval training! When we briefly pulled off the road at an overpass to rest my stomach, jittery from the three bacon burgers, I was shocked by what I saw printed on an Oregon Trail historical sign: We'd gone 9 miles in 30 minutes—more than we normally went in an hour.

I didn't say a word—yet. Something pretty cool was happening here.

Back on the highway 3 minutes later, Joey started counting markers again, louder and louder, pushing harder and harder—20, 25, 30 markers in a row. He was rocking the bike so hard that I had to sit down to control it.

Watching the mileage markers, I could see we were knocking off miles at a 3-minute pace, sometimes less. A long downhill knocked off another one in a couple of minutes. After another 35 markers, we came to another downhill, killing another mile. I made Joe sit on the descents to save his strength for the climbs.

I told Joe that we easily were going to set a new hour record. When he heard that, he stood, rocked the bike, and called out, "50 markers!"

As the mileposts flew by, I did the math. In 50 minutes since the Burger King—including the 3-minute stop—we'd gone 16 miles. We now had a mild tailwind. Could we do 4 miles in the next 10 minutes—24 miles per hour? Could he keep up the pace?

I looked at my watch and kept up the praise. "This is crazy! A new record!" I exclaimed, and Joey kept pushing. "Sixty markers!" he screamed as we tore up the shallow inclines.

With 7 minutes to go before the hour mark, we passed a sign that read, "Watch Out. Gusty winds next 11 miles." That meant tailwinds. I couldn't believe it; this could actually happen!

Joey, seemingly possessed, kept pushing—70, 75, 80, 90 markers.

With five minutes to go, we were at 18 miles. A long climb materialized. Joe rocked like a crazy man. I stood up, too. We needed divine intervention now.

And we got it. At the top we crested a monster downhill, the biggest of the day. A mile and a half gone, just like that. After a flat stretch, all in the big chainring, we had another descent, pushing our legs and lungs to the limit all the way.

At 59 minutes and 34 seconds (including the 3-minute stop), we hit the 20-mile mark.

But Joey, on fire, couldn't stop. He kept counting: "100 markers! 110! 120!"

We went another 2 miles before he conked out.

We coasted to a stop and Joe lay on his back in the weeds, heaving. "I need food," he said. I unzipped the frame pouch, handed him a chocolate Pop-Tart, and leaned over on the concrete railing overlooking the vast fields of green, irrigated by the waters of the Snake River. I took a photo. A very cool moment for both of us.

The last 10 miles into the small town of Glenns Ferry, Idaho, took us 2 hours. Joey, completely depleted now, could barely pedal anymore, and we paused for numerous photo-ops. We stopped in town for gigantic half-pound hamburgers and lemonade at the famous Oregon Trail Cafe & Bar, and then rode in the dark to a campsite at nearby Three Island Crossing State Park, located on bluffs overlooking a precarious Snake River crossing point on the Oregon Trail. We entertained a young couple camped next door with the story of our great 76-mile day, the biggest of the trip.

Over the next few days, we went sightseeing at Twin Falls; overlooked the 100-foot gorge where Evel Knievel tried to jump the Snake River on a rocket-motorcycle in 1974; swam in the Snake; rode through a 10-mile construction zone; lost a pair of gloves, a pair of sunglasses, and a pair of bike shorts; and discovered that little tangerines are the ultimate energy bars. We made it as far as Pocatello, where my wife picked us up. The first thing she actually said to me was, "What happened to your legs? It looks like they've shrunk."

Yellowstone was another 160 miles north. Two more days, maybe three, given the 4,000-foot elevation gain.

Joey and I posed at the "Entering Yellowstone" sign with our bike helmets on and the front wheel of the tandem. The family then did a driving tour of the spectacular national park in three days, which really wasn't long enough.

Joey and I both were bummed-out that we didn't make it all the way to Yellowstone under our own power. When I'd planned the trip, I hadn't factored in enough time for the distance and the conditions. But we gained some perspective from an old ranger one day at Old Faithful.

"When you come to Yellowstone, we sincerely hope that you don't see it all," he said. "Because you always need to have an excuse to come back."

Without knowing it, we'd already taken his advice. Driver's license notwithstanding, Joey told me he wanted to do another tandem trip the next summer.

MOTIVATION CASE STUDY #5:
SEE THE CHAIR

At the BC Bike Race, the slow guys prove you see the most if you stop to smell the roses.

Near Whistler, British Columbia, deep in a forest so dense with evergreen trees that sunlight barely penetrates the canopy, is a chair.

It's a big, puffy, reddish-orange half-loveseat—something you'd think would be hard to miss in a world of green leaves and green moss and green ferns and brown bark. Like the performance art of a demented interior decorator, the chair sits perched at an angle on a four-foot-high tree stump like a drunken throne, regally on display about eight feet off of Bart's Dark Trail, a bumpy, rock- and log-strewn single-track that elicits a loud stream of rattles, groans, and expletives from 400 mountain bikers. They are participants in the 2008 BC Bike Race, a seven-day, 330-mile single-track endurance test from Vancouver Island to the BC mainland that ends in Whistler today. All of the riders are tired—maybe too tired and too focused to look up from the precarious trail to notice the anomalous living-room chair colored like Bozo's hair.

Except for the three of us, that is. "Roy, climb up and sit in it—it'll be a funny picture," says Paul. I look over at my other teammate, Ed, and hesitate. We don't want to risk missing the checkpoint time cutoff, which would deny us official finisher's status after a week of the craziest, hardest riding of our lives. Do we really have time for this?

"Get up there already!" yells Paul. "This chair embodies everything we ride bikes for. It encapsulates our very philosophy of life, our *raison d'être*. It's why we formed the BPA!"

Ed and I look at each other—and burst into uncontrollable laughter. Paul, the most unlikely member of the BPA—the Back of the Pack Association—had completely drunk the Kool-Aid. Just 48 hours before, he'd been a hard-core, front-of-the-pack bike racer; he would have thought that taking 5 or 10 minutes in the middle of a bike race to stop and climb into this funky chair to shoot photos was stupid. He would have thought the BPA—the club Ed and I founded to honor the slow, undertrained, underskilled, or overweight laggards like us who pull up the rear at big multiday team stage races like the BC Race—was ridiculous.

But now, after riding with me and Ed, the speedy Paul had become one of us. In fact, Paul was out-BPA-ing the BPA—and having the time of his life. He'd lost his original teammate. But apparently he'd found his soul mates.

Making the Right Match

Too bad there's not an eHarmony.com for bike teams.

Team endurance events like the TransAlp, TransRockies, TransScotland, and TransAndes are booming these days. I've done a few of them. When you ride, eat, and sleep together 24/7 under arduous circumstances, you'd better have the right partner.

Teammates of vastly different abilities tend to get on each other's nerves—and even wreck their health. My world-class TransRockies

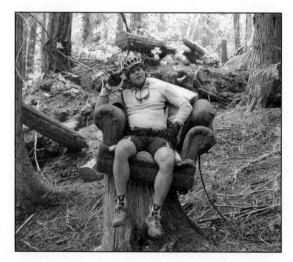

Does a chair in the forest exist if you never see it? At the BC Bike Race, the slow guys saw the sights the elites missed.

partner, chafing at my snail's pace, would ride so far ahead that I'd find him hours later waiting at the checkpoint with his teeth clattering, freezing. He was sick for a month afterward.

But even if you are of similar abilities, different attitudes can sour a team. I like to shoot the breeze at food stops, meet the locals, and take lots of photos, the wackier the better. I don't care if we come in last, as long as we make the cutoffs. More than one teammate at the Eco-Challenge and Primal Quest adventure races told me to keep my eyes on the trail and hurry my ass up. I'd respond, "Hey, we're not going to win anything—and we'll never see anything like this again."

These races are usually held in beautiful places—stunning mountain ranges and rainforests. That's why, as I explained to my BC partner Ed Korb, a local riding buddy of similar ability (who's also organized, a good mechanic, and loves corny photos), I have never considered being a back-of-the-packer as a mark of shame. While some mid-packers and front-packers will screw up their faces and exclaim, "What happened?" when they hear your day's finishing time (usually anywhere from two to four hours more than theirs), their times would make me wonder, "What's the rush?"

Back-of-the-pack means more time to enjoy the ride. Besides, being BP doesn't even have to mean you finish BP. Once, at La Ruta de los Conquistadores, the famous ride across Costa Rica, I finished 100th of 102 official finishers; but since 100 more starters had been disqualified for missing a checkpoint, I finished in the top 50 percent overall.

Bottom line: You can be slow and complete these events and come home with a bunch of good laughs and a great photo album. But you can't afford one bad day.

The Rise of the BPA

The first two days of the BC Race took us through Vancouver Island's lush, primordial forests of towering trees and giant ferns. But at dinner the second night, Ed got angry—and came up with an idea.

He'd found out that the back-of-the-packers missed out on a lot of things that the front of the pack enjoyed, such as being greeted by cheerleaders at the finish line, getting pizzas for dinner, and being given chocolate Honey Stinger bars at checkpoints. All were gone by the time we arrived. In fact, the water had run out at Checkpoint 2, a time cutoff at the top of a long, terrible, sunbaked climb that a bonking Ed and I made by just 30 seconds. Hearing the "What happened?" comments at dinner from faster riders stung him; he felt that there was a systemic lack of respect for back-of-the-packers.

"We need to organize," he said. "Our way is better than theirs. We are more true to what real mountain biking is all about. As of right now, we are officially the Back of the Pack Association— the BPA."

Yes, the BPA. Just a joke, really, but we ran with it—and soon so did everybody else. The BPA struck a chord with our fellow laggards when we announced it at the starting line. By midday, the conversations at the back of the pack had become surprisingly philosophical. To be BPA meant being more soulful, more human, more in touch with the giant ferns of the forest and the beauty of the snowcapped mountains. BPAers stopped to smell the daffodils, to notice the bear droppings, to, as Chris, a heavyset BPAer whom I recognized from the back of the pack at the 2005 TransRockies, put it, "inhale the musky scent of decaying plant matter being recycled in nature like mulch."

A strange pride was building. As word spread, the slow riders began chanting "B-P-A, B-P-A."

Ed epitomized the BPA way. At one point, he stopped and asked a group of BPAers for complete silence while we "listened" to the forest— to birds we had never heard before, snakes slithering on the ground, bears moaning in the distance. Then we let out a couple of cries just to hear our voices echo.

The front of the pack probably did not do this.

For BPAers, being part of a real group rather than independent stragglers seemed to engender a sense of connection, of community, of validation. The bonds grew over the days as the course meandered north up Vancouver Island and ferried over to the Sunshine Coast on the British Columbia mainland. We even developed our own inside-joke routines that made fun of the *front* of the pack.

"Hey, how do you think Tinker did today?" I'd say to Ed whenever we had an audience.

"Tinker *WHO?*" he'd say loudly with his face twisted at the mention of the world's most famous mountain biker, Tinker Juarez, battling other endurance stars up at the front. "Tinker *WHO?*" Scattered laughter would ensue.

"How do we join the BPA?" a team of slow women from Alaska and New York asked at a checkpoint. "Join?" I replied. "If you're riding behind us, you *are* BPA!" The yucks spread as Ed and I dubbed ourselves "The First of the Worst."

All the BPA gaiety and the camaraderie were fine, but ultimately we came here to get a finisher's medal. Miss a cutoff, and we would be NOR—Not Officially Riding—which would shatter the happy BPA world we'd constructed and ruin what little respect we had left from the front- and mid-packers.

Finishing was not a given on Day 5, which socked us with 65 kilometers and 6,490 feet of climbing over some of the most physically and mentally demanding terrain I've ever seen.

It was seven hours of ducking branches; yanking your wheels over logs, roots, and rocks; juking your body every which way to shift mass and keep momentum even on the simplest trails; then swallowing hard and keeping a steady hand on the ubiquitous "aim-and-pray" bridges cobbled from fallen trees and wooden slats. It was a total-body workout, leaving forearms, hands, shoulders, and chest fatigued and aching. This was on the climbs. The descents were so rough that we'd have to stop just to bring our heart

rates down. The demand on your skills was so relentless that it seemed like graduate school for mountain bikers. By the time I was done, I'd never been this exhausted—or this good.

At any team event, you need a partner who can push it into a higher gear when the going gets tough. I've got that gear. Fortunately, as I hoped, so does Ed.

We were the only BPAers to make the 1 p.m. cutoff on Day 5. Ed looked at me when it was over. "Now, we ride not just for ourselves anymore," he said solemnly, without a hint of sarcasm, "but for all of the BPA."

Paul the Moonie

The reaction to our finishing Day 5 brought forth a rush of emotion from the BPA. At the start line on Day 6, two women who were blue-labeled (now riding with number plates marked by blue tape, indicating they were NOR) accused us of no longer being genuine BPA members. That hurt.

Ed and I lamented that our fellow BPAers would not get medals, and wanted to do something special for them. We had begun formulating an idea of presenting a slide show after the awards ceremony the final night. After all, we had pictures of everyone as well as hundreds of scenic and joke shots.

Ironically, as we discussed the show in the starting chute before Day 6 began, we were approached by a rider with an unusual request. "I'm tired of going so fast, so I split with my partner," said Paul Keller, a 49-year-old businessman from Seattle who'd been coming in two or three hours before us. "The word is that you guys go slow. Can I join you for today?"

Ed and I were leery. Did Paul understand just how slow we were, that we stopped to set up repeated auto-timer photos, that we were cofounders of the BPA? And on top of that, already on the cusp of the cutoff times, could we afford to be responsible for somebody else?

"Okay, man, but if you need to go ahead, do it," I said, figuring that he'd most likely get frustrated with our pace and leave us. In fact, I started actively talking about the BPA, figuring the concept would be so repugnant to him that it would scare him off.

But it wasn't. Paul hadn't heard of the BPA, but was intrigued. As we filled him in on BPA history and what it stood for, he grew more and more excited, as if he was having some sort of epiphany. We thought his awakening was an act, because he was out of sight after the first long climb. But at the bottom of the following descent, 15 minutes later, there he was, waiting for us. "I'll get used to this pace," he said.

At one point near the end of a fun day of riding and talking, of Paul posing for pictures ("Notice here how a young tree has grown out of a tree stump," he explained like a professor), riding behind us, shouting words of encouragement ("Great line, Ed!"), and talking about his young family and his booming commercial enterprises, he suddenly blurted out at the top of his lungs: "They just don't understand us! They just don't understand the BPA!"

Ed and I looked at each other with raised eyebrows. Paul had become more BPA than either of us. He had become a BPA Moonie!

At 2 p.m. of Day 7, a surprisingly, terribly hard day in and around Whistler that began with a straight-up, 1,500-foot climb, the three of us stopped dead in our tracks in the forest. "Look," said Paul, pointing eight feet off the trail.

It was The Chair.

Ed and Paul lifted me onto the decaying, red-orange loveseat. It creaked and cracked like it would fall apart any second. Ed snapped off the photos. I jumped off and the chair tumbled over. We carefully replaced it on the stump exactly as it had been, as if not to disturb the cosmic order.

As we rode on, babbling joyously about including The Chair in the slide show, and pondering the concept of finding "Chairness" in everything you do (heavy, huh?), I was suffused with a quiet pride. Ed and I had changed Paul to

the point where *we* were learning from *him*. After all, Paul was the one who insisted that we shoot the very symbol that epitomized the meaning of the Back of the Pack Association: The Chair.

Soon, we rode past a BC race worker who gave us alarming news: The checkpoint ahead would close in 15 minutes. That was impossible; the schedule called for another hour. Riders coming up behind us said the same thing. It was clearly a mix-up; we'd find the organizers and straighten it out at the finish. But as we and other teams stressed and strategized, Paul was silently freaking out; suddenly, wordlessly, like a fish pulling out of a hook, he bolted and was gone. His true nature broke free, like a front-of-the-pack wolf in BPA clothing. We never saw him again.

We rode in to the checkpoint and the finish at a steady pace, gathered together two dozen riders who'd been affected by the mix-up, and met with the race organizers, who admitted they'd made a timing mistake. With our medals around our necks, Ed and I became the very last official finishers of the BC Bike Race. Time: 55 hours and 21 minutes. That was four hours in back of the next-worst times in the general classification category, the 80-plus division and the 100-plus division, and double the time of the winners.

We were DFL—Dead Fricken Last—and incredibly happy. We bro-hugged, grabbed my computer, and headed for the hotel. We had a slide show to finish.

The Epiphany of The Chair

Five hours later in a Whistler bar, before 500 reveling BC riders and their families, with all but a couple dozen BPAers wearing the medals embossed with the Inuit totem-pole carving typical of the coastal British Columbia Indian tribes, we showed our slides, complete with the "Rocky" theme. The picture of me squatting red-faced over a pile of bear poop got a huge laugh. The shots of all the BPA members—including a shot of Tinker *WHO?* thrown in for good measure—got huge roars, and even some tears, I think. This, after all, was the BPAers' four seconds of fame—their finisher's medal. Almost everyone would come up and thank us afterward.

Then the big screen flashed with the shot of me sitting in The Chair. A giant wave of laughter and noise erupted—followed by confusion.

People looked at each other. Did you see that? No, I didn't see that. Where was that? How'd it get there? How in the world could I miss that? The questions never stopped coming at us when the show was over. Where did you guys get that chair?

Of course, it was right there in plain sight. Just eight feet off the trail.

Epilogue

At 1:00 a.m., Ed and I were eating hot dogs at a stand in the middle of Whistler Village when a short Aussie walked up with his entourage. He was a pro rider named Adrian Jackson. He and his teammate had finished third overall. "Hey, you're the guys who did the BPA slide show," he said. "Great work. Funny."

I looked at him. "Do you mind if I ask you a question?" I said. "Did you see The Chair?"

He looked down for a few seconds. "Mate," he said sadly, in his Down Under twang, "I didn't see The Chair. I didn't see the mountains. I didn't see the rivers. I didn't see the trees. I didn't see the people. For seven days, I only saw the ground and the rear wheel in front of me."

There was silence for a moment. Then he added, weakly, "Sometimes I do these things and I wish..."

These mountain bike stage races are all around the world now, and they are spectacular. Crossing the Alps from Germany to Austria to Italy. Crossing the Andes, the Rockies. Traversing Portugal, Crete, the Carpathian Mountains. Riding Pacific to Atlantic in Costa Rica and Mexico. Taking your body to the total-body, bone-jarring limit on the intricate, masterful

trails of British Columbia. They make you feel great to be alive.

Just make sure you have the right teammates along if you want to see them.

MOTIVATION CASE STUDY #6: DON'T LET AGE HOLD YOU BACK
At the Breck Epic, 65-year-old Wendy Skean showed 'em who's boss.

"Hey, you guys just got your ass kicked by a 65-year-old woman!"

Ed and I looked at each other, stunned. Those words, spoken by the timekeeper at the finish line on Day 3 of the 2009 Breck Epic mountain bike race, slammed us like a Mike Tyson uppercut and hung in the air like stale cigarette smoke. Then, as if our thoughts were molten lava bubbling up under a volcano ready to blow, we simultaneously erupted in one primal scream of shock, pain, and humiliation: *"Wendyyyy!"*

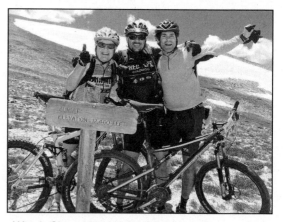

Wendy Skean, 65, caught young studs Roy and Ed near the top of the Breck Epic.

How in the heck did Wendy Skean, the kindly, white-haired sexagenarian first-grade teacher from Idyllwild, California, get ahead of two strapping, super-fit hunks at one of the hardest multiday mountain bike stage races in the world?

This is not to say that Wendy isn't worthy. Not your normal AARP poster girl, she's got a laundry list of off-road accomplishments. In 2002, at 58, she won the women's 45-plus division at the 24 Hours of Adrenalin Solo World Championships by riding 165 miles, including through a torrential storm that scared everyone else off the course. In 2005, she was the first and only woman over 60 to finish the Leadville 100 in under 12 hours, in 11:24; that was 30 minutes faster than she'd done it in 1998, when she became the event's oldest female finisher to that point. She's also the oldest woman to finish Vision Quest, the legendary Southern California off-road 50-miler with 11,000 feet of climbing.

Impressive. But, as the sarcastic timekeeper kept ribbing us, *she was 65!*

I know Wendy's story well. I profiled her in the first edition of *Bike for Life*. She began riding after her divorce at age 42, taking her two teenaged sons on mountain biking–bonding adventures all over the West. "It kept us a cohesive family unit," she said, "and it turned me into a hard-core rider." Over the years, the trio competed from Crested Butte to Big Bear. One boy became a serious bike racer. Both eventually ended up running bike shops. And both were here in Breckenridge, Colorado, at the Breck Epic to support her attempt to "push it to the next level," as she put it, at her first multiday stage race.

She picked a monster: The Epic is an insanely hard, six-day, 240-mile race, with 37,000 feet of climbing and gasping-for-breath elevations that begin in the city at 9,600 feet and top out on the trails at nearly 13,000 feet.

The altitude affects everyone differently. For an Orange County beach boy like me, it meant a desperate gasping for breath. I felt like I was sucking oxygen through a loofah sponge. But I couldn't blame the thin air (or my inability to sleep, or my jumpy stomach, or my constant, low-grade headache) for the Day 3 loss to Wendy. For that, I credit my tried-and-true stage-race philosophy: Goof-off as much as possible.

You see, my friend Ed Korb and I were proudly, unabashedly back-of-the-pack (as described in the previous section). At events like this, we don't worry about our times. Our focus isn't moving up a couple places in the standings; it's on stopping to read every information sign about abandoned mine shafts and gold-dredging machines, shooting pretty pictures, and posing in kooky photo-ops with oddball junk on the trails—abandoned snowmobiles, office chairs perched on tree stumps, and old shacks tipping sideways like amusement park funhouses. Ed and I see these events as tours, not races. But through it all, we still keep our eyes on the prize: the finisher's medal.

We didn't miss any of the cutoffs at the BC Bike Race in British Columbia the year before, and we wouldn't here. In fact, except for one day at La Ruta when my derailleur fell off and I separated my shoulder, I've never missed a cutoff at any other stage race I've done—including the TransAlp Challenge and the TransRockies Challenge. And I've never felt the need to beat anyone.

Still, I was kinda curious: How did a 65-year-old woman get ahead of us?

We rolled back to the condo after Stage 3, picked up a couple of barbecued chickens at the supermarket, and decided to laugh it off. Screw that finish-line worker and his taunting insinuations! Little old Wendy was no threat to our manhood. Besides, it wouldn't happen again, anyway. What she did was a once-in-a-million anomaly; we weren't going to let it cramp our style.

Then, lining up at the start of Stage 4 the next morning, we found out something weird: Wendy had also beaten us on Stage 2.

Again, so what? We weren't changing our style. Then something happened on Stage 4 that made us rethink our thinking.

The Rivalry

Stage 4 put the "epic" in Breck Epic. It featured a pair of brutal, beautiful, high-altitude climbs up French Pass and Georgia Pass to the Continental Divide, then took us home with the stunning and challenging single-track descents of the spectacular Colorado Trail. Our seven-hour ride, featuring 40 miles and 9,800 feet of elevation gain, was jammed with super photo-ops that reflected the unique iconography of the Breckenridge area and its indigenous mining culture. It's also the day that this event became a true mano-a-mano grudge match between me and the 65-year-old woman.

Stage 4 started off with a police escort that took all 110 riders to the trailhead. Even after three days of riding at elevation, I still had a headache, a nervous stomach, and the in-and-out wheezing of a lung-cancer patient on life support. As usual, as the day's initial 3,000-foot climb to French Pass began, we found ourselves in the back of the pack with "Big Jim," a hefty and happy single-speeder; "Complaining Debra," a first-time stage-race rider on a titanium 29er ("It's so hard to breathe"; "My darn gears are sticking"; "I couldn't sleep last night"; "My &%$#@ ass hurts!"); and, of course, Wendy Skean, lurking silently.

I didn't really give a thought to the little schoolteacher as we plowed several minutes ahead of her and the others, then let her pass by as we stopped repeatedly to photograph the awesome scenic views.

But soon Ed gave me some news that dramatically changed my laissez-fare attitude.

At Checkpoint 1, which came about halfway into the 12-mile ascent to 12,046-foot French Pass, Ed pulled in 5 seconds before me and overheard Wendy talking to one of her support-crew sons. "Yesterday, it took me the whole day to catch them, but today, I already caught up to them," she said proudly.

"Could 'them' be me and Roy?" Ed wondered.

Wendy left the checkpoint a few minutes before we did. Without saying anything to me, Ed suddenly bolted ahead, caught up to her after about 15 minutes, and began making casual conversation. "You really want to beat Roy, don't you?" he said.

"Like you can't believe!" Wendy replied.

As I ascended through the thinning air on my way to the pass, my breathing took on the tone of an asthmatic scuba diver. Soon, as the grade steepened, we were forced off our bikes into lurching steps as if we were walking on the moon. After a solid hour of moon walking, we'd passed Big Jim, Debra, and Wendy; passed the tree line; watched the surrounding grassy hills became striped with snow; and finally reached the top—a pile of rocks with an elevation post stuck in the middle. We set about shooting photos and happily greeted the lagging trio as they came up from behind us.

Then came the descent—2,000 feet of pure bliss. About 30 seconds down was a giant patch of snow about 200 yards wide. Of course, Ed and I shot goofy videos of us making snow angels and glissading for the next 10 minutes in the fluffy white wonder.

As we watched Wendy and Big Jim disappear down the hill into tiny specs, Ed decided the time was right to tell me what he'd heard earlier from Wendy.

"What?!" I shrieked. I couldn't believe it— Wendy, the woman I had written articles about, put in my book, and considered a friend, was taking this "competition" seriously! I wasn't quite sure what to do about it. Had I been back-stabbed, betrayed? Was my ego bruised? Would I become a laughingstock on the Internet? Was my reputation—*my manhood*—at risk of being destroyed by a 65-year-old woman?

Ed and I discussed it for a few minutes. Ed pointed out that there would be no shame in losing to Wendy—that she "was no ordinary 65-year-old, with mountain biking in her blood and race credentials longer than your arm."

"Think about it," said Ed. "Whereas you and I have each other to rely on for moral support, little Wendy is out here in the forest doing this crazy six-day event all alone, relying exclusively on her moral fortitude. Whereas this is our second big stage race in a year, she is completely inexperienced. And whereas we stop to eat three or four cans of sardines and several oranges and apples a day, she doesn't appear to require food at all.

"In other words, she *is* tougher than us. Whereas we are completely inconsistent with our riding, dilly-dallying all day and turning up the volume only if we need to make a checkpoint, Wendy is a hallmark of consistency, plugging along relentlessly, the little engine that could. If we stop for 5 or 10 minutes to eat or shoot a picture, she passes us. It's inevitable—we can't beat her. So accept it. Get her out of your mind. Don't let her wreck our fun. Don't get paranoid."

He was right. I had already begun likening Wendy to a hunter, a stalker, to the shark in *Jaws*, even the Terminator.

"Face it—Wendy has earned our deep, abiding respect as a furious competitor," said Ed. "Make no mistake: Give her an inch, and Wendy will kick your ass."

At that instant, something snapped inside me. I turned to Ed, dead serious. "Maybe so," I intoned gravely, "but from now on, she is not going to kick ours."

The Comeback

Wendy has a weakness: She gets scared on steep, technical downhills. We took full advantage of it, leapfrogging her on all the descents. Our downhill skills allowed us to ride through rocky areas where Wendy had to dismount and walk. Watching her from a distance, we marveled at how fast she moved on foot, often breaking into a run. Still, she couldn't hope to catch us.

At one point, we powered through a difficult river crossing with downed trees that acted as a makeshift bridge. The trees were slippery and flimsy.

I said to Ed, "Let's stop and help her."

"Are you sure?" he said.

"Don't worry about it," I replied. "There's still a lot more descent after this."

A second round of climbing began in earnest with a long, laborious, 2,000-foot ascent up Georgia Pass. When we stopped for a quick sardine break, who do you think passed us within a minute? The little white-haired Terminator from Idyllwild.

About 45 minutes later, when Ed and I reached the top of Georgia Pass at 11,585 feet, we naturally spent 15 minutes eating, stretching, doing push-ups, shooting the breeze with hikers, and snapping pictures with the Continental Divide information sign. And Wendy passed us again.

We weren't worried. An easy quarter-mile ride brought us to a monster 4,000-foot descent on the famed Colorado Trail, which became highly technical and even dangerous at times after it crossed back through the tree line. That meant we had a massive advantage. We followed her closely until there was room to pass. Wendy graciously pulled aside and we disappeared down the mountainside.

Ed and I stopped repeatedly on the descent to shake the cramps out of our hands, eat, and shoot more pictures. But now, there was an undercurrent of urgency. "Hurry," one of us would say. "She's coming!"

Actually, we didn't see Wendy for the rest of the day, but for the first time in a stage race, we began questioning one another: "Do we *really* have time to shoot *that* photo?"

When we came out of the mountains into the final stretch of Stage 4, we came across a giant mile-long rock pile, the leftovers from the gold-dredging machines that had decimated the local landscape 100 years ago. I insisted that we stop and shoot a photo. Ed, on edge like I'd never seen him before, nervously said, "No, we don't have time!" I had to laugh. After an entire day of being hunted by a human Jaws-on-wheels who was out to besmirch our collective manhood, Ed was getting paranoid, too!

We finished the day at 7 hours and 9 seconds. Wendy came in at 7 hours, 18 minutes. We'd been waiting for her with Big Jim, who had come in a few minutes before us, cameras ready. We let out a gigantic cheer when she crossed the finish line, and all posed together for a final shot before rolling into town.

We could tell Wendy felt great. And Ed and I looked at each other with unspoken pride, our battered *machismo* restored.

The Final Stretch

Ed and I were feeling pretty smug that night—we'd really showed Wendy who was boss. But at about 4 o'clock in the morning of Stage 5, I was awakened by a blood-curdling scream.

"*Roy!*"

"Ed, what, what, what—it's four in the morning! What the hell is wrong?"

"One word," he said. "*Cumulative.*"

My eyes went wide, and then I nodded in concern. No wonder he'd woken up screaming: She'd beaten us twice and we'd beaten her twice (including by three minutes on the short, steep time trial on Day 1), but we didn't know the cumulative time. Wendy could still be ahead of us in the GC. We didn't know how far ahead she finished on Days 2 and 3. So we could win Day 5 and still be behind overall.

"I know that Day 6, the final stage, is nontechnical, minimizing our advantage over the little Terminator," said Ed. "We need to pound it hard today—a 40-miler with 8,000 feet of elevation gain. Otherwise, we may forever be known as the two guys who lost to a 65-year old woman."

By the fifth day of sleeping at 9,000 feet and riding past 12,000 feet, you are drained. At this elevation, you simply don't recover. Your body moans and groans. You don't think straight.

Stage 5 began with a snail's-pace climb up to the ski resorts and the trailhead of the Peak to Peak Trail, altitude 10,100 feet. Meandering under and over the gondolas and ski lifts, we hit Checkpoint 1 at mile 14, which marked the start of the Wheeler Trail and a horrific 2,700 feet of steep traverses and false summits to an altitude of nearly 13,000 feet.

Ed, cursing the $5.99 eight-piece Chipotle chicken special he'd eaten during our "We-beat-Wendy" celebration the night before, slowed to a crawl on the two and a half hours of hike-a-bike drudgery. Guess who was the first person to pass him on his first of many bathroom breaks?

"Is everything okay?" A disembodied grandmotherly voice called out. It was Wendy, of course.

Pushing a bike on foot for endless miles at the top of the world is a walk-20-steps-and-stop-a-minute-to-breathe torture-fest, but even worse is waiting at the top to set up a photo at the summit sign in freezing, howling, 40-mph winds.

"Hurry up, Wendy, get over here for the photo!" I yelled out when she finally appeared on the horizon after about 10 minutes. The three of us posed with the summit sign, elevation 12,460 feet, as teammates bound forever by this incredible day. Wendy exited quickly and was 10 minutes down the mountain before Ed and I packed up. Half an hour later, we passed her, clearly struggling on the steep, technical, 3,000-foot descent. The endless rock gardens and another 1,000 feet of climbing that followed certainly didn't help her, either.

Ed and I finished Stage 5 in 7:19, hours behind the bulk of the riders. We were tired and beat up, but it could have been worse; we knew that Wendy was up there still fighting her way down the mountain. Ninety minutes later, showered and shaved, we arrived at headquarters for the rider dinner meeting and noticed a tiny white-headed body lying face down on the massage table. Wendy endured 29 more minutes of hell than we did, but you wouldn't have known it by the smile on her face.

"I hope you guys are going to be ready tomorrow," she said, her eyes crinkling with delight. "Because it's not over yet."

Okay, so maybe you get a little delusional at 65. But you gotta like that spunk.

Climbing 5,000 feet in the big and middle chainrings is chump change when you've been granny-gearing twice that elevation gain day after day. Stage 6 was a short day that topped out at "only" 11,500 feet; we finished with Big Jim and Complaining Debra in just under four hours—double the times of the pros. Then the announcer began the countdown: "Wendy, Wendy, Wendy!"

Nobody left the venue as the fluorescent-green-and-pink-clad first-grade teacher descended toward the finish line. When Wendy crossed the threshold, we seated her in an easy chair we'd placed there and handed her a beer. The teetotaler took a swig and posed with curious onlookers as if she were the queen of mountain biking—or at least the queen mother.

Later that night at the Breck Epic dinner and awards ceremony, as Ed and I were sitting at a table with Wendy and her sons, she was called up on stage. "We all want to be like Wendy when we grow up," said the announcer. The crowd gave her a standing ovation.

"I feel honored and humbled," Wendy said to the audience. "I'm not any more special than anyone else here. Mountain biking is just something I love doing and I don't want to stop." She doesn't plan to, expecting to ride 100 miles at age 100, a not-impossible goal given her genes—her mom lived to age 101, her dad to 95.

When Wendy got back to the table, absolutely glowing, she looked at me and smiled. "And by the way, I did want to beat you in the worst way," she said. "But don't take it personally. At every race I do, I always pick someone to beat. You just happened to be there. But I had no illusions. I knew your male pride would kick in eventually."

Full Speed at 70

Five years later, I called Wendy to tell her I was going to put our battle in the book. She was 70. She did the Breck Epic again in 2010 and cut an hour off her time. Setting her sights on being the first 70-year-old to break the 12-hour time at the 2014 Leadville, she did a bunch of races in 2013 and early 2014, including the 24 Hours of Old Pueblo, where she won third place in the overall single-speed category "against women in their 20s and 30s," she says. Having retired from teaching after 34 years in 2012, Wendy was riding every day and was supremely confident. "My skills and engine are better," she said. A new 29er taught her how to plow over rough stuff instead of walking. A single-speed improved her out-of-the-saddle climbing and strength, as did a weight program. Unfortunately, six weeks off the bike in June due to a broken tibia left her undertrained for Leadville 2014. She DNFed at mile 75. "No big deal," she says. "I'll break the 12-hour mark in 2015 at age 71."

"I will always ride, and I will always have goals, no matter what age. When I hit 60, I realized life begins at 60. Now that I'm 70, life begins at 70. After that, it'll be 'life begins at 80.'"

As for me, I'll be 67 by then—and you can bet that I'll be training hard. Because I don't want some punk at a checkpoint razzing me with, "Hey man, you just got your ass kicked by an 80-year-old woman."

MOTIVATION CASE STUDY #7: TURN A BUSINESS TRIP INTO A BIKE TRIP

Tack a few extra days on after a meeting, grab a bike, and get yourself an epic Italian cycling vacation.

One early August day in 2011, I dropped a $12,000 bike.

In the slow-motion, frame-by-frame playback of my mind, the flawless $12,000 bike departs from my grasp, plummets agonizingly to the ground, then rattles on the concrete. I will for 10 days in the 2011 Tour de France, which had ended about two weeks before. Millions of rabid cycling fans had watched this bike on TV every day with lust in their hearts. To drop it to the blacktop of a parking lot, however unintentionally, was pure sacrilege.

To make it even worse, Ernesto Colnago, the legendary bike builder, the octogenarian whose name was on this $12,000 bike, and on the building behind us, was there to personally witness the horror. He stood frozen in silence, too shocked to speak. So were the half-dozen cycling journalists who had just toured his Milan-area Colnago factory with me.

When we got back to the bus, they unloaded. "You're an idiot!" "You're a disgrace to the bike industry!" "You fool! Mr. Colnago himself *gives* you a $12,000 bike—and you not only drop it but put $10 flat pedals on it!"

I had to laugh. They weren't really mad, I decided. They were *jealous.*

You see, I was staying in Italy for four more days, while my press-trip pals were flying home. They hadn't thought to ask the travel agent to change their departure date, or to borrow a bike for a few days, so they could take a bike trip around Lake Como. And now, the reason they were jealous was that, while they were rushing home for no apparent reason, I would be

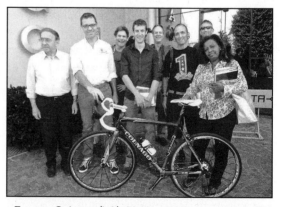

Ernesto Colnago (left) thinking, "What have I done?" as he hands his beloved C59 Italia off to Roy (third from left) for a bike tour of Lake Como.

never forget the stunned faces around me convulsing in horror. For a cyclist, this bike was a combination of the Hope Diamond and the *Mona Lisa.* It was a Colnago C59 Italia, at that moment one of the most sought-after bikes on the planet.

You see, the C59 Italia was the same carbon-fiber dream machine that Thomas Voeckler had just ridden while wearing the yellow jersey heading into the Alps, circumnavigating one of the most picturesque bodies of water in the world, and maybe even running into George Clooney, who has a lakefront home there. I'd also be seeing the bucket-list sight that every cyclist must see in his or her lifetime: the Madonna del Ghisallo, the world-famous "cyclists' church," the little shrine often seen in the Giro d'Italia that was officially blessed by a pope as home to the mystical "patron saint" of cycling.

That I'd be doing it on a $12,000 bike—a $12,000 work of art with hidden cables, 22-speed Campagnolo Record gears, and octagonal-shaped carbon-fiber lugged tubing—was frosting on the cake. It was completely unexpected. During the factory tour, Mr. Colnago had just asked me what I wanted. Of course, I replied, "a C59 Italia."

I was shocked when he gave it to me. I'd expected to rent a cheap mountain bike so I could also go off-road. I never ride trails clipped in, which accounts for the cheap $10 pedals. It was like wearing flip-flops with a tuxedo.

Regardless of the footwear interface and the fact that I suddenly raised my mileage and sightseeing goals, the point of this is not about how awesome it is to ride around the world's most bike-loving country on a super-bike that millions of people had been drooling over on TV—although that is pretty awesome. The point is that, if you're a cyclist, you can easily and inexpensively turn a business trip into a bike trip. The plane ticket is already paid for by your company; just fly home on Sunday instead of Thursday, and you get a three-day cycling vacation. When your business is over, lock your computer and luggage in the Hilton's closet, rent a bike, and go exploring some cool new cycling turf for a few days. For the cost of a few nights at cheap hotels, you get a full-bore cycling vacation.

Forget the hassle of bringing your own bike; any decent rental will work. A brand-new $12,000 Colnago C59 Italia will do in a pinch.

The Passion

Riding a great bike makes any ride better, but riding this bike in this country was a whole different story. About 25 miles north of my start at the famous Duomo, the cathedral in central Milan, I stopped at a McDonald's in the town of Lentate. There, as I laid out my map of the Lombardy region on a table to check my route, I was approached by a boisterous 70-year-old on a mountain bike.

"*Vedo che hai la passione!*" he boomed, as I gulped a spoonful of pistachio McFlurry.

The kid behind the counter helped translate. "I can see you have the passion," was the English.

I smiled with pride. "*Ah, la passione! Si signor,* you no doubt have noticed my energetic athleticism, my infectious *joie de vivre*, my swashbuckling sense of adventure?"

"No," said the old man. "I noticed your bike." He pointed to the words "Colnago C59 Italia" on the frame, and gave me the thumbs-up.

That's how it was the rest of the ride. Whether on the road or stopped at a market, heads would turn and fingers would point at the Italian uberbike they'd all seen on TV. Actually, I got paranoid, keeping the bike cable-locked even within touching distance, and never out of my sight. Imagine the look on Mr. Colnago's face if I called with news that his $12,000 bike had been stolen.

Another 20 miles brought me to Lake Como, a vacation wonderland since Roman times. It was easy to see why: The southern edge of the Alps plunge down to a shoreline teeming with red-tile-roofed villas, soaring bell towers, and intricate sculpture gardens. Fishermen and windsurfers ply the waters while everyone from middle-class families to Ferrari-driving plutocrats crowd miniature golf courses, kiddy parks, campsites, and resorts. Even the cheapest accommodations had class. It was only 17 euros (about $24) for a bunk at the famous hostel, the Ostello della Gioventu, situated high on a hill over the highway in the western-shore town of

Menággio. Its best feature is a gigantic dining-room picture window with stunning panoramas of two-legged Lake Como, which is shaped like an upside-down Y. A ferry ride away, in the crotch of the "legs," were the shimmering lights of Bellagio, the storied playground of the rich and the starting point for the big climb to the Madonna del Ghisallo.

With three days to ride, I was saving the church, the highlight of the trip, for last. So on Day 2, I headed west and made a big climb over to Lake Lugano in the Italian-speaking part of Switzerland. After circling Lugano, I headed back to Italy and went around the north end of Lake Como, arriving at the ferry landing in Bellagio at dinnertime.

Bellagio is like Beverly Hills with boats, a glittery glam-fest of jewelry shops, five-star restaurants, $8 gelatos, and $500-a-night hotel rooms. After a fun 100-mile day, I sat down on a lakeside park bench while waiting for the ferry back to my hostel in Menággio and retrieved a gigantic Toblerone chocolate bar from Switzerland out of my backpack. Then I surveyed the lake and craned my neck at the mountain behind Bellagio that led to the Ghisallo, which I'd be climbing the next day.

Prayers Are Answered

Visiting the various castles and museums lining the Lake Como shore could keep you busy for a year. But now, on Day 3 of the trip, I was here to see only one building—the little cyclist church on the mountain. So about 10:30 a.m., I took the ferry back to Bellagio and started up the hill. And I mean up: grades of 8 to 14 percent.

An elevation gain of 1,811 feet in 6.6 miles won't kill you. But it does earn you the same bragging rights as Giro di Lombardia riders, who do it every year (it's in the Giro d'Italia frequently, but not always). And it leaves you at one of the cycling world's most unique and venerated shrines.

According to medieval legend, a count named Ghisallo was saved from an attack by bandits on

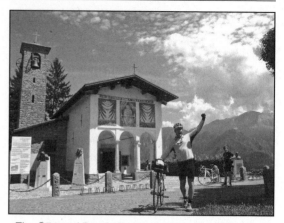

The C59 and Roy at the iconic Madonna del Ghisallo, the church of the "Patron Saint of Cycling."

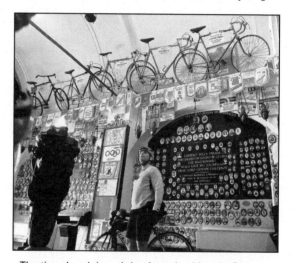

The tiny church is a shrine featuring historic Giro d'Italia and Tour de France bikes and memorials to killed riders.

a hilltop by the sudden appearance of the Virgin Mary. As promised, in her honor he built a church on the site. The apparition and the site became known as the Madonna del Ghisallo. In 1949, after the hill became a frequent and much-loved part of the two Giros, Pope Pius XII proclaimed the Madonna to be the "Patron Saint of Cycling." Nowadays, the shrine, barely big enough to hold eight or nine people at once, is a pocket cycling museum and memorial visited by cyclists on training rides and busloads of weekend tourists. A big cycling museum, loaded with a couple hours' worth of photos, articles, and bikes of the greats, was built 50 yards away on the same hill in 2006. When it was completed, Pope Benedict XVI was there to bless the cornerstone.

After about 90 minutes of riding and stopping for photo-ops of Lake Como's spectacular eastern gorge, I crested the peak and saw the tall bell-tower of the tiny church. Slipping under its tall, dramatic portico, I entered the tiny sanctuary, no bigger than 10 by 15 feet. Ten bikes, five on each side, line the rafters—among them those of the famous (Merckx, Coppi, Gimondi), the innovative (Moser's mismatched-disc, hour-record "funny" bike), and the tragic (Fabio Casartelli, who died in a Tour de France crash). On the walls are hundreds of names and dozens of photos of the dead in oval tile frames—all ages, including unknown 18-year-old kids like Simone Soriga and Marelli Paolo, both killed in 2005 while riding. While I was inside, a mother left roses under a photo of her deceased cyclist son. Outside, examining the busts of Coppi and Bartali in the front of the church, I marveled at the steady stream of riders coming up from both sides of the mountain, even though it was a Friday, not the weekend. I'm not Catholic, but I'm a disciple of cycling, a believer in the holy trinity of road, mountain, and tandem. Yeah, I got a bit misty-eyed.

But there was no time for crying. I looked at my watch: 1:15 p.m. I had to get the C59 back to the Colnago factory by 4 p.m., when the company would shut down for the month of August, along with half of Italy. And so began a madcap two-hour dash to the little village of Cambiago, 15 miles east of Milan. I don't know the exact distance because I cannot retrace my seat-of-the-pants navigation methodology, but with the long 1,300-foot descent due south off the mountain and the endless big-ring climbs over hilly roads heading southeast, I'm guessing 45 miles. Totally wired, I did not sit down once, hammering to my limit the whole time. (Only while writing this,

two years later, do I realize that I had backup if the factory closed, as Mr. Colnago lives in a big villa right across the street from the factory.)

I arrived back at the Colnago plant 45 minutes before closing. Mr. Colnago came over and I thanked him. I laid out my Lombardy map on the counter. He speaks no English, and I no Italian, but when I traced my route with my finger and guessed I'd gone maybe 420 kilometers—about 250 miles—he bugged-out his eyes, said "wow," and hugged me on the shoulder as if I were some kind of superman.

Colnago seemed genuinely impressed, but I had to wonder why. After all, pro riders routinely dwarf this mileage over several training days, and an average club rider can pedal me into the ground.

Then I realized that Colnago himself, just like racers, club riders, and my journalist buds, simply can't conceive of riding a bike unless it's for racing, training, or a charity AIDS ride, not just for the sheer fun and adventure of taking a tour to some famous, bucket-list place. I don't know why. Maybe the time and organization required of touring are too iffy. Maybe the stereotype of bike tourists as hippie-granola nerds is too entrenched. Whatever the reason, hard-core roadies don't seem to do it.

They don't know what they're missing. No matter when or where you go, a bike tour is always a cool adventure. But if you travel occasionally for your job, and therefore can trick your company into paying for most of it (I spent about $150), it's even cooler. And if you get ahold of a fast bike to do it on, $12,000 or not, it is truly unforgettable.

MOTIVATION CASE STUDY #8: START A RIDING STREAK
Scott Dickson and Jim Langley have ridden every day for decades.

A lot of people say they've been riding bikes for 20 or 30 years. Jim Langley and Scott Dickson can say that—literally. Rain or shine, sick or well, without missing even one day, these two accomplished, lifelong cyclists haven't let travel or family tragedies or football games get in the way of their daily rides for decades.

SCOTT DICKSON: Almost 40 Years

Riding every day for 30 years, a milestone that 64-year-old Scott Dickson reached in May 2013, doesn't fully explain the scope of his accomplishment, according to the esteemed racer and retired Iowa college professor of environmental geography. The streak should have been 40 years long, he said.

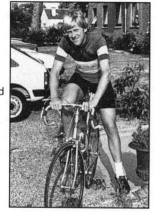

The legendary Scott Dickson has hardly missed a day since he began his riding streak four decades ago.

Two accidents cost him a decade. Hooked on cycling after doing some touring in high school and racing in college, Dickson said that the idea of the streak arose in May 1973. "After a long, rainy weekend in grad school, I felt so terrible from the inactivity that I decided to ride every day the rest of my life," he explained. He rode daily for the next seven years and seven months. Then, during a Texas criterium, he was hit by a truck and suffered a punctured lung, broken ribs, and a broken shoulder. Back in the saddle in 45 days, he rode daily for two years straight until injuries from another crash cost him two weeks off the bike. So the current 30-year streak officially began in May 1983.

Dickson is a veteran of more than 1,000 races and has a legendary résumé. He's proudly done every RAGBRAI (the weeklong ride across Iowa—41 of them as of 2013!) and has won races at all distances, from time trials to ultra-endurance events, including three wins at the 1,200-kilometer Paris-Brest-Paris randonnée (1987, '91, '95). He claims to have ridden 810,000 total lifetime miles, with 660,000 of those coming during his three-decade streak. He averages about 40 miles a day, 300 miles a week, and 10,000 miles a year, down from 500 or 600 a week and 23,000 miles a year in his younger days.

For a day to count as an official ride, Dickson has adjusted his requirements over the years from 20 miles to 3 miles. All the while, one factor must remain constant: The ride must be outdoors.

While this personal rule presented problems in the snow, sleet, and ice storms of wintertime Iowa, the source of most of his dozen or so 3-mile mountain bike rides, his most anxiety-ridden day came in February 2010 after a surprise 27-inch snowfall in Delaware, where he and his wife retired several years ago.

"It was touch and go waiting for the snowplows," he said. "I was getting pretty owly (Iowaese for "grumpy") until they came in the late afternoon." He'll ride with lights if he has to.

"I usually plan ahead," he said. An inveterate Weather Channel watcher, Dickson will often get out after midnight to get in the next day's ride before a storm is set to hit. He often uses the same strategy to handle travel days. For long overnight trips in the United States or to Europe, he'll arrange to have a bike waiting for him.

"The only problem [with maintaining the streak] is that I can't go to Australia and China," said Dickson. "That would require losing a day when flying west and crossing the International Date Line." (He said he was warming up to the idea of someday seeing Asia by traveling east around the world, which wouldn't cost him a day.)

Other than that, there have been no

downsides to the streak. He started it before he married his wife, who served as his crew chief at his P-B-P races. "It keeps me in shape and provides motivation and continuity," said Dickson, who has no children. He mainly rides a carbon-fiber Virtuosity, with another road bike and a mountain bike always ready, as well as a couple of old "beater bikes" for riding around town. "One thing I miss about not racing anymore is that I used to get bikes free," he said.

In a life defined by cycling, Dickson said he will remain a purist to the end. He does no yoga. No weight lifting. No running. No swimming. "It's always been 100 percent cycling. Barring accidents, I will continue the streak to the end."

JIM LANGLEY: Two Decades and Counting

A top Northern California Masters racer well-known to millions of cyclists as a longtime technical editor at *Bicycling* magazine in the 1990s, and since then on the Roadbikerider.com website, Jim Langley completed his two-decade streak on December 30, 2013. It started with a streak of envy.

"In 1990, I got jealous as I watched a couple of my fellow *Bicycling* editors, Ed Pavelka and Fred Matheny, set a record for the fastest relay team crossing of the United States in the Race Across America," he said. "I wanted to do something,

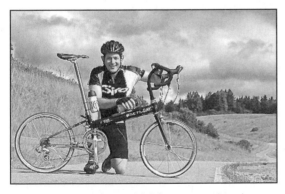

Jim Langley says he wouldn't have a two-decades-long streak without his trusty Bike Friday Pocket Rocket.

too." So he went outside and rode his bike for an hour. Then he did it every day for three years straight, until he hit a patch of black ice, broke his hip, and was off the bike for six days.

"That really annoyed me," he said. "Three years wasted. But since I turned 40 that year, I figured I may as well keep going." He put his bike shorts and jersey on, hobbled over to a stationary bike in the rehab room, screwed a clipless pedal on, and spun with his good leg for an hour.

That set the tone for the next 20 years. Langley's rule is that he can ride indoors or out, but it must be a serious effort of an hour or more. "I never said it had to be hard and that I had to suffer, but it has to be a 'real ride'—not easy," he said. "That means no gym shorts and sneakers; you gotta suit up, with cycling shoes."

"Ten years came and went so fast," he said. "So I decided to shoot for 20." The streak was in jeopardy only twice—both during overseas travel. In 2009, a cancellation and an all-day delay of a vacation flight to Maui with his wife, Deb, finally deposited him at Kahului airport at 9:45 p.m. Raining, pitch black, with the only route a winding, two-lane road all the way to the condo, Langley put together his trusty Bike Friday Pocket Rocket, a custom folding bike, in the back seat of the rental car as his wife fumed.

"You're crazy, you'll die!" she worried. "You don't have any lights!"

He finally convinced her to drive over to a 7-Eleven, where he bought a flashlight, batteries, and duct tape. By 10:30, he'd fashioned his own handlebar lighting system.

"I was almost run over by 18-wheelers twice," he said. "But I got the hour in, with 30 minutes to spare. My wife was fine in the morning."

Langley's closest call came in England in 1997 on a trip to interview Alex Moulton, engineer of another collapsible bike that has now morphed into a whole series of models sold under his Moulton brand. Arriving bike-less with just two hours left to ride, Langley was so jet-lagged that he nodded off for 45 minutes. Just in time, he woke up and frantically started knocking on doors until he found someone with a bike he could borrow. A terrifying hour on a narrow, heavily trafficked country rode left him shaken, but he'd kept the streak alive. After that, he never traveled without his Bike Friday. ("It flies free as regular luggage," he said. "It's saved me thousands over the years.")

Despite the occasional family stress, equipment breakdowns, and necessary 5 a.m. rides in Las Vegas during the annual Interbike convention in September ("It's frightening—everyone out then is drunk," he said), Langley said his streak has lots of great benefits. "You get sick a lot less, get multitasking time to watch movies and listen to NPR and audiobooks, and it makes you very optimistic, because you always have something to look forward to." he said. "And there are real performance benefits: You never lose your biking mojo, like you do when you're off the bike for a while, and you get great active recovery."

If pure performance is any guide, Langley's streak is a grand success. A lifelong cyclist who owns 70 bikes and set the 1-mile record on a big-wheel Penny Farthing at the Stanford track, he has podiumed frequently in NorCal district Masters races, including a third place in the 55-plus age group in the 2012 40K time-trial championship (in 55:13, or 25 mph) and a second place in the 2013 road race 60-plus division.

Langley gets his recovery from hard races and training days while watching movies on his trainer, follows a rigorous stretching routine, and for strength does step-ups, push-ups, and crunches. He loves mountain biking, but finds that it "de-trains" him because it is too hard for recovery but not hard enough to elicit gains.

When his streak hit 20 years in December 2013, Langley thought about ending it—then decided to go for another 20. "In life, you have to pretend you're 80, and look back and ask, 'Am I going to be disappointed that I stopped when I was 60?' If the answer is yes, then push on."

MOTIVATION CASE STUDY #9: DO GOOD
John Wordin gives hope to disabled vets with adaptive bikes and Ride2Recovery.

The rocket-propelled grenade that hit Matt De-Witt in Iraq in 2003 at age 26 didn't just blow off his hands and forearms. It blew away eight years of joy. "I loved mountain biking, but couldn't do it with the Civil War–era hooks I wore below my elbows," he said. "I tried once in 2005, and I crashed after two seconds on my driveway. I couldn't brake or switch gears." So the resident of Weare, New Hampshire, went to school, bought a house, had a son, ballooned 40 pounds (up to 210), and got more depressed every year until 2011—when a tip from the Veterans Administration led to a surprise phone call that changed his life.

"Ride with us," said John Wordin. "We have a bike for you."

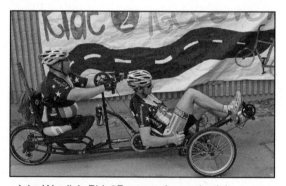

John Wordin's Ride2Recovery has revived the spirits of thousands of wounded veterans.

Wordin is the founder of Ride2Recovery, an organization that stages rides for disabled vets and supplies them with adapted bikes. He sent DeWitt a ticket to R2R's Fall 2011 Honor Ride in Las Vegas, and there he greeted him with a road bike with a special butt-brake actuated by a bar on the back of the seat and an electronic Di2 shifting set-up that featured paddles connected to the top tube that shifted gears when pushed by the knees.

"This thing's a rocket!" DeWitt remembered thinking. He was off the back on the 40-mile ride but exhilarated as he learned how to ride again. "I immediately felt my life returning." Within two years, he'd lost 40 pounds and was competing in one of the world's toughest mountain bike events, the Leadville 100.

This kind of metamorphosis was exactly what Wordin hoped would happen when he founded Ride2Recovery. "I got into cycling from a rehab point of view myself, so I knew about the sport's mental and physical healing power," he said.

In 1985, Wordin was a 6-foot-5, 260-pound defensive end on the Cal State Northridge football team who was told by his doctor to lose weight or risk destroying his knees. Within six months, he had lost 60 pounds and had taken second place in his first bike race, the Rose Bowl Road Race, as a Category 4 amateur. By the 1990s, he was founding the NutraFig and Mercury professional teams. The latter eventually became one of the top US domestic squads. Gaining renown for his organizational ability, Wordin was contacted by the City of Los Angeles about starting 5K events for kids, which ultimately led to the creation of the Fitness Challenge Foundation, the organization behind R2R. In the kids' events, which are noncompetitive, participants can run, walk, ride bikes, or even skate.

In September 2007, Wordin got a call from the Palo Alto Veterans Administration about creating a cycling rehab program for vets. A ride with one active veteran taught him about how cycling had changed the vet's life and led Wordin to create the national Ride2Recovery program. "I thought, 'This is what I have to do with my life,'" he said. "By January '08, I was in the VA's national office in DC. That's pretty fast."

Today, Ride2recovery, a 501(c) charitable nonprofit corporation, makes its own adaptive bikes. As of fall 2013, it had staged 35 Challenge Rides, which are weeklong 350- to 400-mile rides of 200 people each, about 75 percent of them

wounded vets. More than 7,000 people overall have ridden routes such as San Francisco to Los Angeles, and Boston to New Jersey. Some 10,000 wounded vets have participated in Project Hero, which uses cycling-based rehab at military bases.

"We've saved a lot of people—many people who would have committed suicide," Wordin said. "We've helped put them on a path to a productive life."

The benefits have been so profound that cycling has become a commonly used therapy for several federal agencies. Governments in France, Germany, and the Netherlands have asked Wordin to help them build similar programs.

Matt DeWitt understands why. "The freedom, the speed, the excitement, and the accomplishment all make you forget your limitations and your troubles," he said. After his first ride in Las Vegas in 2011, DeWitt went home and, with his dad and the local bike shop, put together a Di2-equipped mountain bike, which he rode 6,000 feet up Mt. Washington in the spring of 2012. He then did Ride2Recovery's seven-day Minute Man Challenge from Boston to New Jersey and the Gulf Coast Challenge from New Orleans to Tallahassee, Florida.

Then came the big one in 2013: the Leadville 100. Awarded one of Ride2Recovery's two Leadville slots, DeWitt finished one of the world's toughest off-road races in 11 hours, 6 minutes, earning a silver belt buckle. More importantly, it signaled that he was back, ready to move forward.

"Everyone on Ride2Recovery calls it their therapy, and it's true," said DeWitt. "It changed my life for the better; now I feel like I can do anything." He's finished his degree in landscaping and environmental engineering, is planning to start a nursery, and hopes to serve as a role model for other wounded vets trying to become whole again.

Mike Sinyard

FIGURING OUT THE FUTURE

The Henry Ford of modern cycling—or the Thomas Edison? Time and time again, Mike Sinyard has identified a tiny, under-the-radar trend, mass-produced it, and improved it somehow. In 1980, after six years of importing European components, making touring tires, and tiptoeing into bike manufacturing with several racing and touring bikes, his Specialized Bicycle Components changed the bike world. Sinyard took a new invention for off-road riding called the mountain bike, then offered by a couple of local Bay Area custom-bike makers, and retooled it for the assembly line. He was stunned when 450 Specialized Stumpjumpers sold that year and abruptly changed the direction of an industry. Before long, his small Morgan Hill, California, company had become a colossus, and it stayed that way by pouring millions into mountain bike racing and developing some of the leading dual-suspension designs over the next two decades.

All the while, Sinyard didn't ignore dedicated roadies, who he felt were asking for street bikes with more comfort. Adopting the mantra "Comfort Equals Performance," Specialized has pushed the development of a new generation of comfort road and racing bikes to address the needs of an aging enthusiast base who are a lot like him: over 50 and still hammering. In his case, as he told Bike for Life *in his March 2004 and January 2014 interviews, it's over 200 miles per week during long road*

and off-road rides in the coastal mountains of the Bay Area.

I GREW UP in San Diego on a little farm with a thousand chickens and rabbits; my mom sold the eggs in the front of the house and my dad was a machinist, and he could fix anything. I was very close with my dad. He never made much money; he used to say, "It doesn't matter how much money you make, it matters what you do with the money you do make." Our house stuff was good because he could make anything. We always had a great big shed in the back where we had a ton of old materials, something you could beat into shape. My dad was always the guy who'd walk around and find a bolt on the ground. And he'd pick it up. He'd go, "Hey, I might be able to use this!"

I was seven when he bought me my first bike at the Goodwill. It was a girl's bike—one of those where somebody had painted the whole bike and tires with a spray can. So we fixed up that bike and I rode it around. As for being a girl's bike, I didn't know much difference. The step-through frame made it easy because it was so big, with 26-inch wheels. Just a few turns of the crank and you were flying on this big ole thing. So that's how I started riding. I really used to love it. In fact, as a kid, sometimes I would have some of the neighborhood guys over, we'd get up in the middle of the night and go riding. At night you feel like you're going so fast. We'd sneak out all the time to ride the dirt roads through the canyon. In daylight, we'd make dirt jumps and wooden jumps. I loved that.

Then it just really developed. A lot of working on bikes. My dad got bikes, fixed 'em, I painted 'em, and we would go to the flea market. So that's really how it started.

I almost cannot remember a time when I wasn't intrigued with bikes. There probably was a little time in high school when I had a motorcycle and thought a bike was a little bit pedestrian. That lasted for a year or two. But then I went back to the bike. I used to take bike trips with friends. And then when I went to college [San Diego Mesa College, then San Jose State], and I didn't drive a car around, I really became connected up with bikes again. Out of college, I wasn't into racing, but I had a nice road bike—a Peugeot U-08, which I took apart and painted. A 10-speed—two in the front and the freewheel in the back. That is when I really began to appreciate high-quality bikes. My specialty was long-distance riding—the double centuries and stuff like that. I was okay at those kind of things, and sort of had to be. Because out of college I sold my van, and I went seven years with no car at all.

When I was in school and a little bit after school, I made a living by fixing old bikes to sell at the flea market. I put an ad in the paper. One ad. And I'd make it a little bit generic: "Nice bike completely rebuilt. Real reliable. Call." I wouldn't list the price and I had about twenty bikes. They'd call and I'd say, "Well what are you looking for?" I'd have probably a bunch in progress and maybe five or six that were already done. If somebody wanted something else I could whip it up.

These were pretty basic bikes—kinda college bikes. And I couldn't really afford the more high-end bikes. But as I got nicer bikes I realized there was a great opportunity for high-end bikes. At that time, in 1969, 1970, there weren't really high-end parts available in the US, except for a few shops that imported directly. So I said to myself, "Hey! When I get out of school, I want to go over to Europe and meet these really great companies that make these products." Most people in the US weren't aware of those companies. At that time, when you went around in cycling shoes and black shorts, you looked like a dork.

The Big Score in Italy

I WAS SO sick of school. So I went to Europe. Rode the bike around a while. Went to the Oktoberfest. Partied up a little bit. I met this one guy who had a bike shop in Holland. And I went there—just outside Amsterdam. Worked in the bike shop for a couple weeks. Fixed some flats and partying. What a life! Can you imagine working in a bike shop in Amsterdam when you're like 23 or something? Then I rode all the way from Amsterdam down through Barcelona. Over to Bonn. Three months. Only spent $350, because I usually slept outside. Had a fantastic time. All self-contained with a sleeping bag and everything.

And then I went to Milano, stayed in a youth hostel and met a woman. I said I was really into bikes. She goes, "Hey, I met Gino Cinelli before." I said. "Wow! Let's go over there!" I had $1,500 in traveler's checks that I got for selling my Volkswagen van. I bought a suit, so I wouldn't just look like a bum. And I went over there and I said I was pretty impressed with their products, their philosophy, and what they had done. And I told Gino that I knew many of the high-end riders in the US and there was a big demand for high-end products. He said, "Sure, we'll sell ya." And I thought, I can't believe he would sell me.

So that was it. I bought those products. And once I bought that, you know, I came home immediately. I primarily bought Cinelli handlebars, which were in short supply. I shipped them home. That was the start of it.

And I thought, Wow, this is great. Now there's access to all these great parts. I called a lot of the bike shops I knew when I got back. I said, "Hey, I got these great parts." They said, "Where'd ya get that? You steal it?" I said, no, I had contacts in Italy. And then essentially the stores bought those products, and I had a lot of the dealers pay in advance.

I decided to call the company Specialized because I always admired the Italian companies that were really the artisans. Artigiani, they call 'em—really focused on doing beautiful work. And in Italy they say "Spe-ci-al-eee-zed." Which means you are really into it. I thought that's the right name for us. I didn't check trademark or anything. I didn't want to call this Mike's Bike Stuff. That's lame.

Soon, I was importing all those products from Italy, when the idea to make my own tires came up. I was importing some Italian clincher tires that were terrible. They would always get bubbles and snake and stuff like that. I told the factory. They said to me, "You must be doing something wrong. Nobody else has a problem with these at all." At first I said, "Well, maybe that's right." Then I thought, "These guys are pulling my leg!" And I say, "You know what? I am sick of this. And I'm not going to sell products that have this kind of quality." So then I started looking. I'm going to make our own tires.

People know us for the mountain bike. But the tire thing was kinda what Specialized was initially known for. It was the tires that really kick-started the company.

I was 25. I got a little experience with manufacturing about that time when I met Jim Blackburn, a really famous designer now known for his racks. He was doing a master's thesis at San Jose University on how to design and develop a product and take it to market. I was selling Claude Butler European racks. And he says, "Man, I could make a better one than that out of aluminum." I said, "Great! Let's do it. I'll buy the first hundred."

So, I just knew there was an opportunity to make a great clincher tire. I was riding 300 miles a week and I knew other people that were, too. I intuitively knew what would be right on the product. I looked around the world and found the best manufacturer for tires in Japan. I don't know if I want to mention the company. We got the tires and we got started really selling a lot of tires. The company really started taking off. Then the guy from the tire company in Japan came over to visit me—and he said, "Geez, this guy is operating out of a shed. He doesn't even have a typewriter!"

Yeah, I was working in a shed at this trailer that I lived in. It was an 8- by 35-foot trailer. And all the products, when I get 'em, I just store 'em under the trailer until they were sold. I would usually sell out of everything in a couple days and get another shipment.

No creature comforts. I put it all back into the product.

A bigger, rival bike company in Los Angeles got the Japanese company to cut me off. But then I found another Japanese manufacturer that was even better that would listen to my requirements more. I would say that I definitely learned a lot from the different cultures. From the Italian culture and then probably the most from the Japanese.

I really respected the Italians' passion and dedication to the product and design. Everything with the Italians is about how it looks. And what I learned from the Japanese was attention to the smallest, smallest detail. No detail was too small.

I made quite a few trips to Japan—that's what really got the company going at that time. Sometimes we'd get these big shipments of tires in. So many tires I couldn't store it in the warehouse. Just had the container there for a couple days until we sold 'em all.

It Reminded Me of Being a Kid

IN 1976, WE made our first bikes: a sport-touring frame called the Sequoia, and the Allez road bike. The Sequoia, which was really received well, fulfilled a niche that wasn't being addressed. Classic Italian road-racing geometry, but you could ride it on rough roads. You could ride it all day long. Nothing else like this—halfway between a clunky touring bike and a road bike.

I was hooked into the mountain bike early because I supplied tubing, lugs, and fittings and all kinds of components like Briggs and TA cranks to builders like Tom Ritchey, Steve Potts, and Breezer. All these guys. Then I said, "Gee, you know? I see a way we could make, you know, a better mountain bike that uses all the latest technology."

In 1978, I had a Ritchey mountain bike—the one he and Fisher made. Riding it, I said, "Man, this is fun! Road bikes are okay. But this is great!" I used to be an off-road motorcyclist, too. So it reminded me of that. It reminded me of being a kid.

One thing made me realize that this is going to be really something. I was riding around on a street where I lived in San Jose, and I saw this older gentleman walking along. He waved to me; I went over there and he goes, "Wow! What kinda bike is that? I remember riding bikes on dirt roads!" You could see this guy's eyes light up.

Then, a few minutes later, I saw these kids, and they go, "Whoa! That's really cool!" So, I go, you know, "Man, this is it!" Because it relates. The old people like it, and the young people like it. It's really the fun bike for everybody.

I had a guy working doing designs for me, an engineer/frame builder, Tim Neenan, who was famous for Lighthouse bikes. Tim told me that he had ideas how to do a bike differently—even lighter, more of a road bike geometry and clearance. In a few months we had prototypes. Then Tim left and Jim Vers came in and made the bikes even lighter.

As we readied the bike, the issue of the name came up. We were sitting around and said, "Hey what should we call it? Well, it's fun. It's kinda funky. Kinda like...? The Off-Roader?" No. So I said, "Hey, how about Stumpjumper?" At first it sounded pretty funky. But, hey, why not? We want something that's fun. And just like when we picked the name Sequoia, it kinda conjured up an imagination.

The Stumpjumper was really the first mountain bike available in the bike shops. I think that is kind of our claim to fame. It was the first one that really defined the category. But yeah, when I first came out with it at the 1980 bike show and took it around, most of the shops went: "What is that? What are you doing with a big kids' BMX? Man, we're only interested in adult bicycles."

I said, "Well this is an adult bike. C'mon, let's go for a ride. I'll show ya."

Our slogan was "The Bike for All Reasons." And, ah, the concept. I even thought we should include it with poison oak medicine and a snake-bite kit [laughs]. 'Cause I thought that makes it sound fun. Just the fun of it.

The beauty of it is, everything about bikes historically has been defined from road bikes—from Rome. I said, "Hey, this is the one that is defined from California." We can make our own parts. We can define it as we want—use our creativity. We could make tires. Search around and find motorcycle levers from Italy. We made the Stumpjumper tire. The handlebar. The stem. Fork. We used a lot of touring components. Like Mafac brakes, TA cranks, Jerez dual-part derailleurs.

I didn't know if it would take over cycling. But I knew this had huge, huge appeal. This is more than just riding. This is a lifestyle. Kinda like the surfing lifestyle. 'Cause I was a surfer for years in San Diego. I felt this is like surfing because it has a whole lifestyle with it. I thought, Hey, I dunno how big it's gonna be. And it doesn't matter. But I'm into it—personally. I may be riding every day and every weekend go for some crazy long ride through the woods.

A lot of those people who ran the shops at that time didn't ride. Some did, usually the people in the stores. Most just said, "We don't want this."

Four hundred and fifty Stumpjumpers sold that first year, 1980. It was fantastic. The Sequoia and the Allez were 100 or 200 units. The Stumpjumper was like "Whooh!" We had no idea how big that was. Everybody who didn't want 'em before now said, "Hey, we want it! Immediately!"

In 1981, everybody had 'em. And a lot of people didn't really think about how to make 'em; they used plain-gauge steel. The forks were bending [chuckles].

Our first bikes had no frame failures; they were overbuilt, 36 pounds or something. They totally held up. Ritchey probably made the lightest ones. But where we added value was in bike parts. We were the first to use the quick-release [QR] hubs.

Everybody was using the bolt hubs. Everybody worried QRs won't be strong enough. And our engineer, Jim Vers, said, "It is stronger. The hollow axle is stronger!" Then we changed the wheels to 32-spoke, down from 40. We had the capability to make prototypes right there—and Jim would make a bunch of different ones that we could test and compare quickly.

From there, the mountain bike took on a life of its own as a whole new sport. You look at the first poster we put out for the Stumpjumper, and we show people are just riding along in tennis shoes and ragged pants and no helmets or anything. So from there, the whole thing of enhancing the whole ride. The gloves. Shorts. Shoes, and all that stuff. For quite a while we didn't go so much with the Lycra stuff, even though we were road riders. We just didn't. It was kind of a rebellion, if you will. Against the road bikes. So they really developed into different groups. The road people and the mountain bikers.

Mountain-bike people were open to anything. Probably too much, because a lot of stupid things have been put out. We put out our share, like the Umma Gumma tires. Really soft rubber for super traction. A great idea. But it was too soft! It wasn't tested enough. The rubber just kinda melted.

We tried lots of different things. In 1985 and 1986, we came out with the Rock Combo—a cross between a mountain bike and a road bike. Basically a mountain bike with drop bars. We said, "Hey, this is what everybody wants!" Now people say, "Aw, that was such a great bike! Kinda like the Edsel."

We had the Expedition bike around 1984. Kind of a full-on touring bike with all the wiring inside. Four water-bottle fittings. Like a Winnebago bike. That did pretty well during the touring period. Then it just kinda died out.

An Everyman Mindset

I WAS ALWAYS interested in those different areas, because I was never a hot racer. I'm just kinda interested in a lot of different areas. By the 1990s, the Sequoia and the Expedition faded out. I was kinda sad to see those go. But we brought the Sequoia back as a comfort bike. And maybe the Expedition will come back as a bike you could jump out of an airplane with a parachute, then go live in the woods or travel across the country with. Yeah, that's the idea. I like that.

Not being a hot racer gives you an open mind, I think. Because if you're a hot racer, you have a hard time seeing why somebody would want a Sequoia bike with a higher headtube and things like that. They can't get their mind around it. Those types at a bike shop won't bring in that bike, right? They'll say, "Hey, nobody asked for it."

Just like nobody was walking into bike shops asking for a mountain bike. You can't define the world based on the past.

Our philosophy is to make the bike as if it were a custom bike—but make it on a production basis. It was the concept I started the company with. Make bikes for the way you ride. That's what we did with the mountain bike. And that's what we did with the Sequoia and the Allez. And I think essentially that is what we did with the Roubaix—a performance road bike loaded with comfort features. Now some racer people might be kind of scared away from a bike with a tall headtube and shock-absorbing forks. They go, "Oh, that is too pedestrian for me." But, you know, it's not....People are really loving that bike.

The Roubaix is a natural. The old road bikes used to have a quill stem, which you could pull way up, which you can't do with the Ahead stem. The Ahead is lighter and perceived as the current thing, but you lose all the adjustments it used to have. Lot of times people who are riding a bike care more about how they look. But common sense eventually rules if you go out on an event ride and look at how people ride. People on the floor in the shops know. Sometimes friends and neighbors help them get set up on a bike, and it's not right. I could easily see this problem. Well, it is just logical. Andy Pruitt [director of the Boulder Center for Sports Medicine] had a lot of influence on us. "Raise the headtube!" he said.

It's basically ergonomics. Even look at these guys who are riding in the Tour. They are riding in a much more upright position. Look at Lance and the position he has. A lot more upright than they ever had. So, I just thought this was logical. And now that we made the Sequoia, that thing really resonated with people well. In fact, half of our customers probably are women. I think there is an opportunity for the Roubaix and the Sequoia to expand people's ability to ride—just like the mountain bike did.

Our latest idea is an aluminum handlebar with a rubber sleeve in it to absorb shock.

I like to go on these real long rides—seven hours. And go over dirt roads and stuff. And, sure, you can do it with any bike, but if you have something that works better, why not? I'd say that the biggest addition to comfort and performance is suspension for mountain bikes. Why not a fully suspended or fully damped road bike? It solves a real problem.

Getting older, I can relate to other people who are older. And I can also relate to people who are just coming into cycling. That is the thing that sometimes we just don't think about. Like, how can we get these other people into cycling? And not making the bike so intimidating. Make them more comfortable. If you're more comfortable, you can go a lot harder and faster. For Specialized, that's the real opportunity.

Ramping Up His Own Fitness

THE LAST COUPLE years I've put extra effort into really trying to be fit. I just wanted to change the level I was at, and I'm kinda pleased and surprised with myself. I was staying at the same level, and wanted to improve. I've always ridden five to six days a week, probably about 200 miles. Now I do yoga; we have an instructor come in here—it's a nice complement to riding. The way you're bent over and yoga stretches you all out. For the last two years, I've lifted weights in the gym probably four days a week. If I miss a day I feel bad. I just feel mentally bad. Because it makes me feel so good. I got some advice from John Howard and Andy Pruitt about position—I was too far back on my seat. You need an expert to give you some tips. I eat healthy. No particular diet—lot of vegetables, olive oil, a bit of pasta, regular vitamins. No big deal. Exercise really changes your metabolism.

I've really worked hard and can feel the difference. That's the great thing about cycling: what you put in, you get directly back. That is so different than other things in life, which are very confusing—there's not a direct correlation. But this is a direct deal.

What would be the ultimate goal in life? It is, like, you know: great family, being healthy. But you see some of these 80-year-old guys in Italy? On Sunday morning they're out riding on these real cool bikes. I mean, that's the goal, to be healthy like that. And [it] helps you keep perspective. You go for a long ride and you come back and you have a full glass of juice. It's like the best thing ever.

As far as endurance, I'm probably better than

I was even 15 years ago. And I just kept working on it. I kinda surprised myself in a positive way. I can go for a 100-mile ride and I'm not that tired.

I'm 54 and a half. I feel 30, mid-30s maybe. I do feel healthy. I feel like even if I am doing things or I am traveling time zones, I don't have any problem. Even riding with the guys around here, can I go as fast as they can? No, I can't. But I probably never could.

It's a shock when you meet people who stopped doing activity once they got out of college. So it's probably been a long time since maybe they even sweated. If they ask me how to get into cycling, I say go and find somebody to get you comfortable on the bike, then go at your own speed just like you were going on a walk. That is one way to think about it. If you were going on a walk, you could go out and walk for two, three, four hours no problem. Well, think about a bike the same way. Don't push the big gears. Spin. Get set up right. Drink a lot of water. Take a few energy bars or something with you. And that is a wonderful way to start. Once you start doing that, it's huge.

People don't have to feel like they have to compete. Just do your own thing.

This whole thing with obesity and kids. Whew. I was maybe too hard-core with my kids. But I said, "Hey, that Nintendo and all that shit? No way! You're not going to have that stuff. Go outside. Get outta the house. Let's get out on our bikes!" Make it a family-focus thing. If the parents are healthy, the kids are like the parents, right?

Around Christmastime in San Diego, I was riding along with a guy—a good, competitive rider around 35, 38, who told me that he only started riding five years ago. Before that, he was overweight and had high blood pressure and was going to the doctor to get this blood medicine. And he told me, "Nothing was working. And my car was out of commission. So for like 10 days I borrowed this guy's Rockhopper to ride back and forth to work. And I kinda started liking it. And

then it just built from there. Now, I've never been happier in my life. I never have to go to the doctor, and my pulse rate is down to whatever. I am hooked."

The same week I was riding down there and another guy out on that ride said to me, "You from Specialized? Well, you won't believe this. But I used to be addicted to drugs. I wasn't proud of that, but it's a fact. Then I got this mountain bike a couple of years ago. Look at my shoulder. I got a tattoo of your bike! A Specialized! Now I'm a fanatic. I plan all of my vacations around the bike. I'm not a superstar. But I'm not bad. And I changed my whole lifestyle."

Those kind of stories are all over. I have one myself—it's about how I got into long-distance riding. In college, I broke up with this girlfriend who I had lived with for four years—so I was really upset about it. One day I just took off and rode from San Jose and I said, "I think I'll go to the beach." I never rode that far, ever. I thought, Shit, I could do that. That is no big deal. Through that process of working this thing out, I went for these real long rides. I got stronger and stronger and I just couldn't believe it. I was always into bikes, but I was never into going very far. Never had ridden 100 miles in a day. But all of a sudden I went that far, and when I came back, I was clearheaded. I was proud of what I did. I was getting fitter. And that was the real turning point in my life.

Update

IN A FOLLOW-UP with a 64-year-old Sinyard on January 14, 2014, he reported that he was fitter than ever and pushing his company "deeper into everything"—from pro road team sponsorship, to installing a museum at company headquarters, to tripling the size of his product development team. But he mainly wanted to talk about the "transformative" effect that cycling can have on people.

"This year, a guy in charge of operations at American Airlines, based on the East Coast, actually flew out to our offices in California just to shake our hands and say thank you for all the weight he'd lost riding a Specialized bike," he said proudly. "*Bicycling* magazine just had a big cover story on people who'd lost weight through cycling. And two years ago we financed a study by researchers at the Harvard Medical School that shows the positive effect of cycling on people with depression and kids with ADHD. Aerobic exercise of any type is good, but the rhythmic cadence of cycling is a unique, powerful thing. Kids are everything—and cycling is a key tool we can use to assure their health and success.

"Older people are harder to influence, but cycling works for them, too. The *Wall Street Journal* recently did a story on four guys in their 70s who did a coast-to-coast relay, averaging 19 mph. This redefines what a 70-year-old is!"

Feeling "about 50," Sinyard has broadened his off-the-bike exercise palate, doing one yoga class and three Pilates classes a week. "It gives me better core strength and helped my posture," he said. He still rides 12 hours a week—two days during the week and both weekend days, about 70 percent road and 30 percent mountain, with most of his riding in the hills of the coastal mountains. "I know I should do some cross-training—running and swimming—but every spare moment, I ride. Nothing else is this fun. I'm not fast—never was—but I try my best to hang in the paceline and feel very lucky to be healthy."

Sinyard's fitness paid off in a 2007 crash in the hills, when he T-boned a deer at 30 mph. "I did an endo, landed on my back, and was taken to the hospital in an ambulance," he said. "No bones were broken, but my back was so bruised up that I couldn't ride for two weeks. The doctor said to me, 'You're lucky. But you must be doing stuff to keep yourself healthy to take a crash like this.' Yes, people will be living to 100, but will they be *living* those years? Cycling helps you live."

12

ROLLING RELATIONSHIPS

Rules for reconciling significant cycling and significant others

The moment that people hear that my wife and I bicycled 600 miles from Monte Carlo to Rome on our honeymoon in 1994, the accusations begin to fly. "You forced her into it," they charge, contrasting my lifelong cycling obsession with her revulsion of anything more taxing than turning an ignition key. So it's fun to see their jaws drop when Elsa smiles, points to herself, and proudly said, "Wait a minute—it was my idea."

Explanation? Elsa hates riding a bike. But she loved riding a tandem.

In fact, it was her idea that I buy our $3,600 Santana Sovereign. Originally, it was a test bike I'd brought home to review for Bicycle Guide magazine. One ride, however, and she was hooked on tandeming's famed win-win: a fitness fix for me, toned legs for her, and "quality time" for the relationship. Although Santana cut me a deal (hey, I was the editor), it's still the most I've ever spent on a bike. But it paid off. I got the girl.

The Santana soon became covered with cobwebs, but I tandemed more than ever. My bike was a $650 Raleigh Companion. My partner was my son Joey, whose legs perfectly fit on the kid-friendly trailer bike I'd attached to my Raleigh with a Trail Gator Tow Bar. We rode the Raleigh almost every day—to and from his school, up the Back Bay bike path to Newport Beach, on steep local dirt trails, even once on the 38-mile L.A. Fun Ride from downtown to Hollywood, where he was

one of maybe half a dozen kids among 2,000 riders. It was a great workout for me, and a captive audience for Joe; he would talk and ask questions endlessly.

"Why do you love bicycling so much?" he asked me on a ride in August 2004, when he was nine.

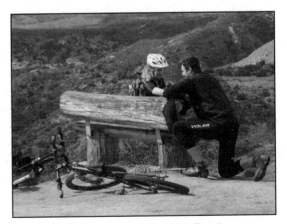

Actual pedaling proposal at Whiting Ranch, Orange County, California, in March 2012.

"It's brought me many good things," I said. "Adventure, health, a career, and…you."

"Me? What do you mean?" he asked.

Joey was born exactly nine months to the day from when his mother and I tandemed into Rome. That led to a discussion of world geography, eggs and sperm, and gestation periods. Soon, he homed in on the delivery system. "How did the sperm get to *the egg? . . . Did a doctor inject it? . . . Did you have S-E-X?" He spelled it out, not exactly sure what it entailed. "Uh . . . s-sex, yeah, we did it," I stammered. Detailed questions followed; soon, my future "birds-and-the-bees" lecture was done, way ahead of schedule.*

We looped the Back Bay, stopped to pet a black Lab (Joey loves all dogs), discussed global warming (he is a rabid environmentalist), and headed home at 18 mph (he always asks our speed). A typical day on a tandem, the ultimate relationship vehicle.

Front side of a T-shirt seen at a Southern California double-century ride: "My wife said if I do one more ultra-endurance cycling event she'll leave me."

Back side of T-shirt: "God, I'll miss her."

John Axtell's first wife used to get so mad when he'd go off on all-day or all-weekend rides with his friends that she'd go out to the garage the night before and let the air out of his car tires. That way, he'd be so late meeting his friends that he'd have to ride alone—or, she hoped, not at all. "So I started parking on the street and putting the sprinklers on all night," said Axtell, a 44-year-old wildlife biologist from Minden, Nevada. He began his marriage riding 2,000 miles a year, and ended it 14 months later, logging 4,000.

"The problem was that she had no friends in the area, no hobbies, and felt lonely," he said. "I used to joke with friends that my divorce really helped my riding."

Cycling can bond you, and cycling can separate you. Axtell's experience will hit home for many. After all, the all-day weekend events, the early

morning rides, the chain lube on the carpet, the travel, the expense, the doctor visits, the all-consuming, round-the-clock focus on the sport, can make the non-cycling spouse (often the wife) feel ignored, abandoned, jealous, and angry. We aren't talking about professionals here; their job requires them to work out all day. But for Masters racers, double-century Death Riders, and mountain bike expeditioners—often Type-A personalities working just as intently on their careers—the cycling lifestyle can include little time for TV, a novel, a movie, or a spouse.

But the issue isn't just cyclist/non-cyclist. There can be similar problems even when both spouses ride, due to conflicting cadences. Take Robert and Sandra Hendricksen of Mar Vista, California, both 38, both athletic. Both enjoy mountain biking. But not with each other.

"I hated riding with him," said Sandra. "We'd start off doing the climb to dirt Mulholland at the top of the Santa Monica Mountains, then I wouldn't see him for 45 minutes. Then, when I get to the top, he's impatiently circling at the trail juncture, and said, 'C'mon, let's go, what took you?' Finally, after a couple of months of this, I just exploded, 'I never want to ride with you again!' I think he was relieved—he felt the same way. Cycling together was driving us apart. But cycling apart, we never spend any time together."

No one knows how many relationships are negatively affected by cycling. No studies have been done. But riders talk about it enough for someone to sell T-shirts about it—and for it to be codified as a recognized condition: the *Cycling Widow Syndrome.*

Although also known as the Cycling Widower Syndrome if the affected party is the man, CWS is clearly weighted toward women, given that roughly 90 percent of the participation in cycling events is male. "It's a very real issue for serious cyclists and others involved in endurance activities," said sports psychologist Kate F. Hays, director of Toronto-based The Performing Edge, a psychological practice specializing in sport, performance, and clinical psychology, and coauthor of *You're On! Consulting for Peak Performance.* "How do we go about balancing individual interests with your needs as a couple?

"If you don't try to reach common ground, rigorous cycling training can become an irritant and source of immense frustration to the non-cyclists," said Hays. "If you want the relationship to survive, you must take steps to prevent your lives from becoming unconnected parallel lines."

One of those steps may be a tandem. Another may be setting up proper expectations. Another may be "bribing" your forlorn significant other with things he or she desires: jewelry, a new hardwood floor, a trip to Mazatlan, dinner at the Sizzler (if she loves cheap, all-you-can-eat shrimp, that is). Those and many more "Anti–Cycling Widow/Widower" tips are outlined in the lists and true-to-life case studies included in this chapter. But be aware that those tips might simply be temporary stop-gap measures if taken in isolation.

According to Hays's *You're On!* coauthor Charlie Brown, a Charlotte, North Carolina, sports psychologist and one of the world's foremost authorities on family therapy as it relates to endurance sports, random Band-Aids may do little to address the deep, long-term fissures that a die-hard athletic lifestyle can impose on a relationship. "But they can work," he said, "if they are used *as part of a systems approach that forces you to pay attention to balance.*"

Systems approach. Balance. Swallowing these unfamiliar concepts in one sentence is difficult. But once you understand them, you may gain the ability to true a wobbly cycling-affected relationship and make a good one even smoother.

First, some background: while most marriage and family therapists hail from the "conflict resolution" school of psychology (that is, they identify a problem in a relationship and try to fix it),

Brown's background is "systems"—a deeper, more macro view. "It's like being a relationship anthropologist," he said. "You dig down through the layers to see how the culture of the marriage turned those problems into a big deal."

Read that last sentence again slowly. You see, as it turns out, resolving conflicts—such as a wife being mad at her husband for going on six-hour rides every Saturday—is not the key to a happy relationship. Conflicts themselves are okay, a part of life. And they're inevitable. No two people agree on everything. Instead, the key to relationship bliss is *not making a big deal out of them.*

"Some of the most compelling research on relationships shows that 69 percent of conflicts in successful relationships are not resolved," said Brown, citing the landmark book *Why Marriages Succeed or Fail, and How You Can Make Yours Last* by frequent *Oprah* guest John Gottman, PhD. "Instead, the couple simply learns how to regulate [lower] the tension of these conflicts."

AIM FOR A 5-TO-1 RATIO

Gottman found that successful couples have three things in common:

1. They know a lot about each other—their opinions, their needs, their perspectives.

2. They maintain respect and admiration for each other.

3. They maintain a high ratio of "emotional deposits" (thoughtful acts) to "emotional withdrawals" (self-centered acts). In fact, the highest predictor of a failed relationship, said Gottman, is a low ratio in this area.

Example: An early-morning, six-hour Saturday ride might be considered an emotional withdrawal to your non-cycling spouse. But its negativity can be canceled out somewhat by positive emotional deposits, such as kissing your sleeping wife on the forehead as you leave (she'll notice), bringing in the newspaper and setting it on the table for her, then bringing home her favorite blueberry muffin from Starbucks after the ride, or just telling her you were thinking about something she said as you were riding. Surprisingly, it doesn't matter how small or big (one muffin or a whole box) or expensive or cheap (a new Lexus or a new sheepskin seat cover) the emotional deposits are; if there is a large ratio of them to the emotional withdrawals, the latter are better tolerated, said Gottman.

So, the big question is, *What is the winning ratio of "good" emotional deposits to "bad" emotional withdrawals?*

Brown found that most men, when asked, think the proper ratio for a good relationship would be at least 2 to 1. Women tend to think the best ratio is 3 to 1.

The correct answer? Gottman found that the magic number is *at least 5 to 1.*

Here's how the math works in practice: "Depending upon the ratio, your significant other may look at the same thing in different ways," said Brown. "Say you walk in from a mountain bike ride tracking dirt on the floor. If you have a good [5 to 1] ratio, your wife will say to herself, 'Poor baby, he was so tired that he forgot to take his shoes off. I'll clean it and bring him a beer.' But if you have a bad ratio, she'll probably blurt, 'Frickin' slob!'"

While there are no known studies of cycling-affected couples, Brown studied the next-closest thing—triathletes. His conclusions were based on a study of 292 responses he received to a questionnaire passed out at three 1995 triathlons, and he presented his findings at that year's conference of the American Psychological Association in New York under the title "The Impact of Training Relationships, or, 'The Trials and Tribulations of Triathloning Twosomes.'" The results were startling: 68 percent of the triathletes and 73 percent of triathlete spouses said that *triathlon training had a positive impact on their relationships.* In fact, triathlete families scored higher for happiness than the general population, even though the average triathlete in Brown's survey worked out 12 hours a week.

How can this be, when tales of broken triathlon relationships are legion? (See Case Study No. 8 in this chapter.)

"It may be that we only hear the horror stories," he said. "Yes, there are a core of 'tri-heads' who don't have much balance in their lives. But they aren't the majority."

Brown's study found that triathlons gave the non-athletic partner many opportunities for supportive, affiliated roles (e.g., family nutritionist, race photographer, training-schedule watchdog) that helped make him or her feel like an important part of the enterprise. Clearly, there are many potential emotional deposits in play here: the bonding of a shared experience, respect and admiration for the triathlete, and compensation from the appreciative triathlete. If, for instance, the race venue is far from home, triathletes might turn the trip into a family vacation, adding to the emotional payoff.

Is the Cycling Widow Syndrome overblown? Even if it only affects a minority, cyclists could clearly improve their relationships by making their families part of their "team." I saw vivid examples of this at the World Solo 24 Hours of Adrenalin Championship in Whistler, British Columbia, in September 2004. Nearly every competitor seemed to rely on a deep commitment from family, extending from training to staffing, feeding, and wrenching for 24 hours at the race site. The support was especially striking from non-riding husbands to competitor wives (see Case Studies No. 5 and 6), wherein the men exhibited a rabid enthusiasm for their wives' interest in the sport.

There's only one problem: 24-hour solos, despite a rapid growth in popularity, are so difficult that no more than a few hundred people a year do them. The Race Across America, arguably another family affair, is annually attempted by a couple of dozen people, max. That contrasts with the tens of thousands of enthusiast cyclists who participate in centuries, double centuries, benefit rides, and Masters racing—activities that generally require no help from spouses, have no common transition or pit area for interaction or even eye contact, and simply do not involve 24-hour-racing-style bonding, support, appreciation, and emotional deposits. In fact, it's just the opposite, some might argue. You train for most cycling events alone or with a network of friends outside the family. You drive to these events alone or with friends, and there is very little that family members can share—other than bitterness over being excluded, forgotten, and abandoned. Therefore, unless you're able to figure out a way to turn a century ride into a family event, your relationship might benefit from developing a strategy to counteract cycling's emotional withdrawals. Here's how to raise your ratio.

A Ratio-Raising Plan

Cycling is a demanding lover, a black hole of passion with an awesome gravitational pull. It can make you feel great about yourself while it sucks away most of your attention and affection from your family without your realizing it. Saul Miller, PhD, a Vancouver sports psychologist and author of *Sports Psychology for Cyclists*, likes to tell a joke that can quickly help put a cycling-affected relationship into perspective: A farmer has a prize cow that is not giving milk. The farmer calls an animal doctor, who finds nothing wrong and suggests that he bring in a cow psychologist. The farmer calls a cow shrink, who comes in and talks to the cow privately. After 10 minutes, the psychologist emerges from the barn and explains the problem to the farmer: "The cow tells me that you keep pulling her teats but you never tell her that you love her."

Miller chuckles at the punch line. "You think that just coming back in a good mood from a ride means it's good for her, right?" he said. "Wrong. There's got to be more."

Gottman calls it emotional deposits. "You," said Miller, "can simply call it *payback*."

Designing a payback scheme that raises your emotional deposit/withdrawal ratio and saves

your cycling and your relationship starts with honesty—with yourself and your partner.

First, if your relationship is worth saving or improving, let your partner know it. "Aretha got it right," said Miller. "R-E-S-P-E-C-T. Show it. Be upfront: 'The first thing is that I love you and want to be in a relationship with you. But keep in mind that as a racer/endurance rider, I need to ride. Are you willing to support me? What can we do?'" This approach immediately works from a public relations and practical perspective. Recognizing the problem in itself is an emotional deposit. And since women often consider themselves "relationship experts," said Dr. Hays, putting the ball in their court "engages their expertise in the issue in a positive way."

Keep in mind, however, that superficial "respect" means nothing; you have to try to understand the non-cyclist's perspective. Look at yourself closely; cycling probably dominates your life a lot more than you think.

"Training triangulates the relationship," said Stu Howard, a psychiatrist and Ironman Triathlon finisher from Cranbrook, British Columbia. "Your passion is seen by the non-cyclist as an addiction, like addiction to alcohol. In fact, it is. Be honest with yourself and call it that."

Echoing 12-step programs for treating alcoholics, Howard advises that you admit your training program isn't just the time on the road—it's the time talking about it, making repairs, buying parts, looking in the windows of bike shops, worrying endlessly about not having the lightest titanium seatpost, and spending large sums on event entry fees, travel, and products that only benefit you, not the family.

"After all, you have to be somewhat obsessive-compulsive to do well in cycling—even competing against yourself," said Howard. "You need to clean your bike, master heart-monitor computer downloads, research power meters. On top of that, many cyclists are Type-A people who push themselves, further draining the energy you have to devote to the relationship. It's very hard for serious cyclists or triathletes to do junk training—even though we read that we should take it easy."

If you add up the sheer hours you spend on the sport, on and off the bike, you may begin to understand why your spouse feels her needs aren't being met. "She has limited hours in a day to relate to you," said Howard. "So whereas you gain self-esteem, fitness, and social bonding from cycling, your spouse views it as, 'I'm losing something.'"

She can't get all that missing time back. But a good start to compensating her is by expressing willingness to compromise. "All relationships on some level are about compromise," said Dr. Hays. "Merely expressing a willingness to compromise is reassurance to the aggrieved party that the relationship is functioning."

Of course, there's a point at which the compromising, the emotional deposits, and the greatest ratios in the world are for naught. "If your significant other isn't sharing some of your passion with you, doesn't understand it, it's more than a minor problem," said Mickie Shapiro, a marriage and family counselor, psychology instructor at UC Irvine, and longtime runner, cyclist, and triathlete. "You aren't sharing a lifestyle."

Shapiro knows of what she speaks. Not long after she got seriously into 10K runs, marathons, and cycling back in her early 40s, around 1980, she walked away from a supportive husband and a rock-solid, 21-year marriage that had produced four brilliant children. Athletics not only gave her a sense of independence and control she'd never before had, she said, but rerouted her from her family's focus on intellectual, academic, and cultural pursuits to a fully athletic lifestyle.

"My husband started jogging, but it wasn't enough," she said. "I didn't want to go to concerts and plays and read so much anymore—because I wanted to work out." The thought of going to Paris to spend three days in the Louvre held no attraction for her anymore. Flying over to do the Paris marathon, then ducking into the Louvre one afternoon at most—that was where she was coming from.

Shapiro felt no guilt over plunging into a sports lifestyle, and you shouldn't either. Passions that lead to relationship problems are not specific to cycling or endurance sports, and they don't indicate that you are uncaring or unintelligent. In fact, history's smartest bicyclist, Albert Einstein, saw his marriage strained as his stature and obligations increased after 1905, but it wasn't because of the bicycle. He'd written four articles that had altered physics forever, including the one introducing his theory of relativity. "I am starved for love," his wife, Mileva, wrote to a friend in 1909. Einstein had sent Mileva a list of conditions that she would need to meet to remain married to him, such as, "You shall make sure . . . that I receive my three meals regularly in my room," and "You are neither to expect intimacy nor reproach me in any way." Albert may have predicted the existence of a space-time continuum, but obviously he didn't foresee the development of Gottman's 5-to-1 ratio.

Remember John Axtell, whose first marriage—and car tires—went flat? For his next relationship, he went out of his way to find a cyclist. But as his mileage mounted, this girlfriend felt abandoned, too, and she left after two years. Today, Axtell's mileage is up to 8,000 a year, including a 100-miler every Friday and numerous double centuries. But he gets no grief from his second wife.

"I learned from my previous relationships that I had to make more of an attempt to explain my lifestyle and lay out my schedule," he said. "So she went into this knowing what to expect." Mrs. Axtell II isn't a cyclist, but she does have a lot of friends and is working on her PhD, so she can find plenty to do on those few weekends a year (14 of them in 2004) when John's out of town. "It's the perfect relationship," he said.

Perfect for him, anyway. Tactics may vary, but a framework of proper expectations, common ground, mutual respect, and a 5-to-1 emotional deposit/withdrawal ratio is a good start for anyone trying to reconcile a cycling lifestyle with the needs of a significant other. Next, check out the dozens of tips, strategies, and case studies outlined in the rest of this chapter. Finding the right mix for your relationship may not come easy, but the payoff can be great.

Ultimately, athletic accomplishments taste that much sweeter when you have someone to share them with. "After all," said former pro triathlete Brad Kearns, whose own marriage barely survived his rocky career, "what if you win your age group and no one's there clapping for you?"

BRIDGING THE GAP: SCENARIOS, STRATEGIES, TIPS, AND CASE STUDIES

There's no right or wrong in a cycling-stressed relationship—just an inevitability that if both parties are not similarly involved in cycling or related sports, vastly different needs will arise. It is hard for the non-cyclist to understand the cyclist's feelings of triumph or pain. It is hard for the cyclist to understand the non-rider's feelings of abandonment. It is impossible to see each other's perspectives without an open dialogue. Therefore, this section begins with communication strategies, follows with tried-and-true tips culled from sports psychologists and athletes, and puts it all together in seven realistic rider/non-rider scenarios and case studies from riders themselves, giving you a wealth of ideas that you can use to bridge the gap in your own relationship.

Communication Strategies

"Communication" sounds cliché, but if you talk the talk, good things happen. In his study, Dr. Charlie Brown found that a calm one-to-one talk about the impact of training, without defensiveness, accusations, or time pressures, did wonders for cycling-stressed couples. Merely agreeing that it *was* stressful helped couples get along better. "Remember," he warned, "training stress causes relationship stress." Here's what a dialogue should accomplish.

Step 1: Get your partner on the same page. Express the passion, joy, and feeling of accomplishment you get from reaching goals in cycling. Over time, make a laundry list: I've lost 38 pounds. I'm proud of my body. I eat healthier. I go to work with more vigor—I see more clients, make more money. This is my window of opportunity to be competitive. I was a nerd in high school and this makes me feel cool. I always wanted to wear tight shorts in public.

Step 2: Find out what bothers her about your involvement in cycling. She may not mind that you ride all day every Saturday. She may be bothered by the fact that you fall asleep immediately when you come home and she can't tell you about her day. Your problem might be solved by a strong cup of coffee. True, you might get an earful of what you don't want to hear: "You spend more time on that bike than you do with me. You are addicted. I am not a priority for you. I feel abandoned, unneeded. I'm overwhelmed by the kids when you aren't here on weekends. The lawn doesn't get mowed. We don't go out anymore. We don't talk. We don't have enough sex. You don't want to be with me anymore. I am supporting you in your goals, but getting nothing in return." But at least she'll feel better getting it off her chest, and a dialogue can begin.

Step 3: Set common goals and proper expectations. Setting common goals shifts the focus to the positive, agreeable aspects of your relationship, rather than the negative ones. Proper expectations allow the two parties to devise a plan that can reduce the emphasis on cycling's negatives and highlight its positives. (See next section for details.)

A HODGEPODGE OF RELATIONSHIP TIPS AND SOLUTIONS FOR CYCLING-AFFECTED COUPLES

Best intentions notwithstanding, you could well fall short of Gottman's 5-to-1 ratio of emotional deposits to emotional withdrawals simply because you don't know the options available.

Below, we've outlined two dozen cycling-relationship stress-busters, divided into cyclist's and spouse's responsibilities, that are designed to help you raise your ratio.

The Cyclist's Responsibilities

1. Make your non-cycling spouse feel welcome in your cycling world: He or she can come to cycling-related events that don't involve cycling per se, for example, such as bike club meetings or brunch after the ride with other riders and spouses. This will provide common ground, plug your spouse into a similar social network, and make him or her feel important to your training and performance.

2. Try to train or exercise with the non-cyclist: In his triathlon study, Dr. Brown found exercising together to be the most effective coping strategy. If cycling is out, consider cross-training activities, such as inline skating, running, and even mixing sports. If she rides more slowly than you, use her as a pacer as you run.

3. Try a tandem, but make it fun: Bill McReady, the founder of Santana tandems, has made a lucrative career out of convincing people that tandems are the best way for a couple of different cycling abilities to secure their relationship—and has hundreds of success stories to prove it. But the non-cyclist can lose enthusiasm and drop out if you move too fast and expect too much. Focus on making tandem rides fun, not serious hard-core riding, until the weaker half pushes the pace.

4. Show appreciation: If you don't provide some attention to your spouse, she'd have to be a doormat not to get mad. Merely conveying appreciation, such as a simple thank-you ("Geez—I couldn't have gotten my PR without your help"), is a good start, as well as bringing a race T-shirt or other special gift home for your husband or wife. Also, you can simply ask, "What can I do for you today, sweetheart?" when you get home. It's a statement of appreciation.

5. Quid pro quo (a.k.a. bribery or payback): Involving your partner in the sport itself may not align with your needs. Many cyclists like to get away from their spouses once in a while—for the solitude, for the camaraderie with other cyclists, or just for the chance to challenge and exhaust themselves. Similarly, many non-cycling spouses have no interest in sports. So, if you go do a century ride, be smart: take your spouse out to dinner afterward. If it's a double century or overnight event, take some time together at a nearby resort town for a weekend soon thereafter.

6. Off-season payback: "I tell pro and top amateur athletes, 'Let your significant other know that you need to be supported,'" said Dr. Ross Goldstein, a San Francisco sports psychologist. "But in the off-season, it's payback time. Basically, you're her slave from October through February."

7. Beware of radical changes in riding quantity: Don't be surprised when sudden spikes in your mileage create strains. Ramp up the payback before your spouse notices.

8. Limit hard events: Monumental events such as the eight-day TransAlp Challenge require a tunnel-visioned focus to do well, but this can be unfair to other family members year after year. So compromise; do the event every other year. For smaller events, like double centuries, limit the compulsion by doing, say, 7 races a year instead of 10. Then take the family camping on those extra weekends.

9. Get your home chores done: If you know in periods of heavy training that the lawn doesn't get mowed, the leaves don't get raked, and the wife gets embarrassed by it, think ahead. "It's not the commitment to fitness that causes family problems," said Dr. Brown, "but whether or not things get taken care of at home." So hire your nephew or the neighborhood kids to do it—you need the help and they need the money.

10. Ride to family events: If your wife wants you to go to her niece's birthday party, don't blow it off because you have a ride that day. Just get up an hour earlier and bike to Chelsea's house.

11. Train in non-family hours: Ride early in the mornings, or before your spouse gets home from work. If it's too cold or dark, see the next entry...

12. Use a bike trainer: Yeah, it can be boring. But with a heart-rate monitor, a favorite TV program, and no coasting, time flies and you pack double the workout in half the time. Triangle trainers are dirt-cheap (some performance models start at $100). Get distracted easily? Pay the big bucks and stay motivated with a Compu-Trainer or similar device that measures and graphically displays pulse, watts, cadence, distance, speed, and more.

13. Make your event a vacation: You can do cycling events anywhere in the world, so make it someplace that your spouse likes. Build a vacation around the Cycle to the Sun hill climb of Mt. Haleakala on Maui, and he or she will eagerly help you train.

14. Reserve special time for the relationship: Make Wednesday night "Date Night," and stick to it. It'll ensure that you get together and function as a couple, regardless of your training schedule.

15. In the end, do the right thing: Be fair and move on if you're incompatible. But don't give up relationships—or cycling. Your cycling/relationship problem may be a manifestation of bigger problems. If the relationship is bad, it doesn't matter if it's cycling or playing bridge. In that sense, maybe cycling provides a valuable service by helping put bad relationships out of their misery.

16. Be honest if you move on: The outlook for a new relationship is probably brighter if the new "significant other" understands how committed you are to the sport and how much time it takes. It may seem ideal to marry another cyclist, a triathlete, or someone else who is very athletic and shares your perspective, so you can share the passion and the motivation. But beware. Don't dive into a relationship with someone just because he or she is athletic. Hard-core cycling may tend to attract addictive personalities. And there is more to a person than the miles they ride or the races they run, like honesty, integrity, and the ability to be nurturing.

The Partner's Responsibilities

1. Get involved in your spouse's cycling world: For example, perhaps you could join the steering committee of the bike club, or help plan events. When you are involved, you will have more friends in common, which will likely lead to social events that don't even involve cycling.

2. Think of ways to be supportive: You might offer to purchase or make special foods that benefit training and race preparation, for example. You could even take a massage class to work on your spouse's battered legs.

3. No name-calling: Don't put down your spouse with labels like "addict," "freak," and "hyper." No one likes to be condemned for an activity he or she loves.

4. Get with it, gal (or guy): Fitness and competition is a good thing for body and soul. If you're not physically active, try to find a sport you love. You may be surprised at how it affects your day-to-day level of happiness.

5. Be positive: Come up with constructive suggestions for ways that your cycling-spouse can get in a workout without wrecking your day.

6. Share a common goal: You have a choice. You can be supportive of your spouse's passions, or you can be antagonistic. Help your spouse to set and reach goals—it'll make you closer. You don't have to ride a bike alongside your spouse, or hand him or her a special energy drink at the turnaround on race day. But if you stop at Trader Joe's, why not pick up a dozen $0.99 Clif Bars in that Carrot Cake flavor she likes?

7. Develop some hobbies: You need a feeling of accomplishment, too. What better way to fill eight hours on bike-ride Saturday than learning Chinese, taking a guitar class, joining a book club, volunteering to help teach the homeless interviewing skills, even stamp collecting—or all of the above?

8. Stay socially active: Spouses can create stories to share by spending time apart. You should both be developing your own sense of identity. When your spouse is out riding, get together with a friend for lunch or for a walk in the park. If child care is a problem, hire a babysitter if you can. You can trade child care with friends who have children—or with your spouse: Maybe he gets his long Saturday ride, but you get Tuesday night book club and Friday night out with the girls. Those times can be a special bonding time for the cycling parent and the children.

9. Look on the bright side: There are several advantages to having a cycling spouse: He's out of the house (and out of your hair), can wear shorts at the company picnic without embarrassment, has his time accounted for (just check the training log), is probably a good Type-A person with the income to show for it, has good diet and health habits, and can teach you a nice stretching routine. According to many *Bike for Life* interviewees (see case studies, below), there may be sexual-performance benefits conferred by the high fitness levels, too.

STRATEGY: COMMON CYCLING-RELATIONSHIP SCENARIOS

Wonder how to put the above tips together? Here's are strategies for resolving the following stressful cycling-relationship scenarios, many of which are from Dr. Kate Hays.

Scenario 1: One rides, the other doesn't.

1. Try to engage your non-cycling spouse in some aspect of your training: Have him or her meet you halfway for lunch, and use a tandem for some training.

2. Get your non-cyclist spouse involved in the sport: Take him or her to events. Even take your spouse to the Tour de France (see Case Study No. 2, below).

3. Get the non-cyclist spouse riding somehow: A tandem works—if you start slow and make it fun. Push it too fast, and you risk your spouse hating cycling forever and never trying it again. If your spouse has sports somewhere in his or her past, he or she may quickly learn to enjoy cycling. If your spouse is not already into fitness or athletics, he or she still may find that cycling is more fun than expected. Take your spouse to a bike shop to buy clothing, shoes, etc. It's no fun cycling without the right shoes and breathable clothing.

4. Set up a quid pro quo: Promise to watch the kids on Tuesday and Thursday to balance your spouse watching them all weekend.

5. Beware developing parallel lives: Carve out time together, such as dinner on Wednesday nights. Talk it out and plan, as you would a business. Joint problem-solving is important, because it makes a couple feel like a couple.

6. Use bribery: Maybe she allows you the double without causing trouble, so you reward her with tickets to *Les Misérables* and agree to go antiquing with her next Saturday.

Scenario 2: Both ride, but one is stronger.

1. Faster partner does "recovery day" rides with the slower partner. If you hate waiting for your spouse at the top of hill climbs, stay on a flat beach bike path. Or use the Rich White "sheepdog" method (see his interview following this chapter): When you arrive at the top of the climb, don't wait—turn around, double back, make contact, and climb again. That way, you get to ride more. And it's a good idea to go back and check on your spouse anyway: He or she may not know how to fix a flat.

2. Buy a tandem and use it for hard rides: The stud gets a great workout; the spud gets a thrill ride.

3. Train together, but add artificial difficulty: The cyclist spouse could try pedaling with one leg, ride in too big a gear, or pull a brick-filled (or child-filled) baby trailer.

4. Split the day: The stronger spouse could hammer with the club in the morning, then come back and pedal easily with the weaker spouse in the afternoon.

5. Buy an e-bike: The weaker rider might love riding with the strong one with some assistance on the climbs from an electric-assist bike. These are exploding in popularity now. With an e-bike, the rider still has to pedal to keep the motor on, and can choose between several different levels of assistance or no assistance at all. Just because one spouse is a purist doesn't mean the other one has to be.

CASE STUDIES

Every cycling-affected relationship has its own unique spin. The following eight case studies offer valuable real-life lessons about bridging the gap between your significant other and your significant riding.

Case Study No. 1: The Education of a Widow-Maker: How a Cycling Psychologist Banished the "Cycling Widow Syndrome"

One weekend in late August 2004, Ross E. Goldstein, PhD, made a decision that he said would have surprised him a decade earlier. Not only did the 57-year-old San Francisco psychologist and Masters racer decide not to ride one day, but he decided to do so *without resentment*.

"Both my kids were in soccer tournaments," said Goldstein, who was logging 175 to 250 miles per week. "So I simply did what was best for the family, without complaint. But when I was younger and obsessive-compulsive like many riders extremely involved in the sport, I would have sulked. Back then, racing seemed almost incompatible with my relationship. Living from race to race, it's hard to see that anyone or anything else is important. I couldn't tolerate taking a day off."

The result? In 1993, when Goldstein was featured in a superb *Bicycle Guide* article by Barbara

Hanscome about problematic cycling relationships, he said his wife was a classic "cycling widow," clearly resentful of playing second fiddle to his bike racing. The relationship was on thin ice. "It was a problem," said Goldstein.

But with age came wisdom—and a smoother relationship with the missus. "Over the years, I've learned that it is my responsibility to do cycling in a way that it does not negatively impact the family. In other words, I pull my own weight—even though I actually ride more now. I share the driving to soccer games. I'm there rooting on my kids. I spend more time with my wife. If I have to give up a morning ride with my friends, so be it.

"Besides, I've learned that if you give concessions, you get back more in the long run."

A Harvard PhD and author of *Fortysomething: Claiming the Power and the Passion of Your Midlife Years*, Goldstein has spent the bulk of his career analyzing generational trends and consumer behavior. Applying his expertise to cycling, he offers the following tips to those who hope to keep their relationships as healthy as their riding.

1. Don't be rigid: "Know when to back off. You make yourself crazy and your loved ones angry if you don't make time to be with them at important times," said Goldstein. "I used to train every Saturday and Sunday morning, but my wife felt that I was giving the best hours of the day to cycling. There are times when trying to do both is like pushing a rock up a hill. I solved the weekend problem by getting up early and riding three days during the week."

2. Adjust according to your life stage: "Look at your life as a series of episodes," said Goldstein. "And fit in as much cycling as is appropriate for the times. When my kids were very young, I actually had to be around more [to watch them]. Now that they're teenagers, I actually ride more."

3. Think quality, not quantity, in your training: Goldstein's shorter weekday rides, more often than not, make up for his longer weekend rides, because he makes them count. "You can get a lot done in 90 minutes if you're focused," he said. "Keep in mind that training programs are guidelines. They don't necessarily have to be followed to the letter to work."

4. Don't abuse others' time: Give your significant other a reasonable estimate of how long you'll be riding. "If you tell your partner you'll be gone for two hours when you know you'll be gone for four, you insult them," said Goldstein. "They feel as if they've been stood up."

5. Negotiate and communicate: It doesn't matter if your thing is cycling, golf, or coin collecting, said Goldstein. "Together, negotiate the boundaries. Tell her what you'd like to do and see how it fits with her plans. Don't be stubborn and insist on getting your way all the time. Since I learned to do that, my cycling is no longer an issue."

6. It's all about balance: "You don't have balance between your cycling and your family all the time," said Goldstein. "But if you recognize it, you can easily get back in balance before your significant other realizes it."

Widows and Widowers: Read this . . .

Goldstein said the onus for curing a cycling-impacted relationship is not only the cyclist's. Cycling widows and widowers, remember this advice:

1. Don't diss his or her passion: Your partner's commitment to cycling may ebb and flow over the years, but for now it is important to your spouse's life. Your spouse will resent it if you demand that he or she give it up. If you make him or her choose between you and cycling, you're likely to lose.

2. Don't nag: It'll make your partner happier to ride away from you.

3. Figure out what bugs you: Are you upset because you don't spend enough time together, and feel left out and undervalued? Or do you simply want to discuss other things besides cycling? "Most people don't resent their partner's

involvement in the sport," said Goldstein. "It's the feeling that they don't matter that bothers them."

4. Be honest: Can you handle it? A relationship with a serious cyclist may be too frustrating for you. You might be happier with someone else.

Case Study No. 2: Bribery, Le Tour, and Killer Sex

"My cycling was an issue with my first wife," said Mike Miller, a 53-year-old electronics engineer from San Diego. "I biked on-and-off my entire life, but got serious in 1989, when I started hitting 5,000 to 6,000 miles a year and going on two- to three-week cycling camping trips with a friend of mine. My wife really didn't like those, but they are the cheapest, most fun vacations you can have. In 1992, we went 3,200 miles in 28 days, averaging 114 miles a day, and spent less than $1,000, including the airfare home from Virginia Beach to San Diego. I figured the trips were good for her, too, because I subscribed to the theory that absence makes the heart grow fonder. You're full of joy and energy to see her after a couple of weeks. Still, it was a balancing act. The complaining and whining wouldn't stop. She was starting to battle breast cancer, while I was doing double centuries. I got a lot of flak for doing a 150-mile prep ride on the Saturday before the double.

"My solution to the problem? Bribe her. I'd take her out to dinner, flowers, clean up around the house—all the things I wouldn't normally do."

Miller's wife passed away in 2002 after 28 years of marriage, and he remarried in the summer of 2004. He upped his mileage to 8,000 per year, yet reported fewer problems despite her being "not into cycling or athletic." She went into the marriage knowing what to expect: "I explained my lifestyle to her up front," he said. Also, a couple things worked on her.

"We bought a tandem right after we got married. She loves it," Miller said. "Then I took her to the Tour de France and didn't bring my bike. We'd see the race for 30 seconds going by then watch it that night for an hour on TV. She really got into the excitement. I guess I brainwashed her."

Is everything rosy all the time? No, but there's a lot more positive than negative. Miller reported: "My wife gets jealous if I spend too much of the weekend cycling. But overall, I think my cycling helps the marriage, since when we're together things are great, and sex is out of this world. My wife jokes about my prowess. And her friends are jealous of my condition. I get a lot of compliments on my looks. I'm 53, have seven grandkids, but look 43. I have only 6 percent body fat. People are amazed. I lift weights. I don't look like the other cyclists.

"I do tough doubles in 13 hours. I did the 24 Hours of Adrenalin event in Idyllwild with my sister. My most difficult challenge: finding time to ride. I'd cycle a lot more if I wasn't happily married."

Case Study No. 3: Tandem Family Affair: Building Bonds with the Kids

"Relationship" isn't just male-female; it's also parent-child. This old story from the March 1993 issue of Bicycle Guide *received a flood of letters and actually changed my life. As soon as my son was old enough, I bought a tandem that we used for a decade.*

"Hey, Butt-head," said 10-year-old Kirsten Von Tungeln to her dad, Jim.

Instead of reprimanding his daughter, however, Jim just laughs and replies, "What, brat?" In this case, *Butt-head* is simply a term of endearment between two riding buddies, and it makes perfect sense from Kirsten's view of the world: sitting behind her father for hundreds of hours a year on the stoker seat of their tandem bicycle.

In 1992, Kirsten, a red-haired fourth-grader from Irvine, California, became the youngest tandemer to have ever completed the L.A. Wheelmen Grand Tour double century (in 17 hours and three flats) and to have soloed the popular Solvang Century (9 hours). That paved the way for her toothy, blonde-haired sister, Allison, who was 7. She did her first century at age 5 on a tandem with their mom, Cindy, and went on to many solos.

Traveling without the girls along was not a consideration for the bike-crazy Von Tungelns, whose garage once housed 12 bikes, including Trek, and Nishiki front-suspension mountain bikes; Fuso, Bertoni, and Specialized Epic Comp road bikes; and a Mongoose Iboc mountain bike with fenders, slicks, and touring bags, which Jim uses to commute 23 miles to work every day.

"Hey, in the long run, doing this was cheaper than a babysitter," jokes Jim, pointing to the two Santana tandems with the wooden blocks taped to the rear pedals. "But in truth, I just don't believe in babysitting at all. You need to spend quality time with your kids."

Jim speaks with authority. A 38-year-old teacher of juvenile delinquents, he holds a doctorate in theology and family counseling. "There is no quality time like traveling together," he explains. "No interruptions. No phone calls. No TV. No superficial two-minute conversations after work quickly asking them 'How'd it go at school today?' and getting a clipped 'Okay' as a response. It's all about being together, having an open ear, letting them lead. The conversations are on a deeper level.

"It enables you to be a friend to your child, because it's just you and the kids having full, uninterrupted talks for hours."

One long conversation that Jim remembers fondly lasted for one and a half hours during the fall Solvang Century. The girls were so impressed with the beautiful green hills and rolling pastoral countryside between Solvang and Santa Maria that they repeatedly asked, "Why don't we buy a home and move up here?"

"That gave me a chance to explain a little about economics," recalls Jim. "I told them, 'There are no jobs up here—that's why no one lives up here.'" Kirsten and Allison asked questions on the subject of their parents' occupations—Cindy is a nurse—for the next 30 miles.

Riding teaches them a lot more, too. Jim ticks off self-confidence, knowledge of time and distance, understanding of grades—as in steepness, not report cards—and even food and diet.

"When we say the ride is 30 miles long, they immediately know that's about one and a half hours," said Jim. "When we say 9 percent grade, they groan. And when we go shopping, they automatically read the nutritional labels and figure out how much fat and carbohydrates are in it."

Not surprisingly, the girls' favorite food and drink are PowerBars and Cytomax. They are exceptionally fit, said Jim, and quite knowledgeable about regional terrain and sights.

Allison's favorite place is the Back Bay of Newport Beach, an ecologically protected area the family rides through on one of their 50-mile Saturday loops. "We always stop and see the ducks," she said. "They are so beautiful."

Kirsten's favorite moment of her life came when she and her dad went for a long ride on a densely foggy day, then struggled up an 8 percent grade in nearby Dana Point harbor. "When we got to the top, we all of a sudden popped through the fog into bright, bright sunlight and pure, blue sky," she remembers. Father and daughter just stood together speechless for 10 minutes looking at the stunning carpet of fog over the Pacific Ocean.

The funniest moment for the Von Tungelns came on a 350-mile biking vacation they took last Easter vacation to Borrego Springs, in the desert east of San Diego. "Little did we know that we had to climb up Montezuma's Grade—12 miles at an 8 percent slope," said Cindy. "It took Allison and I four hours. During that time, someone called the sheriff's department and told

them that some crazy lady was climbing up the hill with a baby."

Speaking of crazy, Kirsten's friends at school don't know what to make of her hobby. "They think I'm weird," she said. "Half the time, they don't believe me." Sometimes, Jim said that Kirsten, an "A" student and acknowledged teacher's pet, gets a little depressed by her classmates' taunts and talks about giving up bicycling to concentrate on her flag football, roller skating, Girl Scouts, and peer tutoring, where she helps teach the special-ed kids. But even though her parents don't push her, Kirsten keeps on stoking. "Sometimes when I ride I feel so good I could just ride 5,000 miles," she said. Her goal for 1993 is to do another solo century: the mountainous Ride Around the Bear from the desert floor to Big Bear and back. (She wanted to do it on a new bike, Klein's diminutive "Kirsten" model, and was disappointed when she learned that Klein changed the name of the bike to the gender-neutral "Panache" to attract small male riders. Luckily, Gary Klein said he has a few Kirsten stickers left over.)

The family's next goal together will come this summer [1993]: to San Francisco and back on the tandems—three weeks and 1,000 miles. The girls shake their heads and say in grade-school parlance, "I don't think so."

But they'll surely be there on Highway 1, singing their old standard, "99 Bottles of Beer on the Wall" and telling the corny elementary-school jokes that have been passed down through the generations. "Why did Santa Claus have only seven reindeer?" asks Kirsten. "Because Comet stayed home to clean the sink." "What did the fox say to the owl?" challenges Allison. "Howl you doin'?"

And then it's Jim's turn to chime in—and teach his kids a little about the real world at the same time. "What animals can open an IRA?" After a brief discussion of tax-deferred retirement plans, Jim finally gives the answer: "A deer, because it has a buck. And a skunk, because it has a scent."

Epilogue

Eleven years later, I followed up with the Von Tungelns.

"When you have kids, most people drop out of cycling," said Cindy Von Tungeln in October 2004. "People feel awkward taking their kids to events, as we did. But they shouldn't. My kids got a number of benefits: they have no fear of talking to adults, who treated them as peers on those rides. They became star basketball players in junior high, high school, and college due to their strong legs and lungs. They learned to never give up when it gets tough, like in the last 50 miles of a double century or the last five minutes of the fourth quarter. And we have some great memories of riding down the coast from Seattle to San Diego over three summers."

The Von Tungeln girls, as their parents expected, "did their own thing" and dropped out of cycling when junior-high activities took precedence, but not before the family racked up an amazing 93 double-centuries between them.

Cindy finished the California Triple Crown series (at least three double-centuries in a year) for six consecutive years (1992 to 1997); oldest daughter, Kirsten, finished it five times (1993 to 1997); and younger daughter, Allison, won the coveted T-shirt three times (1995 to 1997). Jim, a two-time president of the Orange County Wheelmen, was the first person inducted into the Triple Crown Hall of Fame; rode a career total of 50 double-centuries; completed the series every year from 1990 to 1998, including all 11 of the 1997 events; completed Paris-Brest-Paris (750 miles with 31,000 feet of climbing) twice; and is one of two people to have completed the L.A. Wheelmen Highland Quad Century of the Grand Tour (400 miles in 24 hours) four times.

Unfortunately, all the riding affected Jim's health and his relationship. Injuring and reinjuring the nerves in his hip when he refused to rest, he underwent five operations and had to give up cycling in 1999. "The pain was 24/7," said Cindy. With Jim unable to bike, and his source of achievement gone, the marriage became stressed. The Von Tungelns' divorce became final in 2003.

Tandem Gear

The Von Tungelns used two adult tandems with wooden blocks on the pedals to accommodate their kids' legs, but the market in 2014 offers a few dedicated kid-friendly tandems with lowered stoker seats. (Incidentally, these telescope up to accommodate an adult, too, so they can be used by a couple.) Models include:

1. Raleigh Companion ($929; uses 26-inch mountain bike wheels)

2. Bike Friday Family Tandem ($1,198; uses 20-inch wheels and folds up for easy transport)

3. Co-Motion Periscope Scout ($3,395; uses mountain bike wheels); and Co-Motion Periscope Torpedo ($4,695, fits into an airline-legal suitcase due to four take-apart couplings)

A less expensive way to get the tandem experience is by using one-wheel trailer bikes, made by Adams, Burley, and Trek, that connect to the adult bike. The least expensive option (which I used with my son from age four to seven) is an ingenious telescoping tow-bar called the Trail Gator ($99.95; www.trail-gator.com), which attaches the headtube of a regular kid's bike to the adult's seat tube in ten seconds. It lifts the front wheel of the kid's bike 3 inches off the ground, giving the "captain" (front rider) complete steering control while allowing the "stoker" to contribute real pedal power.

Case Study No. 4: Get a Sugar Momma

Dan Cain, a 46-year-old bicycle retailer and consultant from Borrego Springs, California, has advice for any man who dreams of riding as much as he wants—even to the point of giving up work to ride: "Fall in love with an independent woman who makes a lot of money," he said. "That's usually an older woman."

He's only partly joking. Living a cycling fanatic's fantasy life in this mountain community south of Palm Springs, Cain is essentially a kept man happily supported by a woman with a full-time career. "Jody's the breadwinner," said Cain. "She lets me ride 20 to 30 hours a week, race every other weekend. She's my Sugar Momma."

She's also his second wife. The first one, a state parks worker to whom Cain was married from 1990 to 1994, "wasn't as permissive of my time," as he put it. She bailed when he refused to buy a house. The couple had been living cheaply in a state park property.

"I was already working full-time at my bike shop, which I founded in 1985 hoping to combine business and pleasure," he said. "Trouble is, there wasn't enough pleasure. I only had time for one all-day ride and a half-day ride a week. I didn't want to work more."

But sometimes life, like cycling, takes an unexpected route. After the divorce, he met Jody, whom he described as "very attractive, five years older than me, no kids, a runner, a well-to-do investment-relations writer." She came into his shop one day, he said, "and I ended up taking her on a tandem ride." More rides led to marriage. Ironically, he did end up with a home, one that Jody purchased in Borrego Springs in 2002. Jody made a high income, so, with her permission, Cain closed the shop he'd run full-time for 14 years, moved it into his garage as a part-time operation, and dramatically ratcheted up his cycling. During the week, when Jody lives 150 miles away in an apartment in Los Angeles and commutes to work, Cain rides for up to 30 hours per week. He races every other week, including three team 24-hour races and one solo in 2004. He finished at the top of the Masters and fourth overall at the 24 Hours of Temecula. At all other times, he's with Jody—fit, attentive, eagerly providing her with what he calls "endless sexual pleasure."

Ironically, Cain and Jody don't ride the tandem anymore. "She took one too many falls, and she's such an independent-thinking woman that she actually doesn't like being on the back of a tandem too much," he said. He rides alone for the most part, except when ex-Yeti pro racer Russel Worley comes out to visit.

Does Cain mind that he might be called a "trophy husband"? "Hey, I get my freedom to ride and she gets her city ya-yas out and a fit man happy to see her," he said. "We both get what we want out of our situation. Isn't that the definition of a good relationship?"

Case Study No. 5: The Lady and the Guinea Pig

"We need to start exercising."

Tammy Darke said "we" because she was too nice a girl to say "you." The registered dietician from Mission Viejo, California, then 27, was a triathlete and marathoner with boxes full of medals. Her husband, Mark, was fat, plain and simple. What else could you call 210 pounds on a 5-foot-9 frame? "I was resentful," said the audio-video shop owner, then 32. "But I immediately started thinking, 'Now, which of the sports that she does is the coolest?'"

It was mountain biking, he decided. But that would have to wait six months. You see, it took that long for the man that Tammy now refers to as "my guinea pig" to slowly work himself into shape. The step-by-step plan they laid out together called for walking, then jogging, then running, but no biking until Mark hit a threshold—185 pounds. On that joyous day in the early spring of 1997, he, Tammy, and mutual friend Tony picked up a new Raleigh M600 hard-tail mountain bike at Sports Chalet and headed to Aliso Woods Park in Laguna Beach. Then wife and friend patted Mark on the back, left him at the bottom, and rode off up the steep hillsides of the Cholla Trail for two hours.

"After three months, I climbed Cholla," said Mark. "After a year, I finally rode with my wife.

That was a cool day. For the first time, I could actually say, 'I'm a mountain biker.'"

After three years, the mountain biker was riding a dual-suspension Rocky Mountain Element and out-riding his wife. At his urging, they entered a team in the 2000 24 Hours of Adrenalin relay race at Idyllwild, California. Their team, The Chick and 4 Nuts, enjoyed the round-the-clock scene so much that they did four more races, once winning the co-ed division. Then Tammy broke up the team.

"I'm not getting enough laps," she told her husband in 2003. "I wanna do a solo."

Today, the former fat man is the pit crew of the woman who nurtured him to fitness. Tammy took second at the 2003 Idyllwild solo. She qualified for the 2004 worlds in Whistler, British Columbia, where I met them. She took twelfth place.

The Darkes weren't satisfied. "We're in this together," said Mark, "and we're going to train harder next time." This time, of course, "we" really means both of them.

Case Study No. 6:
Twenty-Four Hours of Love

In 1993, after a year of marriage, Barbara and Bill Kreisle were stressed out. As a social worker, she'd bring home depressing stories from her job. As an oncologist treating terminal cancer patients, he'd carry home the weight of the world. "I knew we had to do something fun, something fit, to bring happiness into our lives," said Barbara. "We had no money. But we did have two old bikes in the garage. The guy at the bike shop said, 'Try mountain biking. Lotta good trails here in Phoenix.'"

That changed everything.

Barbara, who had never been athletic, immediately discovered that she was a good rider. So good that the guy at the shop said, "Why don't you race?" By 1995, she was on the podium. By 2000, she turned pro. And after a few years, Bill, who had enjoyed riding with her, began to say, "Hey, there's more to life than mountain biking."

That's when it hit Barbara: "Our mountain biking was all about me-me-me—so I became more supportive of his needs," she said. "It seemed unfair that I had a very happy lifestyle while he was holding people's hands in death. . . . He needed to get out and pursue his own hobbies. So I take the boys [their two sons], and urge Bill to go do his fly-fishing, his skiing, his backpacking."

When the family moved to Boise, Idaho, Barbara discovered round-the-clock racing. While on a vacation, she and Bill flew to England's biggest 24-hour mountain bike race, the Red Bull Rampage. She competed in the 2003 World Solo 24 Hours of Adrenalin Championships at Whistler, British Columbia, in 2003, taking eighteenth place. She and Bill went back again to B.C. in 2004, where I ran into her husband manning the pits.

"We ride together once a week, and I keep up with her," said Bill. "I know her friends. I'm in the network. But I'm really happiest in this role—as her manager."

"Bottom line? I'm happy if my wife's happy. And she's happiest on a bike."

Case Study No. 7:
Triathlon Relationships:
And You Thought Cycling Was Tough

When Denise Berger of Mission Viejo, California, then 39, arrived home from the 1992 world duathlon championships in Frankfurt, Germany, with a bronze medal around her neck for her age group (35–39), her husband of two years, Tim, excitedly congratulated her. That seemed strange, since he'd grown increasingly antagonistic toward her devotion to racing and training. But it soon made sense.

"Now that you've won a medal, this is it—no more training, right?" he asked, hopefully.

"Absolutely not!" Berger responded, flabbergasted. "This is who I am. I've been athletic my whole life—and into this sport way before I met you. Give it up? I want more medals!"

Tim took off his wedding ring and threw it at her, then stormed out the door, five years together gone forever. Another multisport relationship kaput.

If dedicated cyclists think they've got a hard time balancing their sport and their relationships, how about training for three sports? No one actually knows if the triathlete divorce rate is any greater than that of the general population, but speculation is rife. "It seems like it's astronomical," said Triathlon USA chief operating officer Tim Yount, who talks to American triathletes and duathletes at dozens of races all over the world. "When I go to events, I inevitably hear, 'Oh, her? That didn't work out.'"

The worst imbalances of all may involve those trying to qualify for the Hawaii Ironman, composed of a 2.4-mile swim, 112-mile bike, and 26.2-mile run. "Like cycling, triathlon triangulates a relationship, but Ironman is worse," said Canadian psychiatrist Stu Howard, a two-time Hawaii finisher. "Ironman can be like an addiction, like alcoholism."

And like an addiction, Ironman training can go on for years. "Once you go to Hawaii, you gotta go back," said Ray Campeau, a New Jersey man who made it to Kona by lottery in 1998. "I chose Ironman training over my marriage," he said. His wife had left him a year earlier after he rebuffed her ultimatum to cut back on his heavy training.

"It's like a drug—it takes over your life," Campeau said. "You can throttle back on triathlon if you do the shorter distances, but if you get the Hawaii bug, you're screwed."

Bruce Buchanan, a dentist-turned-personal-trainer from Fernandina Beach, Florida, clearly explained the role triathlon played in his life when he married his second wife. She was proud and supportive of him when he swept the 50–55 age group in 1991, 1992, and 1993. Then, after five years together, they got divorced. The problem was typical: "I didn't make her feel like a priority," said Buchanan. "You get tunnel vision and self-centered training for Ironman. I wouldn't let anything interfere with it—except my dental work. Not her."

Proving that old dogs can learn new tricks, however, Buchanan made amends with his third wife, Lee. "I realized from the previous marriages that you must always put your spouse first," he said. "That's critical for saving the relationship." He now gives up training time for Lee, her projects, and cultural events. He will skip a swim practice to go to a movie with her, or a run to go to dinner. He found that his small sacrifice not only makes her feel important, but does not impact his performance. He won his age group again in 1999, 2001, and 2002, the latter in a new 60–65 age-group record.

"In your first year of Ironman, you can get away with being obsessed," said Buchanan. "But after that, you can't expect [your spouse] to be the only one making sacrifices. Besides, triathletes probably need the time off anyway, since we all train more than we need to."

There's an ah-ha moment: The smart triathlete or cyclist doesn't look at time with his spouse as a skipped training session. He just views it as recovery time.

Rich White

Manufacturers may think they gain new converts by advertising in magazines aimed at cologne abusers from Manhattan. In truth, people get into mountain biking the way they get into anything: word of mouth. And when it comes to riding, Rich White just won't shut up.

—Rob Story, Bike magazine, 1997

because of Rich. When I want to ride somewhere local or international, he's the guy I want along. Rob Story, one of the finest sports/ adventure writers of this era, called Rich "the head cheerleader for mountain biking's 40-million member team." He called the column about Rich excerpted above "The Reverend," and the name stuck.

We all know a Rich White—the guy who makes the calls, maps the route, introduces new people to the sport, makes the ride happen, keeps the tradition alive. But for those people in Southern California and in the bike industry lucky enough to have met him, there is only one Rich "The Reverend" White— our own personal cycling celebrity, a superb athlete with a Bruce Lee body, the outsized personality of a comedian and late-night talk show host, and the blunt, commonsense wisdom of your neighborhood's most grizzled old granddad.

Rich, variously a bike-shop manager, salesman, and mechanic, manufacturer marketing manager, and occasional freelance writer, owns no property and few possessions—except bikes. He lives and breathes mountain biking—all cycling, actually. His passionate pontificating about all things—music and history and culture and books, but especially cycling—earns him sizable real estate in any conversation and press from any magazine editor within earshot. I've written stories about Rich and

A customer walks into the shop. "I'm looking for something with a RockShox and costs no more than $800," he says.

"OK," Rich says, "but what do you wanna do with it?"

"Umm..." the customer ponders.

"Well," says Rich, "next weekend I'm hitting this buff single-track that drops 3,500 vertical feet through four different climate zones. Last time, I couldn't believe how cool that view was, when we were on top of the mountain looking down on the clouds as the sunset turned them red. Does that sound like something you'd do? 'Cuz you're welcome to join us if you want."

In no time the shopper's wheeling a $1,500 bike out the door. Whether he rides with Rich depends only on his motivation. But the offer's genuine. Rich White, like Barry White, always wants to spread the love.

—R.S.

As you'll see in this Bike for Life *interview conducted in December 2004, Rich was on the wrong path in life until the day he found cycling, and it changed him. That was a good day for all of us.*

ME? BEING INTERVIEWED along with the likes of Gary Fisher, John Howard, Mike Sinyard, Ned, Missy—such an esteemed list of heroes and dignitaries? Unbelievable. First, my picture on a magazine cover [*Bicycle Guide*, 1993], next a story about me [*Bike*, 1997], then a few bylines, then crossing the Alps by mountain bike, and now this. In the Library of Congress forever. Pretty good for a guy who hasn't accomplished anything, really, except wake up every morning and shout to the world, "I love riding my bike!"

I was born in 1959, but my life actually began in 1984, on the day I won a bike in a poker game. I wouldn't have believed it at the time if someone had told me that that bike—a Raleigh Traveler, a 21-inch steel road bike, way too tall for me—would change my life. Get me out of an unhealthy lifestyle into a healthy one. But it did.

At that time, I was all about entertainment. Sex and drugs and rock 'n' roll. I was into going to Hollywood and seeing bands and being around nightclubs. After I got out of high school, if I'd had a business card it might have said "part-time gambler, nightclub host, nightclub security, concert security." I was a regular in Vegas at the Dunes poker table and I had a regular game at my house three times a week. You could sit in with 50 bucks. Also, we were into fighting—because that's what we did at our nightclub, as security guards. Scrawny guy like me—I wasn't the bouncer—I was more of a host-diplomat. That means I had the mouth; I was the guy who talked guys out of fighting. I patrolled the line outside to make sure the pretty girls got inside. I don't have a black belt, nothing. What I had was a bunch of big guys kick my ass all the time and teach me how to keep them from doing that.

I worked the L.A. Olympics for two weeks in 1984 as a trained observer. I was paid to walk around just observing people, because they thought there was going to be terrorist activity. I was actually working out at the area where they had the cycling events, and I got into watching it. It was a couple days later when I won the bike in a poker game. A guy owed me money and didn't have it, so I just took the bike and rode it until he paid me, and he never did.

Immediately, I found that I just liked the feeling of riding, traveling from A to B, human-powered. I'd forgotten that I rode as a kid—a lot, actually. I used to ride my bike 17 miles to school without my parents knowing it. I lived in Carson, but I went to this Christian school in Harbor City, down by San Pedro. I'd sneak my bike out of the shed, skip the bus, and ride my bike. But I didn't consider myself a cyclist. I just didn't want to take the bus; I wanted the freedom. I never thought about it as something to compete with or ride for pleasure. But now that I had a bike again, that big-mileage gene kicked in. I was living in Downey, and I'd ride that beat-up old Traveler down the riverbed to the beach and back—40 miles or so. One day, about a month after the poker game, I ran into a friend who I didn't know rode. He was all surprised, and said, "Man, I got to get you a better bike." And he got me a Raleigh USA bike, just like the ones they rode in the Olympics.

I just totally fell in love with it. I instantly knew that that was me. I was addicted. Because I worked at night in a nightclub, I had free time to ride all day.

Before the bike, I hung out by the pool all day and hit on all the strippers getting tanned. I actually married a stripper—in '83, I think. Beautiful Chinese girl with big fake hooters. I met her before I got into cycling. Lilly. After she married me, it was Lilly White, which always got a laugh. But she stuck with me, even when I went to jail five years later....

Why did I go to jail? Because I got involved in the most popular industry of the '80s—selling drugs. I worked in a nightclub, where you can make money being a bartender—or a . . . facilitator. Money's coming in, money's going out, all the time. Rock 'n' roll, gambling, and drugs.

It wasn't prison. It was just jail. Only did five months, but I say a year. I got a job in the jail school. I helped everybody write letters home to their family and friends. I used my diplomatic skills to get along with everyone—all the various races and factions. Once it was over, all I knew was that I never wanted to do anything again that got in the way of cycling.

Jail had a significant impact on me. It was an exit gate from one life and an entry gate to another. I did what I had to do. I paid for it, and I moved on. I knew that I didn't want to do that anymore. I didn't think I necessarily had to do cycling to keep me away from my old life; I just liked it enough to where I didn't want that old life. That's the whole thing about the "Reverend" deal. It's pretty easy to preach cycling when it saved me from the purely low-goals life. I could have done other things for a living I guess, but I didn't have anything that I liked more than that. I had options; I just didn't know what they were. Everyone has options; that doesn't mean you want to take 'em. If people are out there having problems, and they don't go out and find what's them, they're just flailing, right? I just got lucky and found what was supposed to be me already.

As soon as I won the bike in that poker game in 1984, I knew where I was going. I knew I was going to get into the industry. But I figured I didn't know anything, and the best way to learn was to go to school, and that school was retail. So about eight months before I went to jail, I worked part-time at Bike Outpost in Fountain Valley—for Bill McReady, owner of Santana Tandems. For me, it was college. I was getting paid dirt, but I was going to school. I had a full plan: I was going to start a bike shop and get out of the security business. I was going to call it Rock Hard Cyclery.

Two days after I got out of jail, I went in to get a tube for my mountain bike, and the manager was a friend of mine, Dave Crosby, who I worked for at Bike Outpost. He hired me on the spot. I didn't ask for a job. He said, "We would love to have someone like you working here. If you don't have a job, I want to hire you right now to sell bikes." He never knew I went to jail. He thought I went away to take care of my sick mom or something. Soon, they fired him, and I was the manager.

The Mountain Dogs and the Reverend

I GOT INTO mountain biking in 1986, two years after I won my bike, two years before I worked in a bike shop. I was always an off-road, dirty kind of guy and thought it'd sure be cool to go off into the mountains. My friend Lance and I went to the bike shop and bought mountain bikes together. It was around the start of the year, I think. It's hard to remember, exactly—that was the decade of decadence. I had long hair like everyone else. Very long, practically down to my ass. Picture Samson with a bad haircut. Anyhow, Lance just got some Christmas cash. I always had money because I was dealing drugs. We went down with $1,200 and bought the bikes, and rode in Whittier Hills. We bought a map, made peanut-butter-and-jelly sandwiches, and rode as far as we could until the sandwiches and water ran out.

Three miles into that first ride, I was obsessed. It felt like my legs were about to cramp up, I was about to pass out. My lungs were fried. Sweat was pouring into my eyes and they were burning. My hands were sweating on the grips. I felt like I was about to fall over and die on the spot. And I figured I needed to go a little bit further.

I absolutely loved it. I was ahead of everyone else, and I thought that was cool. Lance was dying worse than me; he weighed about 80 pounds more. Actually, though, I just liked the fact that when I looked up to the top of something, if I kept going, I'd get there. When I got there, I thought, Now, I just want to go to the next-highest thing.

I loved riding road bikes just as much. But now I couldn't stop riding either one. Every time I was on one, I felt like this is where I'm supposed to be.

Everyone I knew bought a mountain bike as soon as I bought one. My whole social circle instantly converted to mountain biking—a bunch of hippie freaks.

We wanted to get matching shirts so that if we got drunk in a bar we could identify each other. We looked at all the other clubs and they all sounded kind of arrogant, elite, and noninclusive, and we just wanted a name that described our lifestyle—we were just a bunch of dogs that liked running around a mountain, whether it was on a road bike or a mountain bike. So we were the Mountain Dogs.

Roadies invited the Mountain Dogs on club rides, but all they really wanted were people to beat. People to make them feel that they were special. Some people think a bike makes them important, but it really doesn't. It made me start thinking mountain biking is different [from road biking]. People who are willing to go out and get dirty and stuff don't look at each other for the jersey they're wearing or how clean their bike is or how bitchin' it is. They go out and suffer and thrash and get dirty together.

And then there's the ride, the scenery, the experience. Lot of road riders don't talk about the ride. They never ride alone, just to do it. They talk about the clothes, the bike they're riding; they never talk about the simple beauties that they saw along the way. They never stop to take a picture. We did.

I'd like to think the Mountain Dogs and I knew most of the trails in the San Gabriel Mountains. That's because I took a map, I laid it on the ground, I started from the left, and I rode every damn trail that was listed.

The Fine Art of Sheepdogging

By 1990, THINGS were great and getting better. I'm working at the Mulrooney shop in Cerritos. I started racing. Then one day this Asian gentleman walked in and said in a thick accent, "Hey, I want to talk to Moun-Tain Dog." He was all Chinesed-out, and I say that without any bigotry, being married at the time to Lilly. But he's the prototypical Taiwanese businessman, with the blue suit and tie, black shiny shoes, and white shirt—the antithesis of mountain biking. I was like, "Okay, I'll be right with you." He was from a parts maker called Zoom and needed marketing help to crack the US market. He had gone to a couple of bike shops, and they were all roadies. To them, the Mountain Dogs were the only real mountain bike club around, and I was the mountain biker—the only one with a mouth as big as mine, anyway. Truth is, no one had gone to as many places as I had locally. Everyone else did the same old rides, and I went off the map. No question, I'm loud. I don't need a bell. The bears need a bell to warn me of them.

So I began consulting for Zoom and eventually left the bike shop. I went on the road with Zoom for five years. Did their national marketing. Went to most of the NORBA races, went to most of their distributors.

Through a stroke of luck, I was on the cover of *Bicycle Guide* in February 1993. The editor started riding with the Mountain Dogs and he asked us to review 19 of the new $700 front-suspension mountain bikes, at that time a breakthrough price point for the technology. The exposure was awesome. Dream come true. It was one of those weird things where, once you're in a magazine, people think you're important, so then they give you things to do, and give you products, and then because you have all those great new things, other magazines think you're somebody, and then they start putting you in their magazine. It kind of perpetuated things for me, no doubt.

In 1997, I was ordained by the bishop of *Bike* magazine—editor Rob Story, one of my heroes and friends. He called me the Reverend—and the name stuck. He wrote a story about my behavior on the trail that captured me to a "T."

I'd ride a lot with big groups, and everyone has a different pace. It's just as difficult to ride faster than someone can than slower than someone can. So everyone has to get into their own groove. But when you're in the back, you feel a little anxiety that you need to keep up, that everyone's waiting for you at the top.

My style was to alleviate that, so everybody would feel comfortable on rides. Instead of getting to the top first and sitting there and waiting for everyone and cooling down, I didn't let myself cool down. I came here to ride—so I'd roll back down to the last guy, make sure he was all right, give him some encouragement, and in the process get myself more training time. It wasn't just because I was thinking about everyone else. It also gave me more ride. I got to climb it again, work out a little bit more, do more of exactly what I came to do. A lot of guys rode up to the top and then they didn't want to ride down and have to do it again. It's like, well, you came to ride—or you came to sit? It makes everyone feel better. The slower guys feel better. The faster guys ride more, and nobody's waiting on anyone. It just makes sense. It's a simple thing. It's a win-win. Nobody loses. There's nothing worse than being left somewhere and not knowing where everyone is. And then when you ride hard and get somewhere and cool down, you gotta warm up again. I don't blame guys for being bummed out for waiting. I just wonder why they wait.

Today, people who meet me ask me what the whole Reverend thing is all about. It's easy. It's not about preaching about your afterlife; I think your body here on Earth is a temple, and you should take care of it. And my way of taking care of it is through cycling as much as I can.

Fitness Advice from a Lean Machine
HONESTLY, IT'S KIND of weird to have someone say to me, "I want your body." Well, you know what? That means you have to climb into my mommy's womb and come out exactly like I did. I'm the only person who has my body; we're all individuals. Don't judge yourself by the mirror. You don't have to be perfect. You just have to be fit enough to do the things that you want to do. That's the most important thing.

On a daily basis, you have to get up in the morning and kick-start your body. Your metabolism. Soon as I wake up, I do half an hour of light aerobics, rowing machine, or a Tai Chi kickbox workout before breakfast.

Food-wise, remember that the hole up on your head is bigger than the hole in your ass. You can't shove tons in, have a little bit come out, and not expect to have the rest stick on your fat gut.

All these bullshit diets with this trend and that trend, it really always comes around to eat a balanced diet. Eat a lot of fruits and vegetables. Cook fresh food. Avoid anything that says "all you can eat." Just because it says that doesn't mean you have to. Soup is a really good thing. You take a lot of really good things and boil them all together. Eat things you like to eat that you know aren't bad for you.

Then put a lock on the TV for one hour after you eat. Until then, you have to move. Do anything—just don't lay down. I was into that thinking before cycling; it's just that cycling made it easy because it's fun. That's the difference. I don't go to gyms to work out all the time. Find something you like to do, whether it's cycling or hiking or bowling, do it a lot. Work up a sweat. Make yourself suffer. One of the things about adventure racing, which I'm now getting into, is that if you can be comfortable being uncomfortable, you'll be a good adventure racer. Well, to work out in any sport, you have to teach yourself to be a little uncomfortable—just for a little while. Just long enough to burn more calories than you consume.

That's easy to do if you find something you like doing, like cycling. That's fitness in simple terms: Find something you love to do—and do it a lot.

Don't Be Afraid to Be Afraid

IN FACT, I think a lot of the attraction of mountain biking is the joy of overcoming uncomfortable situations—the hard work, the fear of the unknown, the fear of getting hurt. Put them all together and you have incredible potential for adventure.

A bicycle's way more fun to adventure on than to race. I've raced; racing is just going in circles. Mountain biking at its best is exploration, the great unknown, pushing the boundaries. Once I did a 13-hour death hike–bike death march in Jacumba in the Southern California desert along an abandoned railway with no lights through tunnels so dark during the day that you couldn't see your seat, cactus bigger than your entire bicycle, more flats than a year of NASCAR racing. Of course, I didn't do these alone. The TransAlp Challenge—eight days, 400 miles with 60,000 feet of climbing—is one thing, but doing it with one of your best friends brings a whole new kind of sentimental value to it. The TransRockies was pretty incredible.

If there is racing that combines the adventure and the camaraderie, it's 24-hour events. Take the first 24 Hours of Moab, 1995. I've never ridden in a snowstorm in the middle of the night before. Four o'clock in the morning, stoned out of my mind, coffee'd up like Juan Valdez.

But the beauty of mountain biking is that you don't need to travel the world to make epic memories. My philosophy is sort of borrowed from my favorite book, *The Way of the Peaceful Warrior*, by Dan Millman. It woke me to the simple way of thinking that I think is important on bike rides—that *there are no ordinary moments*.

You don't need an exotic place to find a great ride. If you're out there with a friend on any ride, it can be a great ride if you just pay attention to that day, that moment. A lot of people, especially those who come where we come from—the Orange County, city-urban areas—are in such a hurry to do other things that a bike ride to them just fits into their schedule. They rush it; they

have a time frame; they hurry up and ride and go home. They have no time to notice the ride, because they can't stop and really see what's going on—it's just a workout. They did it, they're done. They didn't feel it, enjoy it.

A lot of people I know do loops, these little carved loops. They never go off the loop. They never go somewhere and just ride somewhere—even if it's wrong. They don't ride the dead-end roads, down past where they know where they're going. They don't go if they don't know if there is going to be water or food or a Power Bar or a flat repair station waiting for them.

They are afraid to be afraid.

You ride with guys who only want to take one tube, one patch, because they are afraid of carrying something. "I filled up my backpack, when I'm done I'm coming back." A lot of people have important things to do. They do the ride between important things. The important thing for me to do is to do the ride. I do everything else between rides.

I always liked hiking and tennis and running. But I always wanted to do them and then come home. But when I got into cycling, I didn't necessarily want to come home. That's where I wanted to be the whole time. I just *had* to come home. Come home to get supplies and go out and do it again.

Tai Chi and Single-Track

OF COURSE, SOMETIMES you need a little extra help to go out again. I started doing Tai Chi after my first huge crash in 1987. I knew that I had a problem; my crash put a lot of fear in me, and I knew that I wasn't as focused as I [should be], because I kept thinking about the crash and thinking about the pain. So I went and took a Tai Chi class so I could redirect my focus and learn a couple basic breathing and stretching and focus exercises. No matter how smart you are, no matter how good you are at what you do, sometimes if you just go take some kind of class or good instruction from someone, it helps you have a direct and complete focus, a really regimented focus on a particular goal. Tai Chi gives you principles that teach you about focus and mental preparation, how to move your body very slowly and to feel your every movement.

I was familiar with Tai Chi from my old life. While working at the club, I was having a lot of problems defending—stopping drunk, nasty people from hitting me. My biggest problem was that I was having problems not looking at what I wanted to avoid. Looking right at them, and not getting beyond that. I was focusing on every little obstacle and not the big overall problem.

Tai Chi helped because I practiced focusing. Every minute of Tai Chi you're focusing on your breath, your movement, your position, your next breath, next movement. A particular exercise called "the archer," where you focus on shooting an imaginary arrow at an imaginary target. If you really practice enough, you can almost hear the arrow hitting the target.

How it translates to the bike: It trains you to look where you do want to go and not where you don't. Helps you relax and give a few little things to focus on. Like anything, if you don't practice skills, they don't come to you easily in panic situations or when you're tired and fatigued. Muscle memory is trained to do something—so things happen without your having to think about them. Like instead of me being scared about the trail being gnarly, I focused on exactly where I needed to ride, and get across the gnarly shit no sweat.

One of my Mountain Dog friends, Jim "Popeye" Thompson, an old grumpy bike dude, helped me in this regard. He taught me not to fear anyone. He told me every day to ride as hard as you can. If the trail beats you, it beats you, but at least you didn't give up because you're scared.

Middle Age: What's Next?

I'VE ENJOYED THE Reverend thing, the notoriety. But let's put it in perspective. I'm no visionary or do-gooder. No matter how good you get at riding it, you're still just riding a child's toy. You're doing a real cool thing, it's real exciting, it's real fun, but you're really not doing anything for the planet, except riding a bicycle around, like kids do every day, in every neighborhood. I do it because it's really fun, it's really good for me. Not for anybody else. It's kind of selfish. Cyclists are the most selfish people around, except for triathletes. It's all about me, riding my bike, as fast as I can.

Over the years, I got invited to do a lot of fun things. I got a lot of publicity that other people didn't get. I had a lot of free time to take people on rides, and of course I'd like to think I've spread some joy to others. The coolest thing in the world is when I see people riding bikes and they're going to crazy places, and I remember taking them on their first rides. That's way better than trophies and medals.

After the Zoom thing was over, I went back to the bike shop. Sold a lot of bicycles. It was fun.

But soon it gnawed at me. I didn't want to live at the beach anymore. I gotta live in the mountains. It didn't make sense to be a mountain biker and to have to drive to the mountains to ride my mountain bike, when I could live at the mountains and ride my bike out my door. In 2000, I got a job at Hardcloud.com, a sports website, now defunct. They hired me to be one of the writers. I could now live anywhere I wanted. A buck a word. Supposedly 2,500 words a month, plus reviews and expenses. All of a sudden I was making a lot of money—for me and my barebones lifestyle. It was stupid money. Internet money. Of course it didn't last.

But it got me to move to Big Bear. And now I live at 7,000 feet, two hours from the concrete chaos of L.A., in mountain bike heaven.

I'm 45. Where do I see myself in the future? In my dreams I want to do La Ruta, road-bike down the Pacific Coast, tour across the States, around the world. How long can I keep it going? Well, remember in 1993 when we rode down the Trans-Canada Highway in Jasper and Banff and saw those specks off in the distance? Remember that? And going into Pocahontas where the big totem poles were? And we kept riding, and we caught those little specks on the highway, and they turned out to be old bastards on a bike tour, 70-, 80-year-old men? We were amazed. "Wow, they're still riding at that age!" we said. Right? Well, what the hell? Why not us?

Update

IN A FOLLOW-UP interview in December 2013, White reported that he was fitter than ever, mainly because he'd added more strength training and eliminated sugars and hydrogenated oils from his diet. Cycling-wise, he'd achieved his goals of riding the La Ruta de los Conquistadores mountain bike stage race and doing a road-bike trip down the California coast. A carless 365-days-a-year bike commuter, he worked for many years at a gym as a much-sought-after instructor teaching "RevCore," his innovative core-centric aerobic workout, before leaving to help run a nursery owned by one of his personal training clients. Enthralled by what he was learning, White became a landscape consultant, an expert in "xeriscaping" (the use of native plants that don't require watering), and a self-described "performance botanist" who educated clients on the native flowers and foliage of the San Bernardino Mountains as they biked and hiked through it.

"I feel like the nursery is improving me as a mountain biker, as an outdoorsman, as a person," said White. "Now, more than ever, I savor the journey, not just the high points. Instead of just being a peacock and a rooster who says, 'Look at me,' I work for people who have peacocks and roosters in their yard. It's a much more holistic and beautiful thing."

13

HOW TO SURVIVE

Staying safe amid mountain lions, bike-jackers, lightning storms, careless drivers, poison oak, rabid dogs, and other unexpected dangers

Call it contingency planning, emergency procedures, or just Plan B. Because even if you do everything we advocate in Bike for Life—*ride a perfect bike with a perfect fit with perfect form and a perfect training plan that ramps up your fitness without injury—fate can intervene. Your hard-won health can suddenly be wrecked for the weekend—or forever if you're cut off by a car, attacked by a dog or a mountain lion, bike-jacked, or riddled with saddle sores or poison oak. Your progress suddenly may slow when you're slammed by headwinds, get caught in a thunderstorm, or end up with a flat when you don't have a repair kit. After all, you can't deprogram bad luck, but you can and should be prepared when it happens. This chapter tells how to survive some of cycling's unexpected roadblocks.*

1. HOW TO SURVIVE . . . A MOUNTAIN LION ATTACK

On January 8, 2004, Anne Hjelle of Mission Viejo, California, 30, literally survived the jaws of death. On a mountain bike ride in Whiting Ranch Wilderness Park, just a few miles from her Orange County home, the personal trainer and ex-Marine was attacked by a 122-pound mountain lion that had killed and disemboweled another mountain biker, 35-year-old Mark Reynolds, hours earlier. As Hjelle descended twisty, cacti-studded Cactus Ridge Trail at 15 mph, the animal, also known as a cougar, leapt on her right shoulder and bit hard into the back of her neck.

As Hjelle screamed and punched him, the animal worked his way around to the front of her neck, and clamped down. Cougars, typically 7 to 10 feet long and 65 to 150 pounds, have 300 pounds per square inch of crushing power in their jaws—about six times as much as a wolf. With the right-hand side of her face torn off, and her carotid artery and trachea missed by millimeters, Hjelle blacked out. It took a team to save her: her courageous riding partner, Debi Nicholls, 48, who hugged her friend's leg and was dragged 20 feet with her down the hill, and three male rock-throwing mountain bikers, who pelted the lion from the trail. Soon, the cat released his prey and loped a short distance away. Sitting under a bush next to Mark's body, the killer watched as paramedics quickly arrived to carry Hjelle to the hospital. Rangers killed the cougar later that day. Despite the attack, Hjelle had no internal injuries. A few weeks after undergoing six hours of facial reconstructive surgery, she was back hiking. She was disfigured and would require many more surgeries, but felt lucky to be alive.

The incident shook up mountain bikers around the country, including me. I regularly bike at Whiting Ranch. Wildlife experts speculate that attacks on people in the wilderness are likely to increase as humans' homes and recreational activities continue to impinge on animals' habitats. "It's completely unnatural behavior—their normal prey is deer and sheep, then raccoons, and even other mountain lions," said John Ganaway, a former head ranger at Whiting and then boss at nearby Caspers Regional Park, where in 2003 a cougar almost pounced on a five-year-old boy until the mother threw a shoe at him. "One animal behaviorist believes that seeing us on a daily basis makes them lose their fear of us—and look at us as a food item."

Ganaway arrived on the scene at Whiting with other rangers hours after the attack on Hjelle and surveyed the scene the next morning. "There was blood everywhere," he said. "It was a fight for her life. And it's a good thing she fought; that's one of the first rules of surviving an attack. As we tell our visitors, mountain lions are used to animals running—not fighting back. And they don't have good endurance, so you can tire them out. The mother at Caspers saved her kid because she read the literature that we pass out."

According to the California Department of Fish and Game (CDFG), 19 verified mountain lion attacks on humans have occurred in California since 1890, 14 of those since 1992. Six of the attacks resulted in fatalities—two from rabies, which is common in the animals, especially during summer months. The last death before Reynolds's was in 1994. Here's what the CDFG suggests you do to survive the trails in a cougar habitat.

1. Don't ride alone. Cougars are less likely to attack groups. Ride with a partner, and stay close together. If attacked, you can help one another.

2. Don't run if confronted by a lion. They instinctively chase—and are so fast that they'll catch you in seconds.

3. Stand tall. Cougars try to bite the head or neck, so try to remain on your feet, and don't bend over or turn away. Make yourself look bigger. Raise your arms, move them slowly, and speak in a firm, loud voice. If you're wearing a jacket, open it. Maintain eye contact with the animal.

4. Raise hell. Yell, scream, act aggressive. Whatever you do, don't be quiet. Noise unnerves the animal and is an audible call for help.

5. If attacked, jab the animal's eyes. Use something sharp—sticks, rocks, a bike pump, or your bare hands.

6. Keep fighting. Kick and punch until you can't anymore. Mountain lions have poor endurance. He might think that this isn't worth it and decide to go back to deer and other weaklings that flee.

7. Don't ride or jog after dusk. Sundown in the mountains is near feeding time for cougars.

8. If you do ride after dusk, affix two lights to the back of your helmet. "They look like eyes to the lions," said Dan Cain of Borrego Springs, California, who rides up to 30 miles per week in the desert mountains south of Palm Springs and has run across the big cats on several occasions. Charged by a lion in 1998 on the Pacific Crest Trail, he stood his ground, screamed "like a rock star," aimed his lights into the lion's face, and sighed with relief as the cat backed off.

9. Most of all, don't take the mountain-lion threat lightly. Beautiful, tawny-colored animals with black-tipped ears and tails, mountain lions have been hunted for bounty for decades, were given "protected" status after 1990, and now number 4,000 to 6,000 in California. Half the state is prime cougar country, especially where deer are plentiful. As suburbia marches toward the foothills and mountains, as in Orange County, expect more encounters. "A week before the attacks at Whiting," said Ganaway, "a Fish and Game warden told me, 'It's not a matter of if we have another attack, but when.'"

Even so, Ganaway notes that "you're still far safer riding in the mountains than swimming in the ocean," according to statistics.

2. HOW TO SURVIVE . . . A FALL

Mountain bike legend Ned Overend was one of the rare riders to go a whole career—an exceptionally long one, at that—without suffering a broken bone. That wasn't by accident (no pun intended). His method, below, applies to both mountain and road riding.

1. Balancing act: Practicing track stands and general balancing will help you avoid slow-speed falls. "It'll give you that extra second to clip-out," said Ned. And avoid toppling over on your hip.

2. Slip out fast: Set up your pedals to get out of them easily in a crash. Clean 'em out, keep 'em oiled, and you can pull your foot out quickly and avoid a knee injury.

3. Soft landing: Minimize impact when you hit the ground. Fight the urge to stick an arm out; that'll risk a broken collarbone. Instead, keep your body in and try to let the handlebar and pedal hit the ground first. Before you hit, tuck your arm in and roll, letting your whole body absorb the blow.

3. HOW TO SURVIVE . . . A FLAT TIRE WITHOUT A PATCH KIT

It's happened to everyone—a flat tire when you're alone, without a spare tube or patch kit, and too far out to walk home before nightfall. How do you survive? "I usually wait until other bikers come along and bum a tube off them," said Jim Langley, a former bike mechanic, longtime *Bicycling* magazine technical editor, and now an industry consultant. But if you're in outer Mongolia and yurt drivers only come along every three days, Langley advises the following.

1. Stuff it with grass. This age-old survival trick is so well-known it's a cliché, but it works. Simply jam your tire with grass, paper, rags—anything that'll solidify it—and keep rolling.

2. A slow leak? Pump it up. Even if it lasts 60 seconds, that gets you a long way on a bike. Ride until it's flat and repeat. Great upper-body workout.

3. Ride it. Flat be damned. If it's on the rear tire, keep pedaling. "No kidding. This usually works as long as you watch out for things that might damage the rim," said Langley. "I've ridden up to 5 miles on flat roads and mountain bike tires with no damage to the wheels. Be careful in corners though—it can get pretty squirrelly." Note: Riding a front-tire flat is nearly impossible; swap it with the good rear inner tube.

Here's Langley's fixes for other common mechanical maladies.

4. Broken chain: You can't jury-rig a chain, or carry a spare. So Langley won't leave home without a chain tool and a special repair chain link that can be snapped in place with your hands.

5. Taco'd wheel: A wheel so bent that it takes on a potato chip or taco shape needs to be replaced, but you can temporarily straighten it enough to get home. Here's how: Remove the wheel, find the largest wobble on the rim, then raise the wheel with two hands over your head and swing it down so you smack the bump on the ground. "Wham! Check the wheel," said Langley. "Closer to straight? If not, whack harder. Move on to the next wobble and whack it until the wheel is straight enough to ride."

6. Bent derailleur hanger: If you crash on the right side of the bike and bend the derailleur, your shifting is gone. To get it back, try this neat Langley trick, which works only if the bend is on the hanger itself, the little finger on the frame where the derailleur bolts on: Take off the rear wheel, remove the quick-release skewer, and unscrew the derailleur so that it's off the frame. Now, you can thread the end of the axle into place where the derailleur used to be. If you can, use the wheel to gently coerce that bent piece of metal straight. Then reinstall the derailleur.

7. Broken shift cable: You're stuck in one gear if the shift cable breaks, so at least make it one you can ride comfortably in until you get home. That involves tightening the cable, which you can do by pulling it to the nearest water-bottle-mount screw and tightening it down. If the remaining cable is too short for that, Langley advises tightening the limit screw on the derailleur to force it to stay in an easy gear.

4. HOW TO SURVIVE . . . A BIKE-JACKING

On June 23, 2004, five-time national mountain bike champion Tinker Juarez was putting in big road miles in preparation for the TransAlp Challenge, a 400-mile off-road race across the Alps that was two weeks away. Heading back to his home in Downey, a Los Angeles suburb, the 42-year-old briefly pulled off the L.A. River bike path at Atlantic Boulevard to change his cassette tape—he hadn't yet updated to the iPod, which was only just starting on the upward trajectory that soon made it ubiquitous. "Just as I was about to hop back on my bike, someone tapped me on the back," said Tinker. "I turned around and saw a gang member guy with a gun camouflaged next to his T-shirt—pointed right at me."

"Give me your bike," the man said coolly.

Wordlessly, Tinker handed him the bike. The gunman rode off on the brand-new Cannondale 613, a unique carbon-aluminum mix so light—15 pounds—that it had been banned from the Tour de France the previous summer. The $5,000 road bike moved fast, Juarez guesses, probably selling for a hundred dollars within the hour.

"I wasn't going to question the guy," he said. "There was nothing I could say to him. I knew to say nothing, just living here all my life. I have cousins like that. I live around it, I see it. There's too much senseless killing every day, for a shoe or a watch—or a bike.

"I don't have to live here. I could live in Colorado with mountains and animals, or I can live here [in L.A. County] with my family and millions of other people, a few of them bad, like this guy."

Juarez knows he'd screwed up by stopping on a path located in a crime-ridden area: "Maybe I need to get an MP3 player," he said. "I definitely got a little too complacent." That's putting it mildly; he was bike-jacked in North Long Beach, a low-income area next to Compton, where his brightly colored bike jersey and tinted sports glasses made him conspicuous. "Normally, when I see people on a bike path who look like gang members, I turn off onto the streets, go around them, and get back on the bike path farther down."

Of course, you can't avoid what you can't see. In a case that made the papers in 1993, Oliver Thompson, then the 51-year-old police chief of nearby Inglewood, was deliberately rear-ended on his custom-made Davidson road bike while riding home from work. Three men jumped from the car and demanded his backpack at gunpoint, and he quickly complied. As his assailants ran back to the car, he pulled a .45-caliber service revolver out of his fannypack and fired, wounding one and causing him to drop the pack. "Good thing they hadn't demanded my bike," said the lifelong cycling aficionado. "Somebody would have died."

The last statement was made in jest. Chief Thompson advised that bike-jacking victims keep it in perspective. "Walk through the what-ifs," he said. "Even if you do the right thing—plan your route around bad areas and avoid riding at night—bike-jacking can happen to anyone at any time. Give them what they want, and hopefully your life will be spared."

The day he was bike-jacked, Tinker Juarez stayed cool and survived. Three weeks later, he won the Masters division at the TransAlp.

Tinker was able to call his sponsor and get another bike. But if you want the insurance company to take care of your stolen bike with no hassle, make sure you photograph it when you get it, so it can be identified later, and know your serial number. You can also register your bike and engrave the ID number on the frame. Otherwise, a stolen bike can be hard to get back even if it's found. You can also purchase insurance for your bike. (Find bicycle attorney Bob Mionske's tips at www.bicyclelaw.com/p.cfm /bicycle-safety/about-bike-theft.)

5. HOW TO SURVIVE . . . POISON OAK, IVY, AND SUMAC

East of the Rockies, it's ivy. Down South, it's sumac. Out West, oak. Mountain bike enough, and you'll eventually be exposed to urushiol, the poisonous sap that can make you regret a day of epic single-track. For some, the immune response to urushiol-contaminated skin cells is a tiny itchy spot on the arm that lasts two days. For others, it means three weeks of oozing, burning, seeping, pus-drenched welts spreading all over your body that cause loved ones to recoil in revulsion and make you scratch like you've never scratched before. But that's not the worst of it. About 15 percent of the 120 million Americans who are allergic to poison oak, ivy, and sumac are so highly sensitive that they break out in a rash and begin to swell in 4 to 12 hours, not the normal 24 to 48. Their eyes may swell shut and blisters may erupt on their skin. Considered one of the few true emergencies in dermatology, it requires you to get to a hospital as soon as possible for a shot of corticosteroids to bring the swelling down.

For most people, the sores usually go away on their own in two weeks. But that fortnight of hell has led to a cottage industry of poison-oak remedies, rumors, and urban myths. First step: Immediately after the ride, wash the affected area and all the clothing you wore with soap and cold water; the easily spread oil can persist in crystalline form on clothing or other contacted items (including pets) for several weeks. Then, to shorten the agony, try out some of the following over-the-counter and home-brewed cures culled from www.gorp.com, www.poison ivy.aesir.com, and www.otan.us:

1. Rhuli: This popular medicine, found in Anti-Itch Gel by Band-Aid, leaves a dry, menthol-tinged film over the affected area. Some say washing the area beforehand with soap or dish-washing liquid will speed the effect. Besides Rhuli gel, try Caladryl, calamine lotion, or Benadryl; the alcohol in each cools and dries the area. Possible downside: Some say that the gel can leave chemical burns that are visible as scars a decade later.

2. Tecnu: Firefighters and wildlife rangers prefer to wash off with this popular urushiol-dissolving skin cleanser right after exposure. It's a good idea to keep a small bottle stashed with your tire repair kit.

3. Ocean salt water: Some believe that poison ivy sores will disappear a day or so after you swim in the ocean; you can also apply a salt-water-soaked cloth to the affected areas for 20 minutes twice a day.

4. Hot water: Increasing the shower temperature to near-scalding, a popular remedy, was so painful that one rider wrote on his blog, "I thought I was nuts." But the first dousing dried up his blisters overnight, allowing isolated hold-outs to be mopped up with Rhuli. Possible downside: Hot showers stop the itching for a while (because the nerve cells have been deadened, say detractors), but may cause the itching to spread, possibly due to the opening of pores and increased blood flow in the area.

5. Vicks VapoRub, Clorox, a warm Epsom salt bath followed by calamine lotion, hydrogen peroxide, and dishwashing liquid: Champions of all of the above say they stifle itching immediately and can dry out sores in two or three days. Some say to apply Vicks twice a day; it slightly burns at first, but may work because of the camphor in the ointment. Clorox bleach can cause chemical burns on the skin (though that might not be apparent at first), damages the eyes, and is harmful if swallowed. For those reasons, and the fact that it probably doesn't work against urushiol, physicians do not recommend it. Even home-remedy enthusiasts recommend strongly diluting the bleach (a quarter cup of bleach to a whole bathtub of water). In short, trying this remedy is not worth the risks, and could be dangerous. Some say that laying a peroxide-soaked washcloth on the infected area for 15 to 20 minutes will make the oozing poison-oak bubbles turn white, at which time you can scrape off the dead skin. Others say that rubbing Joy dishwashing liquid onto the skin and letting it dry overnight kills the itch (and also works for mosquito bites). Check with your doctor before trying these or any other "home remedies" found on the Internet.

There are many urban legends about how to cure poison ivy, oak, and sumac: hairspray, burdock-root tea, hemorrhoid ointment—you name it. Some desperate souls have boiled the root of a poke sallet plant into a smelly paste form and rubbed it on the sores until they started to burn or sting. Others, perhaps tired of rubbing goop onto their skin, have made a lead fishing-sinker necklace by pounding a sinker flat with a mallet, punching a hole in it, and threading a string through it. "I live in the country, am very allergic to poison ivy, and have been using this 30-plus years. It really works!" said one old-timer. Some of these things may be useless, but at least harmless; others may cause bigger problems than the one you're trying to solve. (Long-term skin contact with lead, for example, or eating with lead residue still on your hands, can cause lead poisoning; and you could be allergic to a plant paste.) Be careful about following home remedies that sound crazy—they probably are.

The best advice of all? Leaves of three, let them be.

6. HOW TO SURVIVE . . . HEADWINDS

The solution is one word—an *aerobar*. Club riders deride this add-on handlebar extension, which lowers and narrows you into a pointy aerodynamic shape, as "for triathletes only." Pro riders only use it in time trials, not the peloton, because it compromises handling in a paceline. Yet when it comes to surviving headwinds, the speed- and spirit-sapping bane of all cyclists, the aerobar also works for average Joes on the bike path and fully loaded bike tourists pushing cross-country with 60 pounds of gear.

I was one of the latter in June 1989, when my triathlete friend Larry Lawson and I pedaled the length of the Mississippi River from beginning to end for three weeks and 1,987 miles, fighting constant headwinds all the way. I was the more experienced tourist of the two of us, having pedaled all around the world in the 1980s, whereas Larry was on his first trip. But it instantly became obvious that he knew more than I did about handling the headwinds that relentlessly blow north from the Gulf of Mexico. Within minutes of departing Lake Itasca, Minnesota, from which the Mississippi emanates as an innocent 10-foot-wide stream, Larry was out of sight. I struggled to stay in double figures as the gusts whistled in my ears, slowing me to 7 mph on the flat prairie. Larry greeted me 20 miles down the road, having read the first chapter of Mark Twain's *Life on the Mississippi*, then bolted off, establishing a pattern that held all the way to La Crosse, Wisconsin.

The difference? Larry had an aerobar; I didn't.

Over a couple of cold ones at the Old Style Brewery in La Crosse, we decided to switch bikes: my steel Univega touring bike with two panniers—bloated with touring books and camera equipment, a tent, and a sleeping bag, total weight 64 pounds—for Larry's aluminum Klein Quantum with Scott triathlon bars and a round Tupperware cake-container suspended under the seat that held one change of bike clothes, a wallet, and a sleep sheet. Total weight: 21.72 pounds. (He'd weighed it before we left.)

His aerodynamic dream machine made a huge difference. Down in the aerobar tuck, I effortlessly sliced through those headwinds at 14, 15, 16 mph easy—it almost felt like cheating. I could see Larry struggling with my barge, banging into the wall of wind. But I didn't see him for long. Soon, he was ahead again and out of sight.

But the experiment was an unqualified success. When I caught him four hours later on the west side of the Mississippi at a drive-in liquor store in Pikes Peak, Iowa, Larry was so exhausted that he hadn't read a page of Twain. I'd arrived fresh, just minutes back. The point? Aerodynamics counts.

From that point we rode in a paceline, the Quantum first, like the bow of a ship, its arrow-point profile cutting wind resistance by a third, all the while creating a draft for the rear rider to rest in. Aerobar inventor Boone Lennon, who modeled the form after the tuck of a downhill skier, later told me that an aerobar could save a pro rider three seconds a mile in a time trial, but I'm convinced that it's worth far more for bike tourists battling headwinds. The second we flew home from New Orleans, just two weeks before Greg LeMond won the 1989 Tour de France by eight seconds using one, I bought an aerobar, and I haven't ridden without it since.

7. HOW TO SURVIVE . . . URBAN RIDING

The good news is that cycling on American roads is safer than it used to be. In 2012, cyclist deaths in the United States were down by 27 percent since 1975—from 1,003 to 726—despite many times more cyclists on the roads. Experts have speculated that's probably due to increased use of helmets, tougher drunk-driving laws, more bike paths and striped bike lanes, and general awareness of riders as the sport has grown. Now the bad news: Cyclists still die at a rate far beyond their numbers. In 2012, according to the Highway Traffic Safety Administration, road accidents caused 34,080 deaths in the United States, which means more than 2 percent of the people who died on the road were riding a bike,

grossly out of proportion to their numbers and total mileage. But you don't have to be a statistic, say cycling-safety experts like John Forrester, author of *Effective Cycling*, considered the bible of bike-safety, and Dan Dabek, director of CICLE (Cyclists Inciting Change thru Live Exchange), a Los Angeles organizer of rides and riding classes. Their advice, in a nutshell: *Act like a car.* It's simple. If you act like a bike, riding in the gutter, trying to stay out of the way, you're invisible. If you act like a car, you make yourself obvious and give drivers signals they understand. Whether you're a commuter, a racer, or a bike tourist, here are the rules for living to ride another day:

1. Ride predictably, in a straight line. Don't weave in and out of the parking lane. That encourages drivers to drift into your space.

2. Look over your shoulder. Safe merging and turning isn't possible in a car or on a bike without this basic traffic skill. Practice it. And keep your neck muscles stretched.

3. Leave the curb area and ride closer to the middle of the lane. This is a key to survival. The curb area is dangerous—debris, car doors suddenly opening, and right-turning drivers who think they have room to pass you before their turn, but don't, or who never saw you to begin with. You're invisible in the curb. To be seen, move left into middle of the lane so cars won't be tempted to squeeze by you. They can easily move into the left lane to pass you safely.

4. Don't ride on the wrong side of the road. This is the major cause of car-bike accidents. Drivers don't expect you there, especially at intersections and driveways. And it's illegal!

5. Avoid sidewalks. They're dangerous and slow. Besides conflicts with pedestrians, every driveway becomes a new intersection. Being hit by a car while riding on a sidewalk is the No. 1 bike-car accident, said Dabek. Again, you're breaking the law by cycling on a sidewalk (unless a local bylaw allows it).

6. Avoid crowded arteries by taking less-crowded parallels. Be smart. Instead of, for example, taking a jammed boulevard, try a less-traveled road that goes in the same direction, said Dabek, especially one with bike lanes.

7. Beware opposite-direction sideswipes. Being hit by cars turning left across the street into a shopping center parking lot is a common bike accident. So look left (as well as right) as you cross a driveway and be ready to make a hard right turn to avoid becoming a hood ornament.

8. Beware freeway crossings. You are particularly invisible to cars speeding or slowing onto on- and off-ramps.

9. If you lack skills, get off the street. Uncoordinated? Out of shape? Unskilled? If you don't have what it takes to ride in traffic, don't risk it: Safe cycling takes more concentration, alertness, and judgment than driving. If you lack these qualities, stay on the bike path.

10. Gear up with a helmet, lights, and bright clothing. You're a fool if you don't. Most bicycle fatalities are due to head injuries. For best visibility, use a flashing red rear light even in the daytime. And neon green and orange jackets, vest, and reflective piping will get attention day and night.

11. Finally, be paranoid. "Yeah, wear a helmet—and ride like you don't," said Robert Hurst, Denver bike messenger and author of *The Art of Urban Cycling.* "You need to be paranoid. Be ready for disaster. In the era of the cell phone, where distracted drivers are weaving all over the place, you can't assume anyone sees you. Riding 'like a car' will keep you safe from 99 percent of drivers, but do you want to take a chance on the 1 percent who don't pay attention?"

8. HOW TO SURVIVE . . . A LIGHTNING STORM

It was July 5, 1982, US Highway 14, Bighorn Mountains, Wyoming. To avoid the heat, we'd waited until dusk to begin a 6,000-foot climb, the longest of our Pacific-to-Atlantic tour, to the top of 8,950-foot Granite Pass. Everything went perfectly at first. The sky was a cloudless

HOW TO SURVIVE THE INSURANCE COMPANIES AFTER AN ACCIDENT

If you don't meet your maker in traffic, but are one of an estimated 45,000 American cyclists per year who are injured in a bike-car accident, the hassle is just beginning. At least 30 percent of bike-car injury cases go to litigation, compared to 10 to 15 percent in traffic cases involving automobiles only, according to West Los Angeles attorney Bill Harris, who handles several hundred bike cases a year. In other words, insurance companies don't make it easy for injured cyclists to collect for their injuries. In fact, the police and the courts are also, to some degree, stacked against cyclists, Harris adds. "Their thinking is, 'You bikers are doing something as dangerous and as crazy as riding in traffic with a bicycle. You'd better be prepared to stop fast—or be careful!'" Although cycling safety guru John Forrester believes that up to half of all bike accidents may be the fault of the cyclist, the fact is that innocent injured cyclists often don't get a fair shake. To protect yourself after an accident, *Bike for Life* has compiled the following tips from Harris. They'll give you a basic guideline of what to do—and what not to do—when dealing with the driver, the police, the hospital, and the insurance coverage.

1. Insist on a police report. Evidence will vanish and stories will change over time as witnesses move and memories fade. Make sure your claim is investigated at the outset. The first and best evaluation is a police report. Even ask the cop at the scene if you can look at the report to make sure everything you know gets put on it. You have the right to request a copy.

2. Get cops (and paramedics) to the scene by stressing that you're hurt. Police often won't come out unless there's an injury. Make sure cops come out and look at physical evidence, such as: (1) point of

(continues)

How to Survive the Insurance Companies
After an Accident *(continued)*

impact, and (2) where and how far the bike was thrown. This will make them material witnesses to the accident.

3. Collect witnesses immediately. Get the names and numbers of everyone who saw the accident. Many people come to help—then leave. You'll probably never see them again. In our system, you have to prove fault, and if you have no witnesses, it is more difficult to reconstruct the accident.

4. If it wasn't your fault, don't move anything, if possible. Let the driver move the car. Don't move your bike. Let the policeman get a look at the most accurate view of what happened.

5. Get all the facts to show who's at fault. A typical insurance adjuster gets only a few—three or four—bike cases a year. Like the cops, they often automatically assume that the cyclist is wrong, so they won't believe you unless your facts are ironclad. They'll jump on bike cases because they think they can play with liability. This is why a higher percentage of bike-car claims go to litigation than car-car claims: more than 30 percent compared to 10 to 15 percent.

6. Contact is not required to make a claim. If you have enough evidence and witnesses, you may be able to make a claim of damages based on a near-miss. That's because the cyclist may have been rattled enough to fall off the bike and sustain injuries even if an actual collision did not occur. This is a proof problem, a much tougher case, but winnable if you have independent, unbiased witnesses.

7. Don't exaggerate or admit too much to the cops. If you brag that you were going 25 mph, it may make it look like you were going too fast for the circumstances. The speed of the rider will be scrutinized very closely when the claim is investigated. If you say you didn't see the car, that could also hurt your case. The opposing insurance company will say that if you were paying attention, you would have seen it, and you could have avoided the crash.

8. Don't be a tough guy—list all your injuries, take an ambulance, and get quick follow-up care. List even your slightest injuries on the police report. Transportation by ambulance to hospital is safer for you and leads to better documentation of your injuries than if you go with a friend or on your bike. If you ride away, the other side could use that as proof that you were fine. And don't hesitate to seek follow-up care. Insurance people don't believe what you say, necessarily—they only believe medical records. Tough guys don't get points in this business. Seek as much medical care as you need.

9. Immediately photograph your visible injuries. They will begin to heal, so take these selfies when your injuries are still looking at their worst.

10. Use small-claims court. If you are willing to accept $2,500 or less, generally too small an amount for an attorney to handle, try to collect it yourself.

11. Use an attorney for big cases. Don't ever handle a big case yourself. You don't know how to value it. An attorney normally takes a standard one-third for attorney's fees, if you win, but it's worth it. Don't delay. Keep the statute of limitations for personal-injury and property-damage lawsuits in mind. These deadlines vary by state, so check with a local attorney for more information. But don't wait until the time is almost up to bring your suit; witnesses will disappear or forget what they saw, and your credibility will wane in the eyes of the jury and judge. If you sleep on your rights or forget to file, the court will not help you.

12. Collect full replacement value for your bike. Don't allow the insurance company to pro-rate your bike. There is no market for a used, broken bike.

13. Don't rush the bodily injury claim. Settle property claims immediately, but consider waiting a bit to settle a bodily injury claim, so that you will have more information about the long-term damage. Permanent scarring—especially facial—is worthy of a large settlement.

(continues)

How to Survive the Insurance Companies
After an Accident (continued)

14. Count on your own auto insurance (if you have it) to cover you. It's a little-known fact, but almost all cyclists are covered by their own auto insurance policy. Look under the section entitled "Medical Pay Coverage." It may be $10,000 to $20,000. If you paid your premiums, you absolutely have the legal right to get your own benefits. If the guy who hit you isn't covered, you are covered under "uninsured motorist." But don't expect much cooperation on this; remember that your own insurance is still an adversary. You may have to demand arbitration.

15. Don't be overly nice to the driver of the car who hit you. Don't make any gratuitous remarks or any statements of admission to the driver; just trade names and addresses. Get the driver's registration information, driver's license number, insurance-company information, and phone number. Don't be nice, and don't be mean, just businesslike. In car-bike accidents, nice guys often lose. If the driver is rattled and upset, you can be a steadying influence without saying anything that would compromise your position for an eventual lawsuit.

---

blanket of black velvet, embroidered with tiny, glistening pearls. It was like a dream, looking out 25, 50, maybe 100 miles and seeing no cars and no city lights—only stars. Off in the distance, tiny, silent lightning bolts flashed every 10 seconds. It was a storm, but so far away that I got out my camera, set the shutter open, and shot time exposures. What a concept: photographing a storm as if it were a tourist sight, watching it like a movie.

Before we knew it, however, we were movie actors. The storm turned, raced closer and closer, and pinned us against the mountainside. Howling winds knocked us sideways. Plum-sized raindrops pounded us. Lightning splattered on the ground

100 feet away, making my skin tingle and hair stand on end. My god—we were human lightning rods, ready to fry! We threw our steel bikes down, sprinted downhill a ways, and squatted down like forlorn gargoyles. For an hour we gazed at the electric light show around us with amazement and horror, wondering if this was the end.

All these years, I've wondered: Did we do the right thing, or was it just luck that we survived?

The US National Oceanic and Atmospheric Administration (NOAA) publishes a preparedness guide for severe weather that the League of American Bicyclists adapted for cyclists. Here's a summary of the advice it gives for handling a thunderstorm.

1. Thunder = trouble. If you can hear thunder (it sounds like a loud crack close-up and a low rumble farther away), get shelter; you are close enough to the storm to be struck by lightning. To estimate your distance from the storm, remember that light (traveling at 186,000 miles per second) is faster than sound (around 750 mph); every five seconds between seeing the flash and hearing the thunderclap equals a mile. If the time grows shorter, take cover in or under a nearby building or underpass.

2. Shorter is better. Don't be the high point on flat terrain. Lightning always takes the quickest path to the ground and usually strikes tall, isolated objects such as trees or tall buildings; the Empire State Building is hit about eight times a year. If you are in the woods, take shelter under the shorter trees.

3. Avoid trees in open areas. If you are exposed, find a low spot away from trees, fences, and poles. (But get to higher ground if flash flooding is possible, such as near a creek bed.)

4. Get downhill. If you're on a hill with exposure to the sky, head downhill and seek an overhanging bluff or a valley or ravine to lower your exposure.

5. Get off the bike. If you feel your skin tingle or your hair stand on end, dismount and get away from your bike. Metal attracts lightning, and rubber-soled shoes and rubber bicycle tires *do not* provide protection from it.

6. Squat down. In the middle of a storm, crouch low to the ground on the balls of your feet. Place your hands on your knees with your head between them. Make yourself the smallest target possible, and minimize your contact with the ground.

Up on Granite Pass that night long ago, it seems that a rare occurrence came to pass in my life: the right decision. After the lightning moved on, we walked the bikes uphill in the drenching rain—cold, soaked, and scared. Three miles up, we came to the Shell Falls Interpretive Site, a nature display with an attached restroom. Inside, high and dry in sleeping bags, were two other bike tourists we'd last seen at the bottom of the mountain eight hours earlier. They didn't like riding at night and left early. And they didn't seem to appreciate being awakened, or to hear us endlessly recount our tale of survival in the eye of the storm.

9. HOW TO SURVIVE . . . SADDLE SORES

As Ethan Gelber, director of the peace-through-cycling organization BikeAbout, put it on Gorp .com, "Being saddle sore and having saddle sores are two different things." The former is a complaint from anyone who hasn't ridden in a while that diminishes as you ride more, while the latter is the "bitter result of steps not taken that let a minor problem get worse."

Saddle sores, cyclists' most common complaint, can wreck a ride. These dreaded pimples, boils, and raw skin are caused by saddle friction incubated in the hot, moist, bacteria-laden environment inside your bike shorts. Saddle sores have stopped RAAM riders, first-timers, bike tourists, and bike racers. According to www .roadbikerider.com, famed men of steel like Eddy Merckx and Sean Kelly had to abandon races when saddle-sore pain became too great, and old-time riders would put slabs of raw steak in their shorts to cushion the tender area. Modern methods are more convenient, but by the time you use them, it may be too late; your ride's over. Here's what to do to stop saddle sores before and after they begin.

1. Correct your saddle position. If the seat is too high, your hips rock as you pedal, creating excess rubbing against the nose of the saddle; the same is true if the saddle is too far forward.

2. Numb it, shrink it, corn-pad it. Dull the pain with Ibuprofen, knock it down to size with Preparation H (Hey, it shrinks swollen tissue, right? Apply it before putting on your shorts.), and cushion it with corn pads, the donut-shaped adhesive pads found in the foot-care section of drug stores.

3. Stand up. Standing while pedaling relieves the pressure on your crotch, restores circulation, and lets you shift things around. Roadbikerider .com recommends standing for 15 to 20 seconds every few minutes. Use natural opportunities such as short hills, rough pavement, or accelerating from stop signs. Stand and stretch when you're at the back of a paceline or group.

4. Keep shifting your position on the saddle. Sit mostly toward the rear, where your sit bones get maximum support and take pressure off your crotch. But also move farther back on seated climbs, and more to the middle when bending low, to make good time. Each shift relieves pressure points.

5. Change your saddle and shorts. Your saddle sore may be isolated in one small area, and changing your saddle and/or shorts could reduce the pressure where it hurts. Chronic sores may mean you have too wide a saddle—which is possible if you are a man using a women's saddle.

6. Lube it up. If you've noticed irritation on previous rides, reduce the friction by dabbing petroleum jelly, Chamois BUTT'r, or Bag Balm on your crotch and the chamois (the material in the crotch of the shorts).

7. Get a fresh saddle. To reduce the transfer of

dirt and bacteria, buy a new saddle when yours wears out. And bring your own saddle or a saddle cover if you're planning on renting a bike out of town.

8. Keep clean. Always wear clean shorts for each ride. If you seem susceptible to saddle sores, you may find it helpful to wash your crotch with antibacterial soap and warm water before lubing up. Dry your skin well before applying the products listed in #6 above.

9. Chuck your undies. Not only can underwear irritate skin like fine sandpaper and trap moisture against the body, but its seams can dig into your crotch. Good bike shorts have seamless padding where it is most needed, reduce sweat where you should be dry, and cut down on chafing. Yes, they are skin-tight and make the self-conscious feel even more so. But they work. If you really don't want to show it off, use the baggy, mountain bike–style shorts with the chamois-lined padding hidden inside. Look for shorts with a one-piece liner or one that's sewn with flat seams.

10. At day's end, strip and clean up quick. Don't give bacteria time to invade saddle sores. Get out of your shorts, wash them out with TLC and a gentle soap, and sleep naked to allow everything to dry.

11. Stop riding and medicate. If it's too painful, you're doing damage. Get off the bike. Go swimming. Wear loose clothes. Take some time off the bike to let it heal. It's far better to lose three days now than a week or more after infection sets in. If you continue to ride on an open sore, it may eventually form a cyst that requires surgery. Whatever you do, don't scrub and clean sores with alcohol, which will only dry out the skin and irritate it further.

12. If sores are chronic, go recumbent. The laid-back 'bents take the stress off strategic spots that a traditional bike might bother. And they're faster, too.

10. HOW TO SURVIVE . . . NUMB HANDS

A loss of sensitivity in your paws, caused by reduced circulation, usually stems from the following: a too-forward body lean, a too-stretched-out position, and/or an unchanging hand position. In theory, some simple fixes apply.

1. Raise the handlebars gradually. Too-low bars (and/or stem) put too much weight on your hands. An ideal, balanced fit distributes your body weight more evenly across your seat, bars, and pedals.

2. Lower the seatpost and/or level the seat. A too-high and/or too-tilted saddle throws your upper body weight forward and puts more pressure on your hands' contact areas with the bars.

3. Slide the seat forward or shorten the stem. If you're too stretched out from the saddle to the handlebars, sliding the seat forward may do the trick. But be careful not to move the seat forward too much. The changed position vis-à-vis the cranks could cause back or knee problems.

4. Switch hand positions often. Especially limit time in the top-of-the-bar position. Carpal tunnel syndrome, a crimping of the ulnar nerve, may result from the hyperextended wrist position of the top bar. Shift from the top of the bar to the hoods and the drops. The hoods will put your hands in the wrist-safe "handshake" position.

5. Kill the "death grip." Squeezing the bar too tightly can cut your circulation. So relax, and gently rest your hands on the bar. As long as one thumb is always under the bars, your hands can't slip. You can steer and control the bike, even when riding fast, with only a very gentle touch.

6. Use mountain bike bar-ends. Although they're out of style, they position hands for better climbing and a wrist-safe "handshake" grip.

7. Shake out your hands. Centrifugal force pushes blood out to the fingertips and capillaries.

8. Wear the right gloves. If your current gloves aren't working, try a pair with more padding.

You can also use gloves with full fingers for cold weather. Avoid gloves that are so tight they restrict the blood flow in your fingers.

11. HOW TO SURVIVE . . . DOG ATTACKS

By Bill Katovsky

I had 30 more miles of Wisconsin farmland to ride before reaching the Mississippi River and Dubuque, Iowa, when it saw me. A maniacally barking mutt, loping beside some kids riding motorcycles along a fence, suddenly changed directions and headed for my right ankle. No problem—I'd outrace it, I thought. But as I pressed hard on the pedals, the sudden torque dislodged the out-of-true rear wheel (it was missing a spoke), yanked it out of the rear dropout, and tangled it in the derailleur. The frame now a limp, metallic pretzel, I collapsed on the ground in a bloody mess. So much for Dubuque, so much for the bike, so much for my 1978 cross-country trip. Its work done, the dog stopped barking. The kids on their bikes came by and eventually brought over their mother, who drove me to Dubuque. My father wired me $300, which I used at the only bike store in town to buy a frame from a brand-new company based in a Wisconsin barn called Trek.

They say that Iowa is all corn. How about pig farms and dogs? As I biked across the Hawkeye State, canines seemed everywhere, and once bit, twice wary. Having already demonstrated the folly of *(1) standing up and out-sprinting them* (the logical first option for most riders, given that most dogs are merely defending their territory and lose interest when you're off the property), I tried to reason with them. In other words, I'd *(2) scream!* They'd hesitate, surprised, aware of what can happen when a human is angry with them; escalating if need be, *(3) I'd raise my hand threateningly* as if it contained a heavy object, because dogs understand the meaning of a throwing gesture. If I had had time to prepare, I'd play *(4) drench the dog.* Seeing your water bottle in hand,

even before squirting it, may make Fido stay away. When none of that worked, especially with big dogs, I would deploy *(5) the bike barrier*—dismounting quickly and holding my bike between me and its chompers, swinging it or a bike pump like a weapon and yelling out for help.

Tired of being understanding, I eventually decided to go on the offensive and buy *(6) a boat air horn* and *(7) Halt! pepper spray*—the latter the weapon of choice for US postal carriers. Unfortunately, it only works if you hit the target in the eyes—a difficult enough feat when you're standing still, much less riding. I taped the Halt! to one side of my handlebars. On the other side, I affixed the small high-decibel air horn. I was ready for battle. But I never used the Halt! And the air horn was more often used to ward off dive-bombing redwing blackbirds nesting in roadside ditches. As I headed farther west, and Iowa's farms gave way to the cattle ranches of Nebraska and then the dry wastes of Wyoming, I gratefully encountered fewer and fewer dogs. I didn't mind this at all. I never liked dogs, though years later, a golden retriever named Rockee entered my life—and ended up staying for 14 wonderful years. The day before this rambunctious, loving animal died in my arms at the veterinarian's from a ruptured spleen, I had towed him up Mt. Tam in Marin County in a Burley children's trailer behind my Klein mountain bike. I was his beast of burden.

12. HOW TO SURVIVE . . . A BEAR ATTACK

By Bill Katovsky

First mountain lions. Then dogs. Now grizzly bears? On August 29, 2004, a quick-thinking mountain biker in Wyoming's Shoshone National Forest fought off a grizzly that repeatedly charged him until a companion drove the animal off with pepper spray. Kirk Speckhals, 46, escaped being mauled, though he sported these trailside mementos: four dirt marks from the bear's claws on his forearm, a punctured bicycle tire, and a bent rim.

The encounter took place during a ride around Pinnacle Buttes, near the Yellowstone ecosystem, where the grizzly population has increased from 200 to 500 over the past 30 years. Riding with pepper-spray-carrying Tom Foley, Speckhals, a ski patroller, had been ringing his bicycle bell at regular intervals to warn possible bears of his approach. For some reason, he had stopped ringing his bell, when he saw a grizzly off in the distance, about the length of a football field, in full charge, coming right at him. "He charged six or seven times," Speckhals later told an Associated Press reporter, but each time was deterred at the last moment by the bicycle. "Finally, he grabbed my bike out of my hands. He started stomping on it." With the bear distracted, Speckhals started creeping away, but Yogi immediately left the bike and put its front paws on Speckhals. "This time he just took me out—drug me to the ground," Speckhals said. "I knew I was in trouble. I rotated and got on my chest." Foley, arriving to find the bear sitting on top of his friend, grabbed his pepper spray, aimed for the bear's eyes, and yelled as loud as he could. The grizzly ran off.

Fear factor, indeed. Grizzlies have been known to attack campers and hikers in Montana's Glacier National Park. It is not a pleasant way to die; hence their Latin name, *Ursus horribilis*. If you happen to go mountain biking in areas known to support grizzlies—Alaska and British Columbia have significant bear populations, including brown and black bears—here's some practical advice to heed, according to *Safe Travel in Bear Country*, by Gary Brown.

1. Start off clean: Since pots often smell and food odors permeate your tent, sleeping bag, and panniers, wash or clean all of them before you begin your trip—especially the fabric items if you've cooked near them.

2. Shower: Food, body odors, and human sexual activity all may attract bears. So keep as personally clean as possible; wash up after cooking, eating, and sex and again before retiring for the night.

3. Eliminate fragrances: Bears are attracted to sweet-smelling products such as perfumes, deodorants, cosmetics, lotions, shampoos, soaps, suntan lotions, and toothpaste; some first-aid items and medicines (such as Campho-Phenique); lip salves and balms, insect repellents, pot scrubbers, vinyl, foam rubber, and motor oil.

The Alaska Bureau of Land Management field office offers these pointers.

1. Look and listen. Bears are active both day and night and may appear anywhere.

2. Don't surprise them. A startled bear may attack.

3. Make noises. Let bears know you are in the area—sing, yell, or clap your hands loudly. Bells may be ineffective. Be especially careful in thick brush or near noisy streams.

4. If you encounter a bear, don't try to run or bike away. They've been clocked at speeds up to 35 mph, and running may elicit a chase response. If the bear does not see you, backtrack or detour quickly and quietly. Give him plenty of room. Back away slowly if he sees you, speaking in a low, calm voice while waving your arms over your head.

5. If a grizzly makes physical contact, play dead. Lie flat on your stomach and lace your fingers behind your neck.

6. If a black bear attacks, fight back. In Alaska, you can protect yourself with firearms if you have a permit. In the lower 48 states, you need to make do with pepper spray.

Most bears tend to avoid people. Seventy percent of the killings by grizzly bears are by mothers defending their cubs, said wildlife biologist and black bear expert Lynn Rogers. "But nobody's ever been killed by a mother black bear defending her cubs. Black bears are not territorial toward people and are usually afraid of being attacked themselves," Rogers said. "Their most common aggressive displays are merely rituals that they perform when they are nervous. Most likely, bears will run away or seek safety in a tree. A bear will break off its attack once it feels the threat has been eliminated. Remain motionless for as long as possible. If you move, and the bear sees or hears you, it may return and renew its attack. In rare instances, particularly with black bears, an attacking bear may perceive a person as food. If the bear continues biting you long after you assume a defensive posture, it likely is a predatory attack." Rogers also urges fighting back.

13. HOW TO SURVIVE . . .
ROAD RAGE AND LOUSY DRIVERS

By Bill Katovsky

Over the years, I have been swerved at by young hot-rodders in California, honked at by malicious cretins in Montana, made the object of thrown beer cans and firecrackers by Michigan motorists, knocked off my bike by a drowsy elderly man outside Ann Arbor, and nearly run over by a feckless 15-year-old in Nebraska who was learning to drive with his mother as his passenger.

One of the most bizarre incidents occurred near my home in Mill Valley, California. I was riding about a foot to the left of the white shoulder line to avoid roadside trash when a late-model Cutlass swerved at me. The driver then stopped in the middle of the road, got out of his car, and blocked my path. Naturally, I was forced to halt.

Fiendishly puffing on a cigarette, he began yelling at me, standing just inches from my face: "All you foreigners coming to my state are ruining it. You're not a native, I am!" I didn't say a word during his insane tirade. Nor could I follow his logic, except to speculate that he might have equated cycling with foreign imports such as Brie and Perrier.

As he spewed angry nonsense, I silently weighed the pros and cons of defending my roadside rights and possibly getting into a fistfight on a glorious Saturday morning in the middle of the road on busy East Blithedale Avenue. When he was done with his roadside rant, he got back in his car and drove off, his broken muffler making throaty, bronchial noises.

Why is everyone in such a hurry? I might scold motorists if they are driving too close to me, or if they cut me off. But with road rage being all the rage these days, I've learned to look before leaping into an altercation. A bike is no match for a 7,000-pound SUV—or a driver carrying a gun! A study by the AAA in 1997 found that 37 percent of road-rage drivers used firearms against another driver, and 35 percent used their car as a weapon.

The rules of the road? The League of American Bicyclists once offered an Emily Post–like guide to sensible riding when faced with road rage: "Remove yourself; make every attempt to get out of their way; yield lane position by turning or slowing down and getting behind them; be prepared to execute emergency maneuvers; do not return any gestures or shouts; do not make eye contact; do not push for proper lane position to avoid challenging the driver."

So swallow your pride. You can't change the behavior and driving habits of distracted or ill-mannered drivers. All you can do is keep your own eyes on the road, both hands on the handlebars, and your ego tightly fastened underneath your bike helmet. And report the miscreant's license plate and description to state and local police as fast as you can.

THE JOURNEY

Centuries. Touring. Hill-climb challenges. 24-hour relays. Cross-state rides. With its immense variety, cycling offers motivation for everyone.

When I was in my early 30s, I used to think that there were two types of bicyclists in this world: the people who like the Donut Shop Ride, and the people who don't. I was one of the latter. I used to think the former were narrow-minded fools, mainly because they seemed unaware that any type of cycling—or anything at all, for that matter—existed beyond their 30-mile neighborhood loop, whereas cycling for me was all about escaping the neighborhood and seeing the world.

I didn't know Donut Shop riders existed until late 1992. One day earlier that year, I had ridden my bike into my new job as editor of Bicycle Guide magazine, a rather ordinary action for the editor of a bike magazine to take, I thought. When I came back from lunch, I saw several members of the ad and editorial staffs, all hard-core racers, gathered around my bike: a Trek 1200 road bike with fenders, huge, triathlon-style Scott aerobars with bar-end shifters, a frame pouch for food, three water bottles, and a special bracket holding lights and a bell. They all wore puzzled expressions and were shaking their heads. "Yeah, rode that thing in Paris-Brest-Paris last year," I said as casually as I could as I went by. "Hardest thing I ever did."

No one said a word. Which was weird, since P-B-P, 750 miles in three and a half nearly sleepless days, from Paris to the Atlantic coast and back, was probably the hardest ultra-distance race in the world, aside from the Race Across America. For the 7,000-plus

endurance riders who show up in Paris every four years, a P-B-P finish is like graduating from Harvard.

Weeks later, my boss called me into his office and told me that several people in the organization had asked him to fire me. Seems they didn't like the idea of a sissy who used fenders being the voice of the magazine. It was at that moment that I realized that none of these hard-core road racers in the office had heard of P-B-P. As I quickly set about explaining to everyone exactly what Paris-Brest-Paris meant and why fenders and lights were required for it, then added that I had ridden my bike 25,000 miles around the world, including through the Soviet Union, and was described as "America's most traveled bike tourist" on my just-published book, the ice thawed. Several staff members invited me to join them on a ride in the South Bay that Saturday morning. And that's when I found out that for many cyclists, the sport is all about the Donut Ride.

Starting in Redondo Beach, they hug the cliffs and zig-zag up and down the steep climbs of the Palos Verde Peninsula for 37 wheel-sucking miles on their aerobar-less road bikes, back then mostly of Italian make. I love the route but hate pace-line riding; it's nerve-wracking. You can't look up for a second to take in the view, much less stop for a photo. Everyone was so serious—and going so fast. We ended up, about two hours after the 7 a.m. start, at a Starbucks, where everybody sat back with

Frappuccinos and muffins and talked about component groups and racing news. New groups of 12 to 20 cyclists came in at a time; maybe 100 all told came by during my 30 minutes. Most had been doing this ride ever since a donut shop had stood on this corner. In fact, for most, the Donut Ride was all they did in cycling. I talked to a dozen people, all hard-core racers or wannabes. Not one had ever been on a bike tour, owned a pannier, or ridden a century, much less heard of P-B-P. No one had ever ridden in the nearby Santa Monica Mountains, full of hundreds of miles of twisty, challenging two-lane roads. That's crazy, I thought. They don't know what they're missing. The bike is a machine of infinite travel possibilities. The cycling world is a huge smorgasbord of events—cross-state rides, double centuries, hill-climb challenges, cross-country touring, and, nowadays, epic mountain bike adventures. How can they get motivated to do this same-ole, same-ole week after week, year after year?

Well, 20 years later, I get together nearly every Sunday morning with two other 50-something guys and do a two-hour mountain bike ride. Nothing epic, just a couple of predictable local Orange County loops in Silverado Canyon, Whiting Ranch, Aliso Woods, Santiago Oaks, and more. Anyhow, Matta and Kennedy aren't interested much in dawn-to-dusk death rides, but they can hang with anyone. We've shared bad crashes, broken chains, and blown tires. They motivated me to get up at 6 a.m., instead of sleeping in. On the way home, we always stopped at Starbucks for 45 minutes of shooting the breeze about cycling and politics and technology and the Clippers.

I still draw a lot of my motivation to ride from planning and training for big epic adventures in far-off places. The bike is, first and foremost, a vehicle of exploration for me. But after all these years, I've come to see the value of the Donut Ride, too.

GET OUT OF YOUR NEIGHBORHOOD

Cycling is a big umbrella that covers a wide variety of riding challenges, from hill-climb events to cross-state tours, mass one-day city rides drawing thousands, multiday mountain bike stage races, 750-mile non-stop endurathons, and epic centuries and overnighters. Experiment, sample a few from each category, push your boundaries; it's one way that cycling can keep you excited for a lifetime. With new cycling events springing up like weeds as charities, foundations, and cities tap the power of the bike to get people out on the streets, the list below can only begin to scratch the surface of what's available. But here are a few good ones to get you started.

I. Road Bike Hill-Climb Events

Fancy aero handlebars, disc wheels, and wind-cheating bike frames won't help you on a hill climb, where fitness, stick-to-itiveness, and some technique and raw pride matter most. Nothing beats the epic satisfaction of conquering a mountain, especially when it's steeped in cycling lore and gives you a finisher's medal as proof, as do the following hill-climb events.

1. ### Cycle to the Sun (Hawaii)
   One of the steepest, longest climbs on Earth—37 miles, 10,000 feet—rises from the sea-level town of Paia, Maui, into Haleakala National Park, passing through several distinct climate zones before reaching the top of the Mt. Haleakala crater.
   When: Late June
   Contact: www.cycletothesun.com

2. ### Bob Cook Mt. Evans Hill Climb (Colorado)
   This 28-mile climb in the Rockies starts at 7,540 feet and tops out at 14,250 feet. It's been canceled twice in 38 years due to snow; be prepared for mountain goats, sheep, awesome scenery, and bitter cold. Pro Tom Danielson set the record of 1:45:30 in 2004.
   When: Late July
   Contact: www.teamevergreen.org/mtevans

3. Bicycle Hill Climb (Utah)
   This 10-miler climbs 3,500 feet up spectacular
   Little Cottonwood Canyon.
   When: August
   Contact: www.bikereg.com/net/19511

4. Mt. Tamalpais Hill Climb (California)
   This classic 12.5-mile climb rises 2,200 feet
   from Stinson Beach and ends with a stunning
   360-degree panorama of the Pacific Ocean, the
   Golden Gate Bridge, and San Francisco. The
   record is 37 minutes, 26 minutes, set in 2003.
   When: September
   Contact: www.goldengatevelo.org/tam

5. Greylock Hillclimb Time Trial
   (Massachusetts)
   This 9.8-miler rises 2,793 feet and tops out on
   3,491-foot Mt. Greylock, the highest point in the
   state.
   When: September or October
   Contact: www.nohobikeclub.org/greylocktt/

6. Mt. Graham Hill Climb (Arizona)
   This 20-mile, 5,600-feet-of-elevation climb
   starts in dry brush and winds up through pine
   forest in 12 hairpin turns to the peak's aspen-
   covered 9,600-foot summit.
   When: September or October
   Contact: www.azcycling.com

7. Sandia Peak Epic Challenge
   (New Mexico)
   Located on the Turquoise Trail, a forested
   national scenic byway between Albuquerque
   and Santa Fe, the climb to the 10,678-foot
   summit of Sandia Crest leaves you at the Sandia
   Peak Tramway, the longest jig-back tram in the
   world.
   When: August
   Contacts: www.nmsportsonline.com;
     www.mountaintopcycling.com/mtb-race/

8. Mt. Charleston Hill Climb (Nevada)
   This 17-mile, 5,700-foot climb begins on the
   parched desert floor 30 miles north of Las Vegas
   and ends in cool (sometimes freezing) pine-tree-
   studded, snowcapped mountains. Pack a fleece
   vest.
   When: September
   Contact: https://www.facebook
     /MountCharlestonHillClimb

9. Mt. Washington Hill Climb
   (New Hampshire)
   This ultra-steep 7.6-miler averages an
   otherworldly 12 percent grade while gaining
   4,727 feet, with the last 50 meters maxing out at
   a tendon-tearing 22 percent. Beware of harsh
   weather, high winds, and occasional subzero
   wind chills near the top of the Northeast's
   highest, steepest mountain road.
   When: August or September
   Contact: www.mwarbh.org/

10. Mt. Diablo Challenge (California)
    You won't be lonely on this 10.8-mile, 2,751-foot
    climb, which gives great views of San Francisco
    Bay from the summit. It regularly draws more
    than 1,000 participants.
    When: October
    Contact: www.facebook.com/MountDiablo
      Challenge; www.savemountdiablo.org
      /activities_events_chal.html

11. Western Montana Hill Climb
    Championships (Montana)
    A tradition for nearly 43 years, this 4-mile,
    840-foot romp in Missoula to the 4,000-foot
    finish has a division for everyone: tandems,
    unicycles, recumbents, and even high-wheelers.
    When: October
    Contact: www.missoulabike.org/hillclimb

12. Mt. Equinox Uphill Bike Climb (Vermont)

The 5.2-mile, 2,800-foot-high route up this Carthusian monastery toll road offers a spectacular view of four states.

When: August

Contact: www.gearupforlyme.com

13. Bogus Basin Hill Climb (Idaho)

Starting in dry brush near Boise, the nation's oldest hill-climb contest travels 17 miles through 3,500 feet of elevation to a ski resort, which is named "Bogus" after the work of two prospectors, who sprayed a little gold dust into the cave walls with shotguns and sold the worthless land to fortune seekers in the 1860s.

When: August

Contact: www.GeorgesCycles.com

14. Mt. Lemmon Hill Climb (Arizona)

Soar above Tucson to get spectacular views on this 27-mile climb to 8,400 feet. The longest climb in the state rises through seven climate zones.

When: May

Contact: www.bikegaba.org

15. Mt. Ashland Hill Climb (Oregon)

The climb from downtown Ashland at 1,900 feet to the Mt. Ashland Ski Lodge, elevation 6,500, is one of the toughest climbing events on the West Coast. A twist: it pits road cyclists (going 24 miles) against mountain bikers and cyclocrossers (going 18 miles on fireroads). All start at the same time.

When: September

Contact: www.mtashlandbike.com/

II. Mountain Bike Multiday Stage Races

"It is in doing the hard things that you learn the truth about yourself." So says Roman Urbina, whto created the now immensely popular mountain bike stage race genre with his La Ruta race across Costa Rica in 1992. Now there are dozens of these epic events around the world. Averaging around 50 grueling off-road miles per day, riders typically spend the night in gymnasiums or tents (or hotels, in the case of La Ruta), then head out at 8 a.m. to do it again the next day for another 6 to 10 hours.

1. La Ruta de los Conquistadores (Costa Rica)

What: Three days, 250 miles

Where: Costa Rica

When: Mid-November

Contact: www.adventurerace.com

From Pacific to Caribbean, tracing the route of 16th-century Spanish conquistadors, this granddaddy of mountain bike stage racing snakes through rainforest, over 11,000-foot volcanoes, and past banana and coffee plantations, blasting you with heat and humidity or drenching you with freezing high-elevation rain.

2. TransAlp Challenge (Germany to Italy)

What: Eight days, 400 miles, 61,000 feet of climbing

Where: Germany, Austria, Switzerland, and Italy

When: July

Contact: www.epic-mountain-bike.com /transalp-challenge.html

From the south German pre-Alps to Italy's Lake Garda, you and a partner traverse jagged, beautiful, and daunting portions of the eastern Alps and Dolomites.

3. Singletrack 6 (Canada)

What: Six days, 200 miles

Where: Canadian Rockies

When: July

Contact: www.singletrack6.com

Tough routes through lush rain forest, high-alpine ascents, arid desert, and the best panoramas in Alberta and British Columbia.

4. BC Bike Race (Canada)

What: Seven days, 350 miles, mostly singletrack route from Victoria to Whistler, BC

Where: Vancouver Island and British Columbia mainland

When: Late June to early July

Contact: www.bcbikerace.com

This phenomenal point-to-point adventure in the Canadia rain forest takes two-person teams through a visual wonderworld of bears, rivers, and ferry rides.

5. Breck Epic (Colorado)

What: Six days, 240 miles of backcountry loops from Breckenridge, mostly at elevations over 10,000 feet

Where: Colorado Rockies

When: August

Contact: www.breckepic.com

This lung-wheezing cloverleaf-format course features 8,100 to 4,800 feet of elevation gain every day on renowned Rockies routes like the Colorado Trail. A daily start and finish in town gets you much-needed rest.

6. Trans-Sylvania Epic (Pennsylvania)

What: Seven days, 207 miles

Where: Spring Mills, central Pennsylvania

When: Late May

Contact: www.tsepic.com

The rugged Allegheny Mountains top out at just 4,000 feet, but beware: the routes are relentlessly hilly and exhausting.

7. Cape Epic (South Africa)

What: Eight days, 560 miles

Where: South Africa

When: April

Contact: www.cape-epic.com

This two-man team race climbs 20,000 feet, passing the plains, mountains, and Big Five Game Reserve of the Western Cape.

III. 24-Hour Mountain Biking and Other Epics

Nothing beats the camaraderie and bonding of 24-hour mountain bike relay racing, which now draws tens of thousands of participants throughout North America. There may be 50 or more races on the continent.

1. 24 Hours of Adrenalin (Canmore, Alberta)

What: One of the world's biggest 24-hour events draws over 2,000 participants to the Canmore Nordic Center in the stunning Canadian Rockies.

When: July

Contact: www.twenty4sports.com; www.24hoursofadrenalin.com

2. 24 Hours of Great Glen (New England)

What: The biggest 24-hour race in New England.

When: August

Contact: www.grannygear.com

IV. Non-24-Hour Epics

1. Leadville Trail 100

What: This thin-air, 100-mile mountain bike ride based in Leadville, Colorado, ranges in elevation from 9,200 to 12,600 feet. Race veterans warn you to race with dark sunglasses during the day because the thin-air sunshine will burn your retinas and leave you with night blindness.

When: August

Contact: www.leadvilleraceseries.com/mtb /leadvilletrail100mtb/

2. Alaska Iditasport Ultramarathon

What: From Knik Lake to Finger Lake, Alaska, this gruel-athon of cold and pain pits skiers, mountain bikers, and runners against 130 miles of the famed Iditarod Trail, site of the Iditarod Dog Sled Race. "Cowards won't show and the weak will die!" once said racer Laddie Shaw.

When: February

Contact: www.iditasportalaska.com

V. Endurance Road-Bike Events

1. Silver State 508 (Nevada)

   A successor to the legendary Furnace Creek 508, this annual destination event draws competitors and media attention from around the world. Solo and team riders cross a huge swath of empty northern Nevada for 508 miles.

   When: October

   Contact: The508.com; adventurecorps.com

2. Paris-Brest-Paris (France)

   The venerabe road-bike 1,200-kilometer randonnée takes you from Paris to Brest on the Atlantic Ocean, then back to Paris.

   When: Every four years since 1891 (the next races are in 2015 and 2019)

   Contact: www.rusa.org (Randonneurs USA); www.audax-club-parisien.com

VI. Multiday Cross-State Rides

In 1973, when *Des Moines Register* feature writer and copy editor John Karras suggested that he ride his bicycle across Iowa in six days in July and write columns about what he saw, a tradition was born. The public was invited, and about 300 riders showed up for the start of the ride in Sioux City on July 26 that year. By actual count, 114 riders made the entire distance, with 500 riding the last day into Des Moines.

Since then, more than 40 other cross-state rides have been established. They have a lot of catching up to do. By 2013, more than 275,650 people had ridden at least some part of the 16,907 total miles covered by the Register's Annual Great Bicycle Ride Across Iowa (RAGBRAI) over the years. RAGBRAI has been routed through every one of Iowa's 99 counties, and 780 of its incorporated towns (80 percent of the state's total), and spent the night in 125 of them. Below you will find contact info for RAGBRAI and some of the other popular state rides. Most are quite inexpensive, considering that riders camp out or sleep in high-school gyms on most rides. If your state isn't listed, try to find it at www.adventure cycling.org or nbtda.com, which has information and links to more than 60 rides, including some in Mexico and Canada.

ALABAMA: Alabama's Magnificent Bicycle Adventure (AMBA)

Seven days, 350 miles

When: Early June

Contact: www.amba1.com

COLORADO: Ride the Rockies

Six or seven days, 350–400 miles

When: Early June

Participation: 2,000, lottery basis

Contact: www.ridetherockies.com

(Also: In late June is BTC, Bicycle Tour of Colorado, www.bicycletourcolorado.com/)

FLORIDA: Bike Florida Spring Tour

Seven days, 350–400 miles

When: Late March–April

Participation: 1,000 riders maximum

Contact: www.bikeflorida.org

GEORGIA: Bike Ride Across Georgia (BRAG)

Eight days, 400 miles

When: Mid-June

Participation: 2,000 riders maximum

Contact: www.brag.org

IDAHO: Ride Idaho

Seven days, 429 miles

When: August

Participation: 150 riders maximum

Contact: www.rideidaho.org

ILLINOIS: Bicycle Illinois
Seven days, 500–600 miles (Cairo to Chicago)
When: Early July
Contact: www.bicycleillinois.com

INDIANA: Ride Across Indiana (RAIN)
Seven days, 350 miles
When: July
Contact: www.rainride.org

IOWA: Register's Annual Great Bicycle Ride Across Iowa (RAGBRAI)
Six days, 450 miles
When: Late July
Contact: www.ragbrai.org

KANSAS: Bike Across Kansas (BAK)
Eight days, 500 miles
When: Early June
Participation: 800 riders maximum
Contact: www.bak.org

KENTUCKY: Governor's Autumn Bike Ride Across Kentucky (GABRAKY)
Four days, 240 miles
When: October
Contact: www.gabraky.com

MAINE: Trek Across Maine
Three days, 180 miles
When: Mid-June
Participation: 1,800 riders maximum
Contact: http://action.lung.org/site/
    TR?fr_id=8070&pg=entry

MARYLAND: Ride Across Maryland
Three days, 300 miles
When: Late May–June
Participation: 1,500 riders maximum
Contact: www.rideacrossmaryland.org

MONTANA: Cycle Montana
Seven days, 280 miles
When: Mid-July
Participation: 170 riders maximum
Contact: www.adventurecycling.org/tours/index
    .cfm

NEBRASKA: Bicycle Ride Across Nebraska (BRAN)
Seven days, 519 miles
When: Early June
Participation: 600 riders maximum
Contact: www.bran-inc.org

NORTH CAROLINA: Mountains to Coast Ride
Eight days
Participation: About 1,000 riders
When: September-October
Contact: cnc.ncsports.org

NORTH DAKOTA: Cycling Around North Dakota Sakakawea Country (CANDISC)
Eight days, 452 miles
When: Late July–August
Participation: 350 riders maximum
Contact: www.NDtourism.com/events
    /candisc-bicycle-tour

OHIO: Great Ohio Bicycle Adventure (GOBA)
Eight days, 350 miles
When: Mid-June
Participation: 3,000 riders maximum
Contact: http://goba.com/wordpress/

OKLAHOMA: Oklahoma Freewheel
Eight days, 400 miles
When: Mid-June
Participation: 2,000 riders maximum
Contact: www.okfreewheel.com

OREGON: Cycle Oregon

Seven days, 380–500 miles

When: September

Participation: 2,200 riders maximum

Contact: www.cycleoregon.com

TENNESSEE: Bicycle Ride Across Tennessee (BRAT)

Seven days, 380–450 miles.

When: Late September–October

Participation: 500 riders maximum

Contact: www.thebrat.org

UTAH: Legacy Annual Great Bicycle Ride Across Utah (LAGBRAU)

Eight days, 400 miles

When: Late August–September

Participation: 130 riders maximum

Contact: www.lagbrau.com

VIRGINIA: Bike Virginia

Five days, 300 miles

When: June

Participation: 2,000 riders maximum

Contact: www.bikevirginia.org

WASHINGTON: Ride Around Washington (RAW)

Seven days, 450 miles

When: Early August

Participation: 150 riders maximum

Contact: www.cascade.org/ride -around-washington

WISCONSIN: Great Annual Bicycle Adventure Along the Wisconsin River (GRABAAW)

Seven days, 490 miles

When: June

Contact: www.bikewisconsin.com

WYOMING: Tour de Wyoming

Six days, 370 miles

When: Mid-July

Participation: 300 riders maximum

Contact: www.cyclewyoming.org

VII. Mass-Participation Road Rides

"Humans have a fascination with transportation and they have a primitive urge to congregate," wrote *Bicycle Guide* staffer Jackson Lynch in 1993. "Put the two together and you've got either a stock car race or a fun ride." This book is definitely not about stock-car racing, and you definitely won't be lonely on these well-populated rides:

1. Le Tour de L'Île de Montréal

    What: 45-mile bike ride around the island of Montréal

    Where: Montréal, Québec

    When: Early June

    Participation: 35,000 to 40,000 riders

    Contact: www.veloquebec.info/en/feria /The-Tour-de-Ile-de-Montreal

2. TD Five Boro Bike Tour

    What: 45 miles

    Where: New York City: from Battery Park to the Bronx, Queens, Brooklyn, then across the Verrazano-Narrows Bridge to Staten Island

    When: May

    Participation: 30,000 riders

    Contact: www.bikenewyork.org

3. Seattle to Portland Bicycle Classic

    What: 200-mile one- or two-day ride

    Where: From Seattle to Portland

    Participation: 8,000 riders

    Contact: www.cascade.org/ride-major-rides /group-health-stp

4. The Hotter 'N Hell Hundred

What: 100 miles

Where: Wichita Falls, Texas

When: Late August (always nine days before Labor Day)

Participation: 8,000 to 10,000 riders

Contact: www.hh100.org

5. Rosarito Ensenada 50-Mile Fun Ride (Mexico)

Where: Rosarito Beach, Baja California

When: Late September

Participation: 9,000 riders

Contact: www.RosaritoEnsenada.com

6. Apple Cider Century

What: 25-, 50-, 75- or 100-mile bicycle tour of the orchards, forests, and wine-making area of Michigan

Where: Three Oaks, Michigan

When: Late September

Participation: 5,000 to 7,000 riders

Contact: www.applecidercentury.com

7. Tour of the Scioto River Valley (TOSRV)

What: 210 miles out and back from Columbus to Portsmouth

Where: Columbus, Ohio

When: Early May

Participation: 3,000 to 4,000 riders

Contact: www.tosrv.org

8. The Moonlight Ramble

What: Longest-running night bike ride in the United States, taking a leisurely pace through the city

Where: St. Louis, Missouri

When: August (2 a.m. start time)

Participation: 10,000 to 15,000 riders

Contact: www.moonlightramble.com

VIII. Gran Fondos

I've done more century and double-century rides than I can remember. But I'd never been led out of town by Lamborghinis and a police escort; timed on an 8-mile, 2,000-foot climb in the middle of one; or treated to a gourmet meal and live music at the finish until I entered a gran fondo—specifically, the 2013 Gran Fondo Giro d'Italia Beverly Hills—one of the hottest new developments in the sport. Created in Italy, like many good things in cycling, the gran fondo (which means "great endurance") reenergizes the age-old century ride, offering long-mileage and short-mileage distances, great food, and a party-like environment at the finish. They've attracted attention in places like Beverly Hills, Miami, and Jerusalem. At this writing, US gran fondos, often co-owned, promoted, and ridden by well-known American riders such as Christian Vande Velde, Chris Horner, George Hincapie, and Levi Leipheimer, are springing up all over the place. Here's a sampler:

1. Gran Fondo Giro d'Italia Beverly Hills

Where: Beverly Hills, California

When: November

Distance: 48 or 90 miles

Highlights: Rodeo Drive, the Pacific Ocean, the awesome Santa Monica Mountains

Contact: www.granfondogiroditalia.com/

2. Gran Fondo Giro d'Italia Miami

Where: Miami and Coral Gables, Florida

When: November

Distance: 25, 54, or 101 miles

Highlights: Miracle Mile, lush gardens and magnificent homes, vast fields of palms and tropical flowers, Biscayne Bay, Miami's Coconut Grove

Contact: www.granfondogiroditalia.com/

3. **RBC Gran Fondo Whistler BC**

Where: Whistler, British Columbia

When: September

Distance: 34, 76, or 94 miles

Highlights: A scenic ride on the Trans-Canada Highway with views of the Howe Sound, featuring 1,700 feet of climbing and 1,000 feet of descent

Contact: rbcgranfondowhistler.com

4. **Cascade Gran Fondo**

Where: Bend, Oregon

When: August

Distance: 22, 53, or 75 miles

Highlights: Mt. Bachelor start/finish, Cascade Mountains, Deschutes Brewery, 6,500 feet of climbing

Contact: cascadegranfondo.com

5. **Echelon Ride to Revel Gran Fondo**

Where: Sonoma and Napa, California

When: April

Distance: 10, 40, or 65 miles

Highlights: Rolling countryside through wine region

Contact: ridetorevel.com/sonoma-napa/the-ride

6. **King Ridge Gran Fondo**

Where: Santa Rosa, California

When: October

Distance: 32, 65, or 103 miles

Highlights: King Ridge Road, Pacific Ocean, 8,500 feet of climbing

Contact: levisgranfondo.com

7. **Gran Fondo Las Vegas**

Where: Las Vegas

When: April

Distance: 70 or 100 miles

Highlights: The Strip, 8,000 feet of climbing in Red Rock (scenic drive) and Lovell Canyons

Contact: granfondolasvegas.com

8. **Golden Gran Fondo**

Where: Golden, Colorado

When: June

Distance: 90 miles

Highlights: 12,000 feet of climbing, Lookout Mountain, Peak to Peak Highway, Continental Divide

Contact: www.granfondonationalchampionship series.com/golden-gran-fondo/

9. **Chicagoland Gran Fondo**

Where: Chicago

When: September

Distance: 50 or 100 miles

Highlights: Kankakee River, Midewin National Tallgrass Prairie, Route 66

Contact: www.christiansgranfondo.com

10. **Gran Fondo New York**

Where: New York City

When: May

Distance: 50 or 100 miles

Highlights: 7,000 riders, George Washington Bridge, Nyack, Bear Mountain, 6,000 feet of climbing, 20 percent grades on County Road 333

Contact: granfondony.com

11. **Maratona Des Dolomites Gran Fondo**

Where: Dolomites, Italy

When: July

Distance: 86 miles

Highlights: 9,000 people, 13,000 feet of climbing in the Italian Alps

Contact: maratona.it/en

IX. Gravel Grinders

Gravel grinding—riding a cyclocross bike, a thick-tired road bike, or even a 29er mountain bike on unimproved dirt and gravel backcountry farm roads, originally in the Midwest and now every-where, seems like one of the newest, weirdest genres to explode onto the cycling scene—until you realize that they've been doing this for a long time. One of the originals, the Dirty Kanza 200, grew from 38 participants in 2006 to more than 1,200 riders in 2014. Cycling celebs like Rebecca Rusch, who won the Dirty Kanza in 2012 and liked it so much that she organized her own 2013 Rebecca's Own Private Idaho, are jumping into the fray. There were some 150 gravel grinders in the country in 2013, according to Mark Stevenson, organizer of the 300-plus-mile Trans Iowa, considered the granddaddy of gravel. See gravelgrindernews.com for a complete roster. Some quick-and-dirty highlights:

1. **Southern Cross**
   Where: Dahlonega, Georgia
   When: February
   Distance: 50 miles
   Contact: 55nine.com

2. **Redlands Strada Rosa Ride**
   Where: Redlands, California
   When: March
   Distance: 62 miles
   Contact: redlands-strada-rossa.blogspot.com/

3. **Barry-Roubaix**
   Where: Hastings, Michigan
   When: March
   Distance: 36 miles
   Contact: barry-roubaix.com

4. **Trans Iowa**
   Where: Iowa
   When: April
   Distance: 310–340 miles
   Contact: transiowa.blogspot.com

5. **Dirty Kanza 200**
   Where: Emporia, Kansas
   When: June
   Distance: 200 miles
   Contact: dirtykanza200.com

6. **Hilly Billy Roubaix**
   Where: Morgantown, West Virginia
   When: June
   Distance: 70 miles
   Contact: abraracing.com

7. **Pisgah Monster Cross Challenge**
   Where: Pisgah National Forest, Brevard, North Carolina
   When: September
   Distance: 70 miles
   Contact: pisgahproductions.com

8. **Rebecca's Private Idaho**
   Where: Ketchum, Idaho
   When: September
   Distance: 50 or 94 miles
   Contact: www.rebeccasprivateidaho.com

9. **Iron Cross**
   Where: Michaux State Forest, Pennsylvania
   When: September
   Distance: 62 miles
   Contact: ironcrossrace.blogspot.com

10. **Three Peaks USA**
    Where: Beech Mountain, North Carolina
    When: September
    Distance: 55 miles (8,000 feet of climbing)
    Contact: threepeaksusa.com

GLOSSARY

Aerobar: Add-on handlebar device that puts the rider in a lower, narrower, wind-cheating shape that adds significant speed.

Anaerobic threshold: The point at which a physical effort becomes so taxing that your body's respiratory system can no longer take in enough oxygen to maintain its speed.

Bonked: When your muscles literally run out of fuel and you must slow down or stop.

Bottom bracket: The juncture of the frame's down tube and chain stays, which holds the rotating pedal mechanism.

Brevets: A series of time-limited qualifiers for Paris-Brest-Paris.

Bunny hop: When a mountain bike rider lifts both wheels off the ground at the same time; useful for clearing trail obstacles.

Century: A bike ride of 100 miles.

Cleat: The metal fastener added to the bottom of a bike shoe that snaps into a companion pedal; this "clipless" shoe-pedal system helps a rider derive more power from all ranges of the pedal stroke.

Crank arm: The lever that the pedal attaches to.

Creep: The gradual, and dangerous, stretching of the spinal-column ligaments, caused by sitting or stretching in a rounded-back position.

Critical mass: Organized rides by cycling advocates that take over city streets during busy drive times to raise awareness about cycling and the need for better treatment of cyclists by motorists.

Cruiser: Low-tech, one-speed, balloon-tire bike typically used to ride slowly on bike paths or in neighborhoods.

Cyclocross: A winter cycling racing sport that is run on a grass and dirt course. Cyclocross bikes with knobby tires are now available.

Derailleurs: The devices, found outside the hub of the rear wheel and at the cranks, that switch or derail the chain from gear to gear.

Double century: A 200-mile ride.

Drops: The section of a road-bike handlebar that loops down in a semicircle, putting the rider in a lower position for sprinting or descending hills.

Fast-twitch fibers: The short, bulky muscle fibers responsible for rapid contractions.

Flat-bar bike: Any bike that uses a straight, mountain-bike-style handlebar.

Flywheel: A heavy, solid, high-momentum wheel used on stationary bikes.

Forkstand: A device that holds a bike in place for repair or for stationary workouts by locking the empty fork of the front wheel in place.

Free radicals: Wayward electrons, thought to be released by exercise and some diets, that shoot through the body and can cause unspecified damage over time.

Freewheel: The ability of the rear wheel of a geared bike to coast when the rider is not pedaling.

Granny gear: The easiest gearing on a bike, typically a combination of the smallest chainring on the crank and the largest cog on the rear hub, that is most often used during steep hill climbs.

Headset: The metal rings and bearings that hold the stem and the fork in place in the headtube.

Headtube: The short vertical-frame tube at the front of the bike that houses the stem holding the handlebar and the support sleeve of the fork.

Heart rate: A measure of the speed at which the heart pumps blood, usually obtained by checking the pulse and expressed in beats per minute (bpm).

Hoods: On a road bike, the rubber coating that surrounds the brake-gear shifter unit; also a common hand position that allows for control of steering, braking, and shifting.

Hub: The axis around which a wheel rotates.

Hybrid: A bike, typically used by casual or fitness riders, that combines the large, fast-rolling "700C" wheels of a road bike with the flat handlebar and more upright seating position of a mountain bike.

Hyponatremia: Water intoxication; drinking too much water without replacing lost electrolytes.

Interbike: The annual cycling industry trade show, typically held in September in Las Vegas.

Leg speed: The pedaling cadence, typically measured in revolutions per minute (rpm). A common cadence is 80 to 90 rpm.

Masters: Older riders, typically 40 and up. Some events consider the Masters category as anyone over 30.

Mountain bike: A bike designed for riding on steep dirt trails that has "fat" (up to 2-inch wide), knobby tires; flat handlebars; and a wide range of gearing.

Neutral spine: Erect, natural, effortless posture characterized by a concave lower-back position, which puts very little stress on the muscles and bones.

NORBA: National Off-Road Bicycle Association.

Off-road: The opposite of on-road; typically a euphemism for dirt trails.

Paceline: Cyclists riding together in a tightly packed line to go faster than one rider could alone due to the effect of drafting, in which the front rider breaks through the wind and succeeding riders pass easily through his wake.

Pannier: A pack or basket hung over the rear wheel of a bike.

Paris-Brest-Paris: Quadrennial 1,200-kilometer (750-mile) timed ride from Paris, France, to the Atlantic Ocean town of Brest and back.

Pedal axle: The horizontal post around which a pedal spins.

Peloton: French name for "bunch," as in a bunch of riders riding en masse, as in the Tour de France.

PR: Personal record, usually referring to a person's all-time best, fastest, or longest ride, run, or other athletic benchmark.

RAAM: Race Across America.

Quick-release: Handled device at the wheel hub that, when twisted by hand, instantly loosens the wheel for removal and repair without the use of a wrench or other tools.

RAD: Rotational alignment device, typically used in a bike fitting.

Recumbent: An unconventional bike, once shunned but now growing in popularity, that has pedals out in front of instead of below the rider and a chair-like back support, placing the rider in a highly comfortable, back-friendly, feet-forward, lounge-chair-like position. The position is also highly aerodynamic, and riders of recumbents own many bicycle speed records.

Road bike: A bike with tall, narrow tires and drop handlebars designed for fast, low-friction riding on paved surfaces. Once known as a "10-speed," it now may come with as many as 30 gears.

Road racer: A competitor who rides a road bike; colloquially called a "roadie."

Sag wagon: A support vehicle that offers food and repair services to riders, typically on a long ride or in an event such as a century.

Slick tires: Low-friction tires, without knobs, used for road riding.

Spin classes: Group indoor-cycling sessions, typically found at health clubs, with an instructor and music—like an aerobics class with stationary bikes—using the Spinner bikes made by Mad Dogg Athletics.

Suspension forks: Shock-absorbing devices with springs and rubber bumpers that hold a mountain bike front wheel in place.

Tandem: A bicycle built for two people with two seats, two handlebars, and two sets of pedals.

Time trial: A solo, timed ride; typically expressed in distance (e.g., a 25-mile time trial, or TT).

Top tube: The tube on a bike frame that connects the headtube with the top of the seat tube.

Triathlon: An athletic contest that is a long-distance race consisting of three phases: swimming, bicycling, and running.

Ultra events: In cycling, usually an event longer than 200 miles (a double century).

Velodrome: A track designed for cycling.

VO_2 max: Aerobic capacity, as determined by the maximum amount of oxygen your lungs can take in, typically measured in milliliters per kilogram. Pro riders usually have an 80-plus VO_2 max.

X-Bike: A novel stationary bike made by Trixter for indoor-cycling classes that has a freewheel and laterally rocking handlebars.

NOTES

INTRODUCTION

1. Richard Corliss and Michael D. Lemonik, "How to Live to Be 100," *Time*, August 30, 2004, http://content.time.com/time/magazine/article/0,9171,994967,00.html.

CHAPER 1: THE CYCLING ANTI-AGING GAME PLAN

1. David Leonhardt, "Olympics: Keeping Score. Athletes Slow Down More Slowly," *New York Times*, August 15, 2004, www.nytimes.com/2004/08/15/sports/olympics-keeping-score-athletes-slow-down-more-slowly.html.
2. M. L. Pollack, C. Foster, D. Knapp, J. L. Rod, and D. H. Schmidt, "Effect of Age and Training on Aerobic Capacity and Body Composition of Master Athletes," *Journal of Applied Physiology* 62, no. 2 (1987): 725–731; US Department of Health and Human Services (HHS), Centers for Disease Control and Prevention (CDC), *Physical Activity and Health: A Report of the Surgeon General* (Atlanta: HHS/CDC, 1996), www.cdc.gov/nccdphp/sgr/pdf/sgrfull.pdf; S. Hawkins and R. Wiswell, "Rate and Mechanism of Maximal Oxygen Consumption Decline with Aging: Implications for Exercise Training," *Sports Medicine* 33, no. 12 (2003): 877–888.
3. Roger A. Fielding, Nathan K. LeBrasseur, Anthony Cuoco, Jonathan Bean, Kelly Mizer, and Maria A. Fiatarone Singh, "High Velocity Resistance Training Increases Skeletal Muscle Peak Power in Older Women," *Journal of the American Geriatrics Society* 50, no. 4 (2002): 655–662.

CHAPTER 5: MEALS ON WHEELS

1. Aseem Malhotra, "Saturated Fat Is Not the Major Issue," *British Medical Journal* 347 (2013), http://www.bmj.com/content/347/bmj.f6340.
2. See USA.gov, "How to Kill E. Coli and Other Bacteria When Cooking Meat," News from Our Blog, June 2, 2011, http://blog.usa.gov/post/6111180790/how-to-kill-e-coli-and-other-bacteria-when-cooking; US Department of Agriculture, "Safe Minimum Temperature Chart," n.d., www.fsis.usda.gov/wps/portal/fsis/topics/food-safety-education/get-answers/food-safety-fact-sheets/safe-food-handling/safe-minimum-internal-temperature-chart/ct_index, accessed July 7, 2014.

BIBLIOGRAPHY

Adamson, Ian. *Runner's World Guide to Adventure Racing* (Rodale, 2004).

Anderson, Bob, and Jean Anderson. *Stretching: 20th Anniversary* (Shelter Publication, 2000).

Baker, Arnie. *Psychling Psychology* (Argo Publishing E-book, 2003).

Brown, Dr. Charlie, and Kate F. Hays. *You're On! Consulting for Peak Performance* (American Psychology Association, 2003).

Cooper, Kenneth L. *Dr. Kenneth L. Cooper's Antioxidant Revolution* (Thomas Nelson, 1994).

Friel, Joe. *The Cyclist's Training Bible* (VeloPress, 2003).

Hurst, Robert. *The Art of Urban Cycling* (Falcon Press, 2004).

Ilg, Steve. *Total Body Transformation* (Hyperion, 2004).

Johnson, Richard, and Patrick R. Mummy. *Symmetry: Relieve Pain, Optimize Physical Motion* (Quantum Media, 1999).

Kolata, Gina Bari. *Ultimate Fitness: The Quest for Truth About Health and Exercise* (Farrar, Straus, and Giroux, 2003).

Maffetone, Philip. *Training for Endurance* (David Barmore, 1996).

———. *Eating for Endurance* (David Barmore, 1999).

Miller, Saul, and Peggy Maass Hill. *Sports Psychology for Cyclists* (VeloPress, 1999).

Pruitt, Andrew L., with Fred Matheny. *Andy Pruitt's Medical Guide for Cyclists* (RBR Publishing, 2002).

Ryan, Monique. *Sports Nutrition for Endurance Athletes* (VeloPress, 2002).

Solomon, Andrew. *The Noonday Demon: An Atlas of Depression* (Scribner, 2001).

Streb, Marla. *The Life Story of a Downhill Gravity Goddess* (Plume, 2003).

Yessis, Michael. *Kinesiology of Exercise* (Masters Press, 1992).

ACKNOWLEDGMENTS

A lot of people through the years helped me get this new edition of *Bike for Life* to the finish line:

Marc Wallack, my brother and my partner on numerous bike trips, including across America from Seattle to Maine to Key West, Florida, in 1982, which led to my obsession with bike touring, my first article for *Bicycling* magazine ("How to Take the Tour of Your Life"), a career change to journalism, and ultimately to my first book, *The Traveling Cyclist*, in 1991, about all my bike trips around the world.

Bill Katovsky, one of the smartest, funniest people I've ever worked with (we were editors together at *Triathlete* magazine in the mid-90s), who called me one day in late 2003 and suggested we put together a book called *Bicycle Sex*, based on stories I'd written about Goldie Hawn, Madonna, Michael Richards (Kramer from *Seinfeld*), and other Hollywood stars riding bikes. Bill had an agent and a publisher lined up and became my coauthor on what became the first edition *Bike for Life*. (*Bicycle Sex* survives as a title for a chapter about cycling-related impotence, but Kramer, Goldie, and Madonna will have to wait for inclusion in the next book.)

Rachelle Berlatsky-Kaplan and Stephen Roulac, respective publishers of *Southwest Cycling* and *California Bicyclist* (both long defunct), who gave me my first jobs in journalism. Rachelle gave a 31-year-old failed MBA a chance to get some bylines as a $100-stipend intern at her local Southern California cycling paper. Roulac let me run his influential statewide magazine after reading three of my articles. Without them, I might have ended up writing about global warming, presidential campaigns, invasions of Iraq, or other less engaging and less fun subjects.

Jean-Claude Garot, the Belgian publisher who let me run his *Bicycle Guide* and *Triathlete* magazines and didn't fire me in 1993 when Raleigh pulled its $200,000 ad schedule because they disliked my review of their new $700 mountain bike—even though they quickly fixed the defect I pointed out.

Stuart Dorland and Roman Urbina, founders of the 24 Hours of Adrenalin and La Ruta de los Conquistadores, respectively. Their round-the-clock and multiday endurance events, which I covered and raced in year after year beginning in the late 1990s, tapped a joyous, adventurous side of mountain biking that has enriched the lives of tens of thousands of people. They gave me personal benchmarks to shoot for the rest of my life, provided tons of fodder for stories, and kept me networked with a vital and dynamic new part of the sport.

Chris Kostman, who at one time was the youngest man to finish RAAM (at 19), helped Johnny G launch Spinning and has created many innovative events of his own, such as Team RAAM, the LA Marathon bike ride, Furnace Creek 508, and the Death Valley Century through his company AdventureCORPS. His invaluable friendship and creativity has gifted me with endless cycling-world connections, expertise, and insights that are threaded throughout this book.

Bob Babbitt, the always-upbeat founder and former publisher/editor of *Competitor* magazine, cofounder of the Challenged Athletes Foundation, and a genuine force for good in this world, who gave me a steady stream of great assignments and let me write any stories I wanted to about my various adventures, some of which ended up in these pages.

David Olmos, former Health section editor at the *L.A. Times*, who in 2002 gave me a biweekly gear column in one of the world's most important newspapers, providing me the opportunity to write big-picture features about cycling and fitness to an audience of millions for many years.

Rich "The Reverend" White, who taught me how to mountain bike, challenged and changed my view of life, is one of my best friends, and joins me on cycling adventures near and far.

Bob Forster, L.A.'s physical therapist to the stars, who's spent hundreds of hours educating me about stretching, strength training, diet, and periodization, cowrote a book with me (*Healthy Running Step by Step*), and has joined me in mountain bike events around the world.

Christopher Drozd, erudite L.A. personal trainer who has schooled me in the finer points of muscle and culture and frequently graced my articles (and this book).

Dr. Chris Powers of the University of Southern California, who opened my eyes to the power of proper form during an invaluable session at the USC human performance lab.

Mark Sisson, best-selling author of the *Primal Blueprint* books, and Jacques Devore, trainer of top athletes, who respectively taught me about the benefits of two important new additions to this edition of the book: primal-paleo eating and the unique "Maximum Overload" strength routine.

Ed Korb, my good friend and partner in some of the craziest cycling adventures of my life, some of which are recounted here.

Finally, my son, Joey, my loyal product tester, photo model, story reader, and partner in mud runs, stand-up paddleboard yoga, 4,000-mile Australian drives, and 800-mile cross-country tandem bike trips.

INDEX